Complementary Therapies

Edited by Mario Bernardo-Filho, Redha Taiar, Danúbia da Cunha de Sá-Caputo and Adérito Seixas

Published in London, United Kingdom

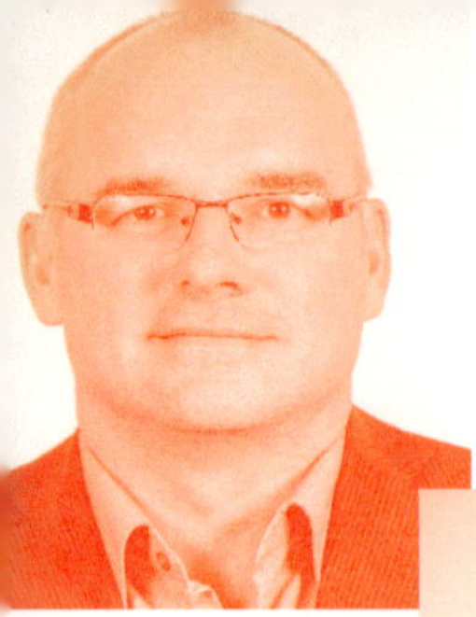
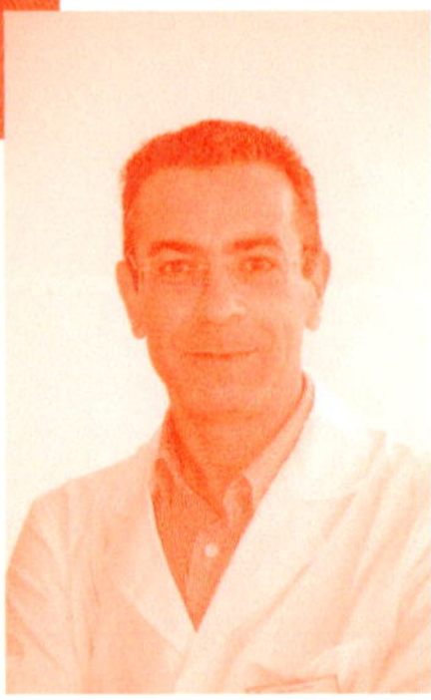
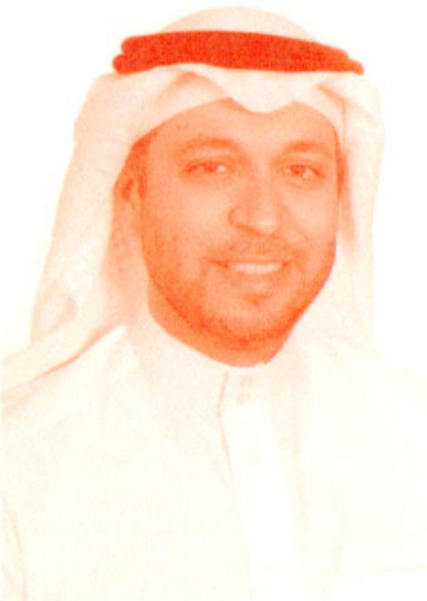
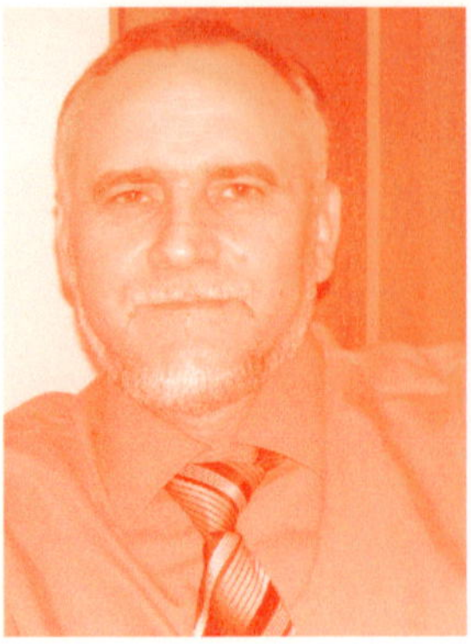
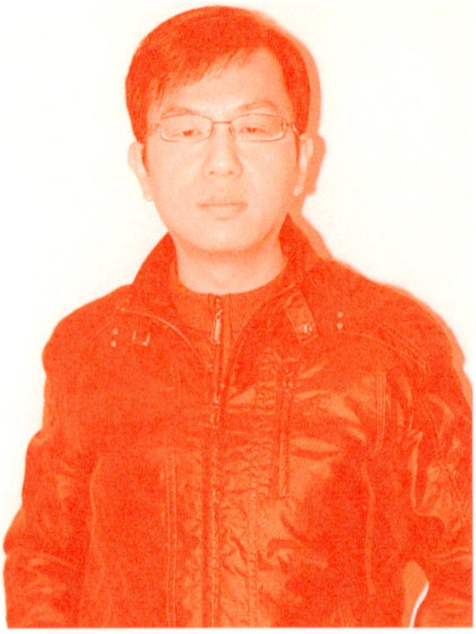
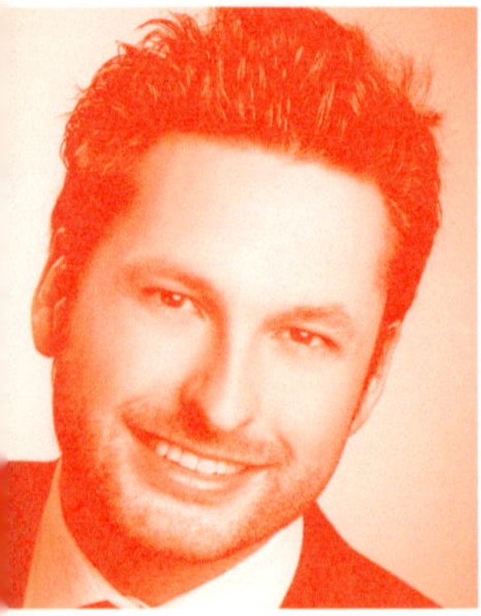
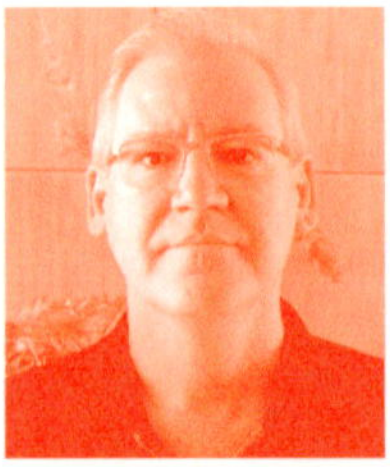

IntechOpen

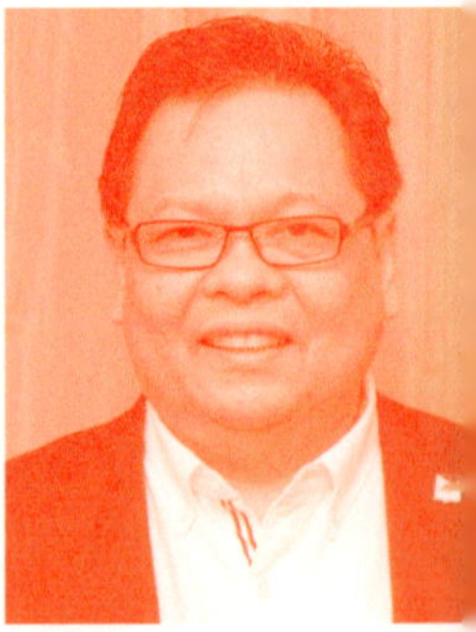
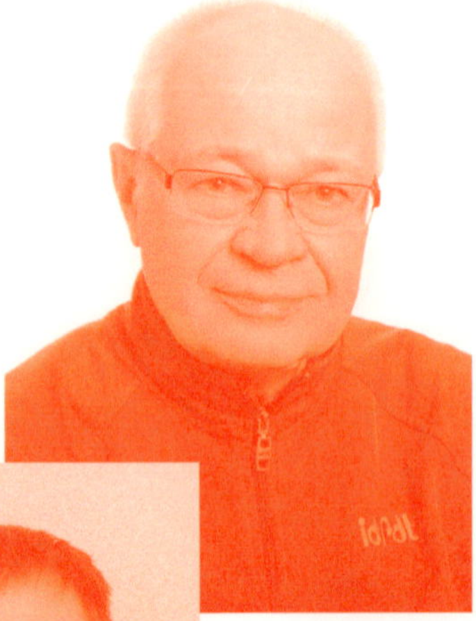
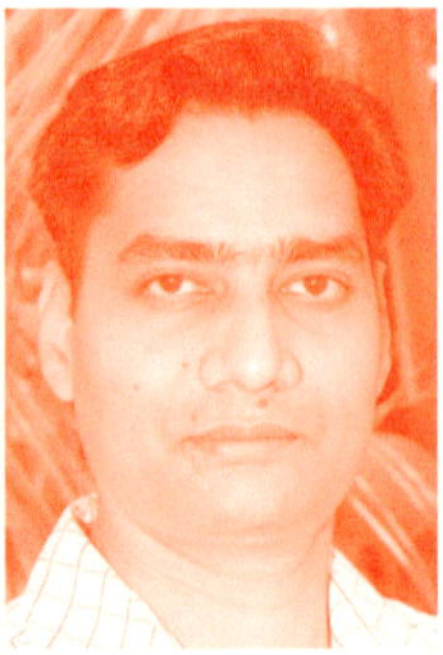
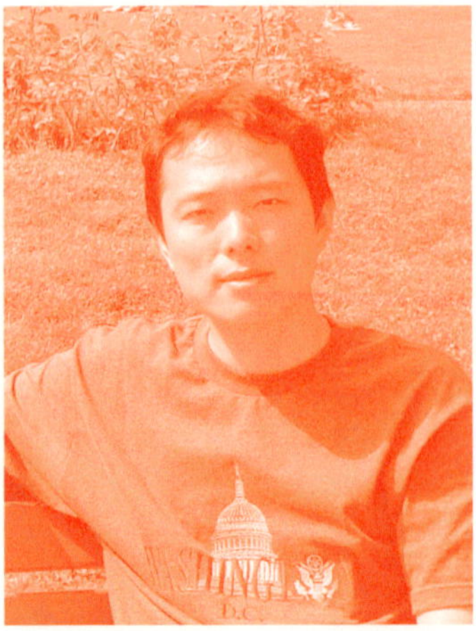
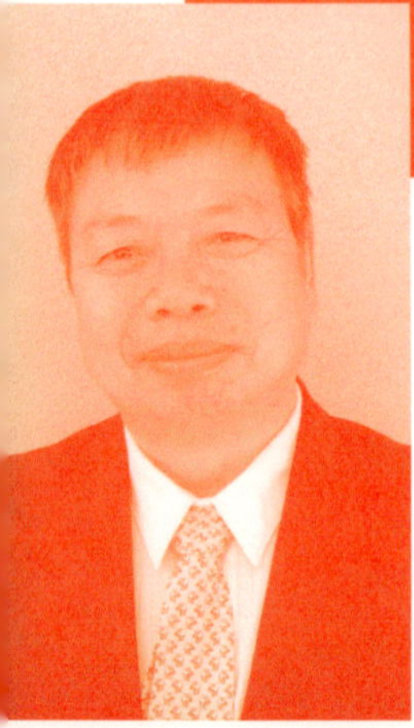
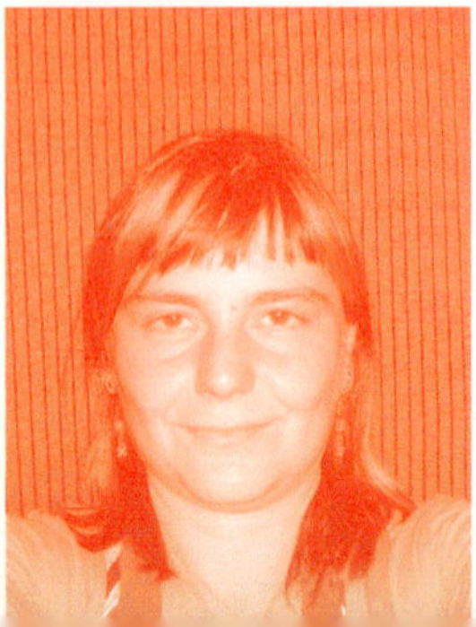

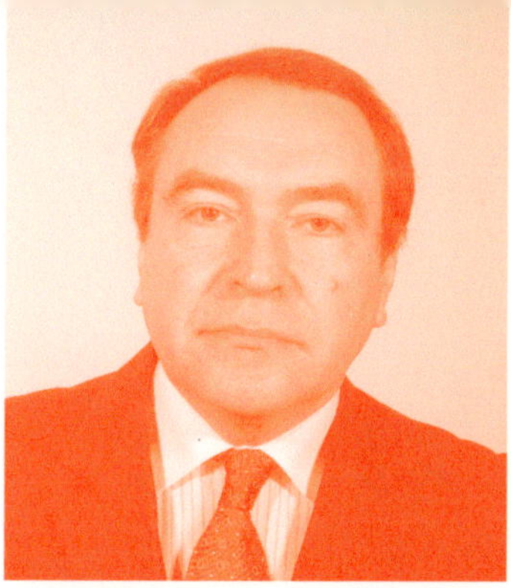
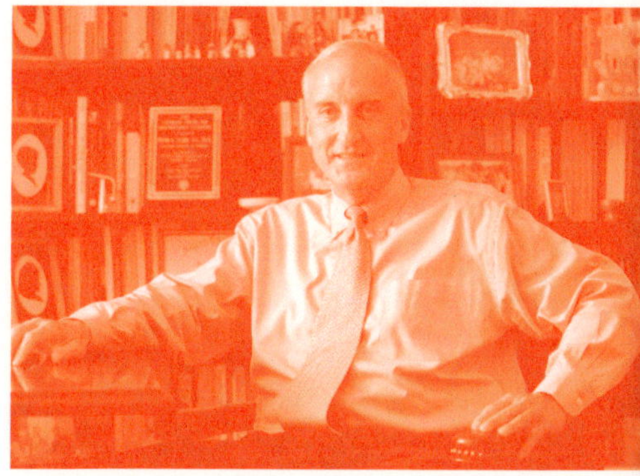
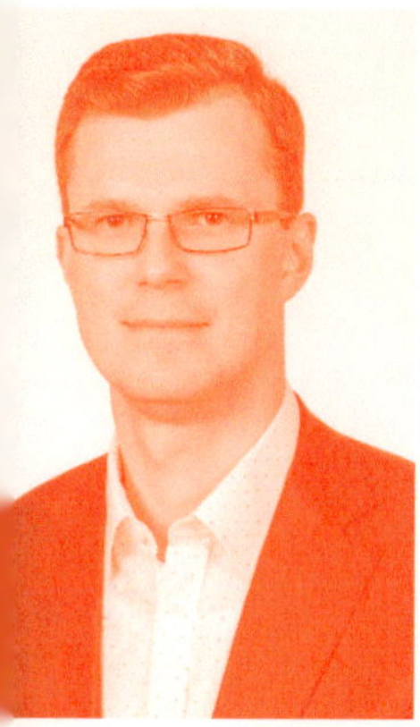
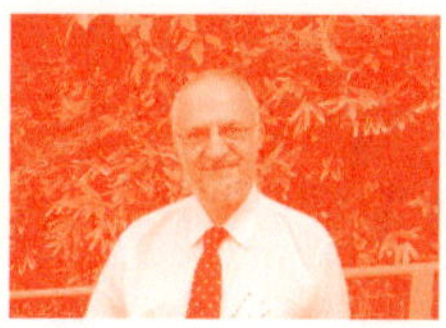
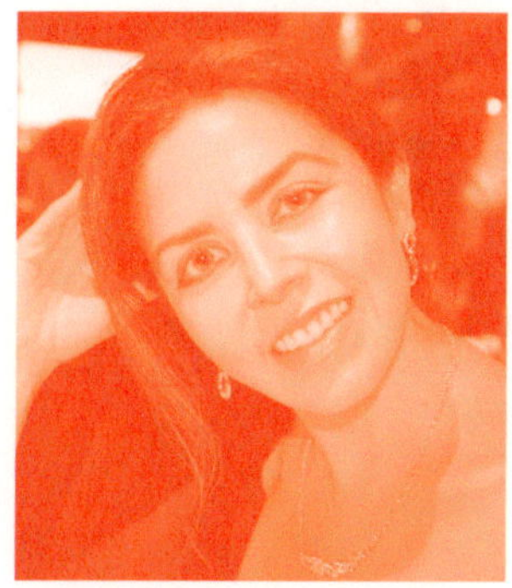

Supporting open minds since 2005

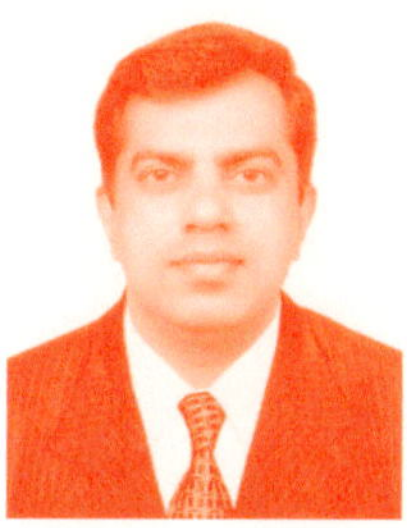
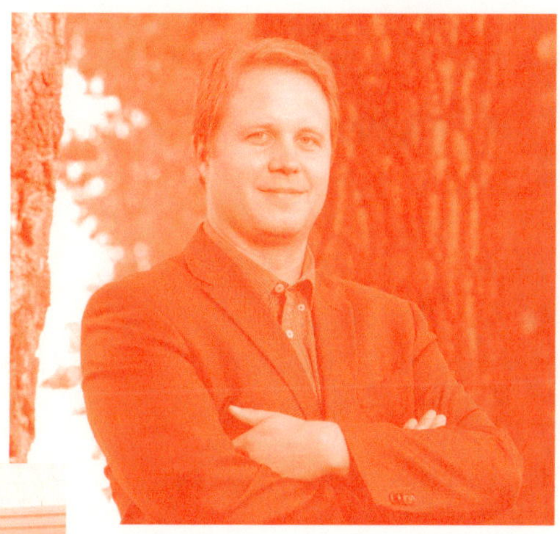
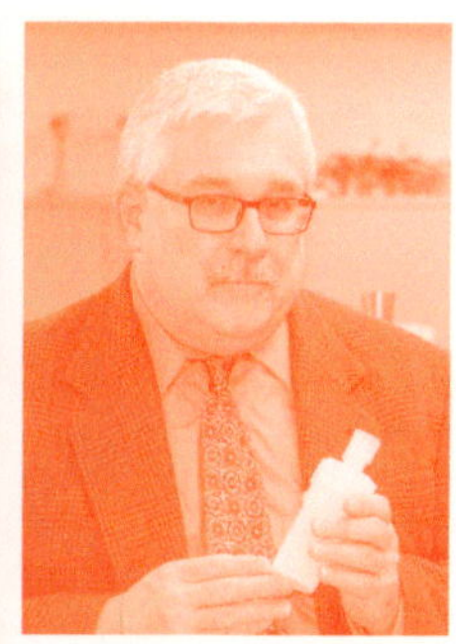
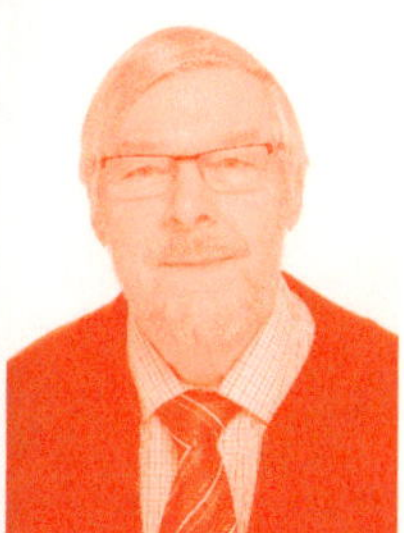
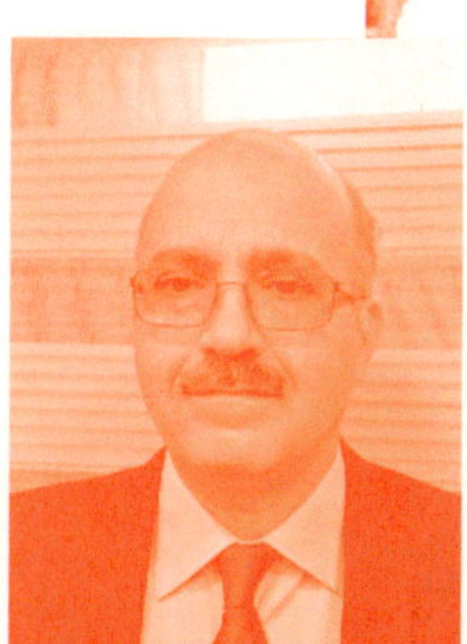
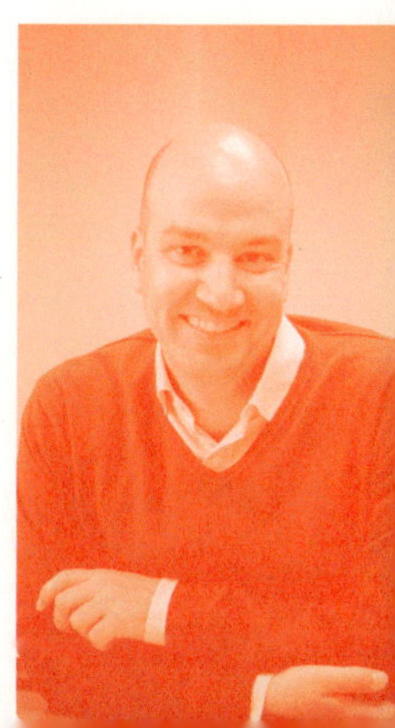
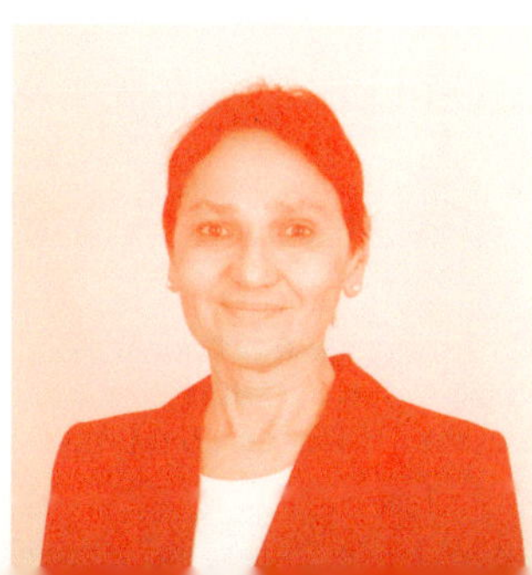

Complementary Therapies
http://dx.doi.org/10.5772/intechopen.95741
Edited by Mario Bernardo-Filho, Redha Taiar, Danúbia da Cunha de Sá-Caputo and Adérito Seixas

Contributors
Tetsuya Konishi, Chandra Nanthakumar, Andrés J. Ursa Herguedas, Dedi Ardinata, Sunday Oritsetimenyin Otimenyin, Lydia Doosuur Ior, Josephine Ozioma Ezekwesili-Ofili, Anthony Okechukwu Ogbonna, Guida Veiga, Graça Duarte Santos, Elizabeth Brooker, Bhagawati Saxena, Sahabjada Siddiqui, Shivbrat Upadhyay, Khursheed Ahmad, Aditi Srivastava, Anchal Trivedi, Ishrat Husain, Rumana Ahmad, Mohsin Ali Khan, Afsana Khatoon, Md Arshad, Paul A. Oakley, Deed E. Harrison, Kamala Pashayeva, Namiq Abdullayev, Mario Bernardo-Filho, Danúbia da Cunha de Sá-Caputo, Adérito Seixas, Redha Taiar

First published in London, United Kingdom, 2022 by IntechOpen
IntechOpen is the global imprint of INTECHOPEN LIMITED, registered in England and Wales, registration number: 11086078, 5 Princes Gate Court, London, SW7 2QJ, United Kingdom
Printed in Croatia

British Library Cataloguing-in-Publication Data
A catalogue record for this book is available from the British Library

Additional hard and PDF copies can be obtained from orders@intechopen.com

Complementary Therapies
Edited by Mario Bernardo-Filho, Redha Taiar, Danúbia da Cunha de Sá-Caputo and Adérito Seixas
p. cm.
Print ISBN 978-1-83969-011-2
Online ISBN 978-1-83969-012-9
eBook (PDF) ISBN 978-1-83969-013-6

For EU product safety concerns:
IN TECH d.o.o., Prolaz Marije Krucifikse Kozulić 3, 51000 Rijeka, Croatia, info@intechopen.com or visit our website at intechopen.com.

Meet the editors

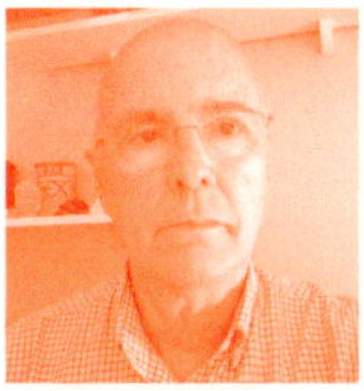

Mario Bernardo-Filho is the head of the Laboratory of Mechanical Vibration and Integrative Practices (LAVIMPI), Department of Biophysics and Biometry, Biology Institute Roberto Alcantara Gomes and Policlinic Piquet Carneiro, Universidade do Estado do Rio de Janeiro (UERJ), Brazil. He completed his academic course in Biomedicine in 1974. He obtained his Ph.D. in 1988 in experimental models using radiopharmaceuticals in studies with rats and *Escherichia coli* cultures. After that, he began investigating the biological effects of chemical agents (mainly stannous chloride) and extracts of medicinal plants in *E. coli* cultures and DNA plasmids. In rats, he evaluated the effect of synthetic and natural products on the biodistribution of radiopharmaceuticals and on the labeling of blood constituents with technetium-99m. In 1999 he participated in a competition to be a Full Professor at UERJ. He finished his academic course in Physiotherapy in 2006. In 2010, he began new research involving integrative and complementary medicine (auriculotherapy and acupuncture) and systemic vibration therapy (SVT). Dr. Bernardo-Filho is a member of the World Association of Vibration Exercise Experts (WAVex).

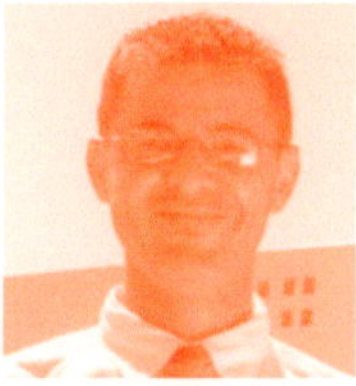

Prof. Redha Taiar obtained a Ph.D. in Biomechanics and is a professor at the University of Reims, France. He has held various positions, including head of the Master of Biomechanics; head of the University diploma of Podiatrics; head of the University diploma of Ergonomics; head of the Laboratory of Biomechanics, Reims; vice head of the Department of Sport Science; head of the Redha Taiar Biomechanical Engineering Society (RTBE) developed for sport and medical advice for industry; and vice head of the Congress of Physical Medicine and Rehabilitation Society Reims, France. His research focuses on engineering for medicine and sport. He is an engineer for different industrial organizations, including Arena, Sidas, and Medicapteur. He previously worked for NoTrax, a manufacturer of anti-fatigue mats. He is a member of the World Association of Vibration Exercise Experts (WAVex).

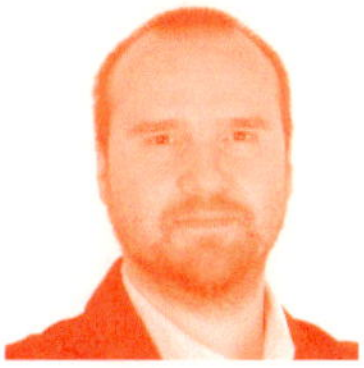

Dr. Adérito Seixas graduated with a degree in Physiotherapy with a specialization in neuromusculoskeletal rehabilitation. He received his MSc from the University of Porto, Portugal, for a thesis on the assessment of sensorimotor skills of blind athletes. He also specialized in data analysis at the same university. He is a member of several scientific societies. Currently, alongside his work as a full-time professor at Escola Superior de Saúde Fernando Pessoa, Portugal, Dr. Seixas is carrying out research for his Ph.D., focusing on the biomechanical and thermophysiological assessment of the foot in diabetic patients at risk to develop foot ulcers. He has supervised more than seventy graduate and master's students in research activities. His research interests include evidence-based practice, assessment of the neuromusculoskeletal system, and the role of cognitive assessment in human adaptation to performance situations.

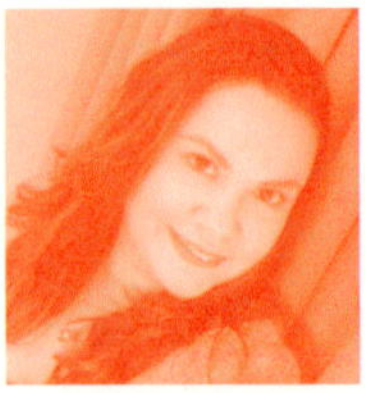

Prof. Danúbia da Cunha de Sá Caputo graduated in Physical Therapy in 2004 and obtained a Ph.D. in 2016. She has been researching mechanical vibration and integrative practices since 2013. She is a professor and researcher at Universidade do Estado do Rio de Janeiro (UERJ). She is a specialist in physical therapy, exercise, and rehabilitation. She is on the editorial board of the Journal of Education and Sport Management, Brazilian Journal of Health and Biomedical Sciences, and Fisioterapia. She is a member of the World Association of Vibration Exercise Experts (WAVex) and Associação Brasileira de Biociências Nucleares and vice president of Associação Brasileira de Fisioterapia Integrativa e Práticas Integrativas e Complementares, Brazil. She completed a post-doctorate at UERJ in 2018. She is a supervisor of MSc and PhD students and is the coordinator of the scientific projects of the Laboratório de Vibrações Mecânicas e Práticas Integrativas, UERJ (LAVIMPI-UERJ) in the Policlinic Piquet Carneiro.

Contents

Preface

Traditional, complementary, and integrative medicine are terms used to try to define practices used in the maintenance of health as well as in the prevention, diagnosis, and management of physical and mental conditions. These practices are based on the knowledge, skill, theories, beliefs, and experiences acquired by different cultures in the world throughout the years. In this book, we use the term "complementary therapies" to refer to these practices. Various complementary therapies have been used in different clinical situations worldwide. It is important to highlight that these therapies are effective and, in general, without side effects or complications when properly performed.

This book provides a better understanding of the qualities and uses of some usual complementary therapies, as well as their proximity with other therapies that are increasing in clinical importance. Complementary therapies vary according to region, culture, and habits. As such, three chapters in Section 1, "Complementary Therapies and Knowledge of Some Cultural Practices," discuss Islamic herbal medicine, African traditional and complementary therapies, and Mibyou care.

Complementary therapies have proven effective for clinical as well as mental disorders. Section 2, "Complementary Therapies and Mental Disorders," includes chapters on cognitive hypnotherapy and eye movement desensitization and reprocessing, which are effective psychodynamic therapies for the rapid reduction of cognitive anxiety, and yoga as an intervention to reduce levels of stress, anxiety, and depression. There is also a chapter on the use of medicinal plants to manage psychosis.

Chapters in Section 3, "Complementary Therapies and Clinical Rehabilitation," address non-pharmacological therapies in integrative rehabilitation and physiotherapy, a new rehabilitation technique called Chiropractic BioPhysics (CBP) for reducing spine deformities, and an integrated psychomotor therapeutic treatment for women with breast cancer.

Finally, Section 4, "Complementary Therapies, Technologic and Science Perspectives," includes chapters on evidence-based acupuncture, vibration therapy for health promotion, and methods and tools for assessing muscle asymmetry in the analysis of electromyographic signals. There is also a chapter devoted to the role of complementary and alternative medicine in COVID-19.

We wish to thank Author Service Managers Ms. Marina Dusevic and Kristina Kardum Cvitan at IntechOpen for their confidence and assistance. In addition, we would like to thank the contributing authors for their excellent chapters.

Danúbia da Cunha de Sá-Caputo and Mario Bernardo-Filho
Universidade do Estado do Rio de Janeiro,
Rio de Janeiro, Brasil

Adérito Seixas
Escola Superior de Saúde Fernando Pessoa,
Porto, Portugal,

Redha Taiar
University of Reims,
Reims, France

Section 1

Complementary Therapies and Knowledge of Some Cultural Practices

Chapter 1

Traditional Islamic Herbal Medicine and Complementary Therapies

Sahabjada Siddiqui, Afsana Khatoon, Khursheed Ahmad, Shivbrat Upadhyay, Aditi Srivastava, Anchal Trivedi, Ishrat Husain, Rumana Ahmad, Mohsin Ali Khan and Md Arshad

Abstract

Herbal products found abundantly in several plants are the rich source of phytochemicals with a wide range of pharmacological activities and few adverse effects. Medicinal plants contain active ingredients that assist the body in reestablishing its natural balance and healing itself. Various herbs, which are commonly used in traditional Islamic medicine, can have an impact on human body systems. Natural products are primary sources of effective drugs with novel structures and distinct mechanisms of action for the treatment of various types of complications as well as the drug discovery process. The various pharmacological properties such as antimicrobial, anticancer, antioxidant, antihypertensive, immunomodulatory, anti-inflammatory and anti-diabetic properties of several natural products are well documented in the Ayurveda and Unani system of medicine. Some of the natural products' active ingredients have been documented, but the majority are still being researched as complementary medicine. As a result, more research is required to investigate their complementary medicine system. The present chapter provides a comprehensive update on selected traditional Islamic medicinal plants and their bioactive products mentioned in Islamic scriptures as complementary therapies to various diseases. The chapter also provides an in-depth update of pharmacological and clinical studies of natural products with special emphasis on cancer and diabetes.

Keywords: traditional Islamic herbs, complementary therapies, herbal products, pharmacological properties

1. Introduction

According to the World Health Organization, an estimated 80% of people around the world use herbal medicine. Studies show that certain herbs effectively treat several health issues, like allergies, premenstrual syndrome, chronic fatigue, cancer, diabetes and many more. India is one of the big resources of medicinal plants and natural products due to its geological diversity. In recent years, various researches have been conducted on medicinal plants and spices worldwide. Plant-derived chemicals have attracted the attention of the scientific community for their various potential positive qualities. Studies have shown that polyphenols are anti-oxidants, anti-inflammatory, cardiac and neuroprotective, as well as having anti-cancer properties [1, 2]. Some of these natural chemicals have been included in clinical trials due to their inherent biological activity in a variety of disease models [3, 4], as they exhibited promising benefits in terms of boosting the anti-proliferative response and reducing the toxicity of conventional treatments.

Islamic medicine, often known as Arabic medicine in medical history, is the science of medicine developed during the Islamic Golden Age, which lasted from the ninth to thirteenth centuries. Although the main medical tradition was Greek, it was influenced by Islamic or Prophetic Medicine, as well as folk medicine to a lesser extent. The Holy Quran has provided the knowledge for a variety of crops, including grains, seeds, and fodder, as well as their germination and growth processes in several Surah. Plants are considered a gift from God, and the Quran mentions various plant names such as Date palms, figs, olives, ginger, grapes, miswak, onion, barley, garlic, pomegranates, camphor, Christ's thorns, bottle gourds and other significant therapeutic herbs and plants utilized as food [5, 6].

Various medicinal plants and nutraceuticals derived from different natural resources, as well as their products such as polyphenolic components, flavones, flavonoids, and antioxidants, have been found to provide significant protection against a variety of diseases [7]. Epidemiological observations show that various traditional Islamic medicinal plants have powerful disease inhibiting properties [6, 8]. Currently, developing a preventive/therapeutic drug that reduces the particular disease without harming normal cells, is the primary goal of the research performed. For instance, in the case of cancer treatment, some of the methods used by the experts to cure the condition include tumor debulking, chemotherapies, radiotherapies, targeted treatments, immunotherapies, stem cell transplants, and photodynamic therapies [9]. Around the world, researchers are trying to develop new strategies to eradicate the diseases.

The present chapter summarizes the recently reported pharmacologically and therapeutically based medicinal plants and its products mentioned in Islamic scriptures. The chapter also highlights the recent studies of medicinal plants and their natural products based on *in vitro* and *in vivo* and clinical investigation.

2. Traditional Islamic medicinal plants and their products

2.1 Dates palm (*Phoenix dactylifera* L.) fruits

Phoenix dactylifera L. (*P. dactylifera*), often known as date palm, is one of the oldest and most important crops in Arab countries and North Africa. Apart from that, dates are also cultivated around the world and in India, southern California, Arizona and Texas [10]. The date palm tree is a part of the family Arecaceae. Date palm is a multifunctional plant that contains fiber, carbohydrates, minerals, vitamins and various phytochemicals, which were used traditionally because of having great therapeutic properties [11]. Therapeutic benefits of Ajwa dates fruits are well documented in Islamic scriptures such as Hadith and other works of Islamic literature. According to Al-Bukhaari (5445) and Muslim (2047), narrated by Sa'd ibn Abi Waqqaas that the Prophet (PBUH) said: "Whoever eats seven Ajwa dates in the morning, will not be harmed by any poison or witchcraft that day."

Date palm fruit has been described in traditional and alternative medicine to provide several health benefits including anticholesteremic, antidiabetic, anti-inflammatory, antioxidant, hepatoprotective and anticancer effects [12]. According to prior phytochemical studies, Date pulp fruit contains about 80% reducing sugars, including fructose, glucose, galactose, and maltose, as well as flavonoids, glycosides, polyphenols, and phytosterols [13, 14]. Phytochemicals present in dates palm fruits exhibit anti-inflammatory, cardioprotective, antioxidant, hypolipidemic and anti-apoptotic properties [15]. The main bioactive components present dates palm pulp are Carotenoids (lutein and β-carotene), phytosterols and phytoestrogens (β-sitosterol, stigmasterol, campesterol, daidzein, genistein and isofucosterol), flavonoids (apigenin, luteolin, quercetin, isoquercetrin, rutin and kaempferol) and phenolic acids (benzoic acid derivatives; p-hydroxybenzoic acid, protocatechuic acid, vanillic acid, gallic acid and syringic acid, and cinnamic acid derivatives; o-coumaric acid, p-coumaric acid, caffeic acid, and ferulic acid) (**Figure 1**) [10, 16].

2.1.1 Utilization of date palm fruit and its products as complementary therapies

2.1.1.1 Cancer

The ethyl acetate fraction of *P. dactylifera* fruit extract has shown the antifibrotic (expression of fibronectin-1 and alpha-smooth muscle actin) and antiproliferative activity in tumor necrosis factor (TNF) stimulated pancreatic cancer cells *in vitro* [10]. In addition, the ethyl acetate fraction of *P. dactylifera* has shown the anticancer effect against prostate cancer cells [17], ethyl alcohol extract against human hepatocellular carcinoma hepatoma G2 (HepG2) cells and triple-negative mammary carcinoma MDA-MB-231 cells [18, 19] and methanolic extract against human breast adenocarcinoma Michigan Cancer Foundation-7 (MCF-7) cells *in vitro* [20]. In a previous study, an aqueous extract of *P. dactylifera* has shown the anticancer potential in diethylnitrosamine-induced hepatocellular carcinoma in *Wistar* rats [21]. *P. dactylifera* has improved the treatment outcome of pediatric cancer patients clinically [22].

2.1.1.2 Diabetes

Low glycemic index (GI) diets have been proven to be effective in the treatment of diabetes. Dates can be classed as a low GI superfood because of their high fructose content, which is sweeter and less diabetogenic than glucose [23]. *P. dactylifera* fruit based-diets have alleviated hyperglycemia in alloxan-induced diabetic rats [24].

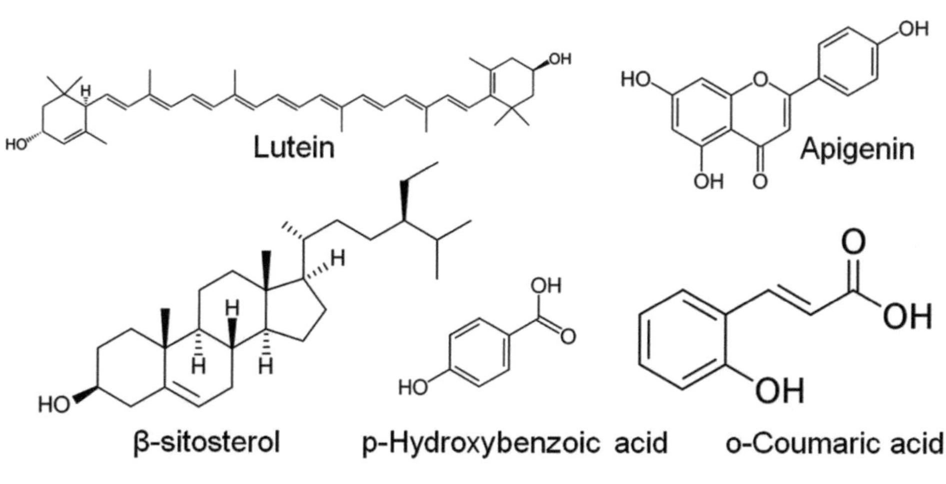

Figure 1.
*Chemical structure of principal bioactive components found in date palm (*Phoenix dactylifera L.*) fruits.*

A previous study has revealed significant anti-hyperglycemic effects of dates fruits in diabetes management of hyperglycemic Sprague-Dawley rats [25] and diosmetin glycosides isolated from the epicarp of date fruits have significantly alleviated the biochemical profile of alloxan diabetic male rats [26].

2.1.1.3 Antibacterial and antiviral

The use of dates is also important for antimicrobial activities. The *in vitro* studies have demonstrated that date fruit exhibits antibacterial, antiviral, anti-inflammatory and anti-angiogenic activity [15, 27].

2.1.1.4 Hepatoprotective and antioxidant

Date palm fruit has shown the protective effect on dimethoate induced-oxidative stress in rat liver [28]. Moreover, date palm fruits have shown anti-hyperlipidemic and hepatoprotective effects in hyperlipidemia and fatty liver male albino rats [29].

2.1.1.5 Pregnancy and delivery

The use of dates is especially important for pregnant and postnatal women. Women who consume dates before and after giving birth might strengthen their uterine muscles by consuming dates [20]. Consumption of date fruit in the last 4 weeks before labor reduced the need for initiation and augmentative labor and resulted in a better delivery outcome [30]. Due to their high fiber, iron and trace element contents, as well as their high energy and low GI, date fruits seem to be the ideal superfood for today's health-conscious age.

2.2 Fig (*Ficus carica*) fruit

One of the largest angiosperm genus, Ficus belonging to the family of Moraceae (Mulberry) are perennial plants comprising of over 800 different species including climbers, trailers, and epiphytes distributed around the tropical and sub-tropical regions worldwide [31, 32]. *Ficus carica* (*F. carica*), a deciduous dicotyledonous tree is the most important member of the genus commonly referred to as 'fig'. Indigenous to Egypt (East Mediterranean region), *F. carica* was initially introduced to different civilizations throughout the world including England, United States (US), East and West South Central, South Atlantic and Pacific [33]. Despite, its origins in the Sub-Himalayan regions of the Bengal and Central Indian subcontinents, it has been widely cultivated all around the globe. However, some of the world's major producers of figs for their dry and consumption were US, Turkey and Greece [33].

Bush/small tree-like appearance with single, alternating and large foliage, deep lobes with three or seven lobes; rough and hairy on the top surface; soft and hairy underneath along with smooth and gray bark. In addition to being cultivated from ancient times, they were found growing in the wild in dry and sunny places with rich and fresh soil, as well as in rocky locations. A reasonably permeable and easy draining soil is ideal for the plant's growth; nevertheless, it can also grow in nutritionally poor soil [34]. The edible part of *F. carica*, the fruit is seed-bearing, fleshy, hollow, and receptacle-shaped. Figs do indeed have a long history of medicinal, mythological, and ecclesiastical applications [35–38]. They are bad cholesterol-free, low in sodium and an excellent source of minerals (K, Zn, Mg, Fe, N, Ca, and P), dietary fibers, carbohydrates, sugars, vitamins (water-soluble—B1, B2, B3 and C; fat-soluble—A), good cholesterol and essential amino acids.

Figs have acquired a considerable amount of folkloric importance and still invite the attention of researchers globally for their pharmaceutical properties to be used as complementary medicine. Ayurveda, Unani, and Siddha are the classical medicine systems of Ayurveda that have acknowledged the medicinal benefits of fig [39]. Therefore, it promises to treat and cure disorders of endocrine (diabetes), ventilatory, cardiovascular, digestive (ulcers and vomiting), urinary, reproductive (menstrual discomfort), and immune systems, as well as infectious diseases of the skin, scabies, and gonorrhea [40].

Phytochemical analysis results revealed a number of secondary metabolites being isolated from different parts of *F. carica* which are phytosterols, anthocyanin pigments, essential amino acids, phenols (proanthocyanidins), essential fatty acids, triterpenoids, coumarins, alcohols, and other volatile counterparts [41, 42].

Linolenic acid (53.1%) was found to be the most prominent fatty acid present in dried figs followed by linoleic acid (21.1%), palmitic acid (13.8%), and oleic acid (9.8%) [41]. Phenolic compounds; 3-O- and 5-O-caffeoylquinic acids, ferulic acid, quercetin-3-O-glucoside, quercetin-3-O-rutinoside, psoralen, and bergapten isolated from the fruit pulp [43]. However, numerous volatile components namely 3-methyl-butanal, 2-methyl-butanal, (E)-2-pentanal, hexanal, heptanal, octanal, and nonanal, 1-penten-3-ol, 3-methylbutanol, benzyl alcohol, (E)-2-nonenol, and phenylethyl alcohol, ketone: 6-methyl-5-hepten-2-one, esters: methyl hexanoate, methyl salicylate, and ethyl salicylate, limonene, menthol, α-pinene, β-pinene, linalool, eucalyptol, α-cubenene, copaene, β-caryophyllene, τ-muurolene, τ cadinene, and germacrene D and β-cyclocitral were found in the *F. carica* fruits (**Figure 2**) [44].

The fruits have emerged as an outstanding complementary medicine that could be used in treating leprosy, nasal hemorrhage, and deficiency disorders as well as are used in various drug preparations [45].

2.2.1 Utilization of F. carica *fruits and its products as complementary therapies*

2.2.1.1 Cardioprotective (hypotensive effect)

F. carica is one of the five plants mentioned in the Quran widely used in the treatment of cardiovascular diseases. Nevertheless, its hypertensive properties are not well documented. However, a study reveals that fruit extract of *F. carica*

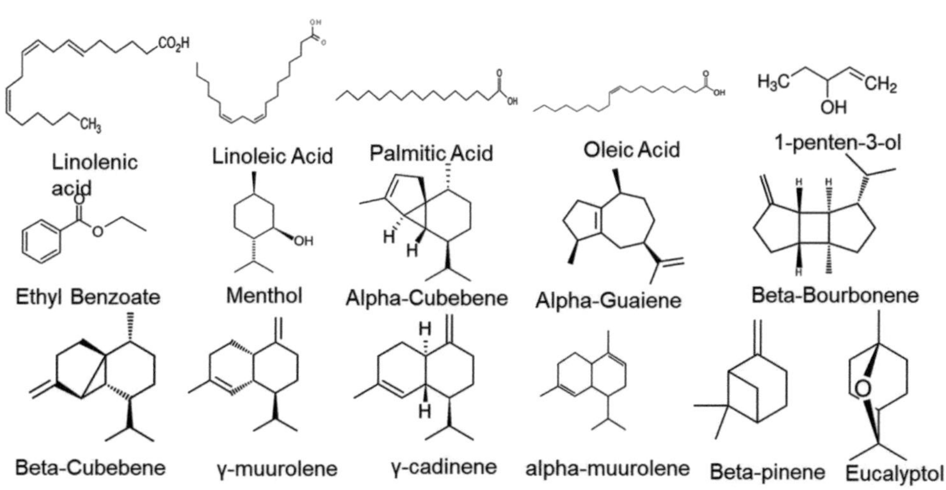

Figure 2.
*Chemical structure of principal bioactive components found in fig (*Ficus carica*) fruits.*

significantly reduced the level of blood pressure in normal as well as glucose-treated (hypertensive) rats. This effect has been attributed due to the presence of flavonoids, phenols and potassium ions which alter the level of glucose/fructose stimulating cardioinhibitory, antihypertensive and diuretic effects [46].

2.2.1.2 Cancer

Methanolic fruit extract of *F. carica* possessed antiproliferative activity against hepatocyte-derived carcinoma cells with an IC_{50} value >2000 μg/mL [47]. Virtual screening, molecular docking and dynamics simulation investigations were combined to give a structural insight into the putative binding mechanism of prospective drug-like phytocomponents of *F. carica* with crucial molecular targets which play a significant role in the pathogenesis of several cancer. β-Bourbonene was found to show the best binding with topoisomerase-I, topoisomerase-II, and Vascular Endothelial Growth Factor-2 (VEGFR-2), thereby, altering their functions to alter the pathogenesis [48].

2.2.1.3 Antioxidant and antihyperlipidemic activity

Methanolic fruit extract of *F. carica* revealed strong antioxidant activity against 2,2-diphenyl-1-picrylhydrazyl (DPPH) dye with an IC_{50} value of 13.402 μg/mL [47]. The most prominent phenolic compounds: quercetin 3-O-rutinoside, dihydroxybenzoic acid di-pentoside and apigenin 8-C-glucoside were most abundantly present in the aqueous-ethanolic extract of Tunisian *F. carica*. Due to these phytoconstituents, improved antioxidant status and lower lipid peroxidation were observed suggesting their protective role [49].

2.2.1.4 Anti-diabetic activity

As a promising nutritional intervention for acute postprandial glucose and insulin homeostasis, *F. carica* fruit supplementation might also be used in the treatment of severe metabolic diseases such as hyperglycaemic condition and type 2 diabetes mellitus to optimize the glucose level in these conditions [50].

2.2.1.5 Antispasmodic and antiplatelet activities

In a previous study, it has been found that the fig seems to have a spasmolytic action that might be mediated by activation of the K^+-ATP channel, which supports some of its therapeutic uses in hyperactive gastrointestinal illnesses, and its antiplatelet effect [51].

2.3 Black cumin (*Nigella sativa*) seed

Nigella sativa (*N. sativa*, family Ranunculaceae), popularly known as black seed or black cumin or Kalonji in Hindi, is an annual herb with various pharmacological properties and a widely used medicinal herb across the world with a rich historical and religious background. *N. sativa* is native to Southern Europe, North Africa and Southwest Asia and it is grown in many countries around the world like the Middle Eastern Mediterranean region, South Europe, India, Pakistan, Syria, Turkey, Saudi Arabia [52, 53]. Black seeds and oil have been used in traditional medicine for more than 2000 years, and Hippocrates and Discroides termed it "the Melanthion" [54]. It is an important drug in various traditional system of medicine like Unani and Tibb, Ayurveda and Siddha. Traditionally, *N. sativa* has been used to treat a wide range of illnesses, diseases, and conditions affecting the respiratory system, digestive tract, kidney and liver function, cardiovascular system, and immune system, as well as for overall well-being [55]. In Arabic, *Nigella* is known as 'Habbatul barakah', which means the seed of blessing. In Islam, It is considered as one of the most effective kinds of curing medicine available as it was stated in one of the Prophetic hadiths that black seed is the remedy for all illness except death. In Tibb-e-Nabwi (Prophetic Medicine), it is suggested to use it on a regular basis [56]. Black seeds have quite a rich history of folkloric use as food and medicine in Indian, Arabian, Southeast Asian, and Middle Eastern civilizations, and have traditionally been used to cure asthma, bronchitis, rheumatism, and other inflammatory illnesses. Extract prepared from black seed is used for the treatment of indigestion, diarrhea, loss of appetite, amenorrhoea, dropsy, and dysmenorrhoea and useful in the cure of skin eruptions and worms [57].

Various therapeutic attributes of black seed and its active component thymoquinone have been shown in *in vitro* and *in vivo* investigations, including anti-cancer [58], anti-microbial [58], anti-pyretic, contraceptive and anti-fertility, anti-oxytocic [52], antitussive, anti-inflammatory [59], and antioxidant properties [60]. Black seed has been shown to have anticancer action in blood, breast, colon, pancreatic, liver, lung, fibrosarcoma, prostate, and cervical cancer cell lines, as well as in animal models of lung, kidney, skin, colon, and breast cancer [61]. Phytochemical investigation of *N. sativa* revealed the presence of hundreds of phytoconstituents, mostly alkaloids, saponins, sterols, and essential oil.

The most important active compounds are thymoquinone (30–48%), thymohydroquinone, dithymoquinone, p-cymene (7–15%), carvacrol (6–12%), 4-terpineol (2–7%), t-anethol (1–4%), sesquiterpene longifolene (1–8%) α-pinene and thymol [62]. Among the various active components reported thus far, thymoquinone, which is a major component of essential oil, is the most bioactive chemical and has a variety of therapeutic properties (**Figure 3**).

2.3.1 Utilization of black seed and its products as complementary therapies

2.3.1.1 Anticancer activity

Thymoquinone, the active compound of the black seed helps to train T cells *in vitro* for adoptive T-cell therapy against cancer and infectious diseases. The cytotoxic effects of different Black seed extracts as an adjuvant therapy to doxorubicin on human MCF-7 breast cancer cells was reported. The lipid extract of black seed was found to be cytotoxic against MCF-7 cells, with a lethal concentration 50 (LC_{50}) of 2.720 ± 0.232 mg/mL, while the aqueous extract was found to be cytotoxic at concentrations as high as 50 mg/mL. *In vitro* and *in vivo* studies showed the

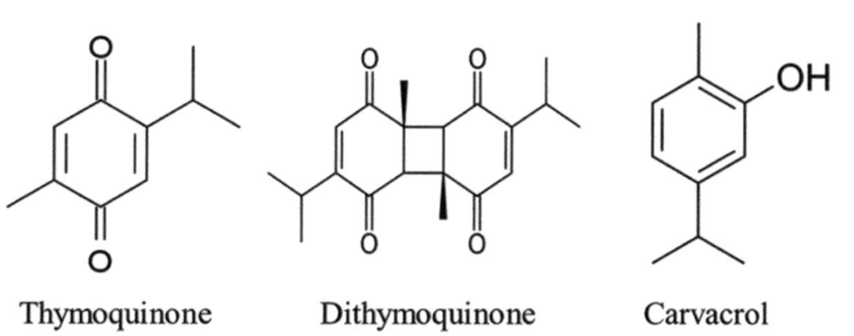

Figure 3.
*Chemical structure of principal bioactive components found in black cumin (*Nigella sativa*) seed.*

antitumor and anti-angiogenic effects of thymoquinone on osteosarcoma [63]. Thymoquinone induced a higher percentage of growth inhibition and apoptosis in the human osteosarcoma cell line sarcoma osteogenic-2 (SaOS-2) and inhibits tumor angiogenesis and tumor growth through suppressing nuclear factor kappa light chain enhancer of activated B cells (NF-κB) and its regulated molecules. Thymoquinone cytotoxicity was also studied in human cervical squamous carcinoma cells (SiHa). Thymoquinone's anticancer effects on breast cancer cells, as well as its potential effect on the peroxisome proliferator-activated receptors (PPAR)-activation pathway, were investigated [64]. It was discovered that thymoquinone had a strong antiproliferative effect in breast cancer cells, and cytotoxicity was increased when thymoquinone was combined with doxorubicin and 5-fluorouracil. Migration and invasive properties of MDA-MB-231 cells were also reduced in the presence of thymoquinone. *N. sativa* volatile oil in the diet of male Wister rats for 30 weeks significantly reduced malignant and benign colon tumor sizes, incidences and multiplicities.

2.3.1.2 Antimicrobial activity

Black cumin is one of the most inspirational medicinal plants, with potent antibacterial, antifungal, antiviral, and antiparasitic properties. Thymoquinone isolated from *N. sativa* seeds showed a broader spectrum of antibacterial activity against gram-positive and gram-negative bacteria, including *Bacillus*, *Listeria*, *Enterococcus*, *Micrococcus*, *Staphylococcus*, *Pseudomonas, Escherichia, Salmonella, Serovar,* and *Vibrio parahaemolyticus*, as well as inhibiting the formation of bacterial biofilms [65]. Different extracts of black cumin and thymoquinone were found to have potent fungicidal activity against dermatophyte strains such as *Trichophyton mentagrophytes* and *Microsporum gypseum*, which was superior to fluconazole but not as potent as ketoconazole [65]. Complete recovery and retroversion of a 46-year-old HIV-positive patient were observed after therapy with 10 mL of black seed twice daily for 6 months, according to a case report done by Onifade et al. [66]. In a mouse model, *N. sativa* seed oil was observed to reduce viral load to undetectable levels in the liver and spleen after 10 days of intraperitoneal injection [65].

2.3.1.3 Antioxidant activity

In vivo and *in vitro* investigations have shown that *N. sativa* possesses potent antioxidant properties [67]. Collagen-induced arthritis was used to test the antioxidant and antiarthritic effects of thymoquinone in *Wistar* rats [52]. After two months of contemporaneous ingestion of *Allium sativum* and *N. sativa* seed, plasma malondialdehyde (MDA) levels were significantly reduced, with enhanced activity in erythrocyte glutathione peroxidase (GSH-Px) and superoxide dismutase [68].

2.3.1.4 Antidiabetic activity

The administration of black cumin seed to streptozotocin-induced diabetic rats for one month resulted in a significant decrease in fasting plasma glucose, serum MDA, interleukin-6, and immunoglobulin A, G, and M, as well as a significant increase in endogenous antioxidant enzymes such as SOD, Glutathione-S-transferase, and catalase expression. Diabetes-induced elevations in tissue MDA and blood glucose were greatly reduced in rats treated with *N. sativa* extract and oil, as well as thymoquinone, and serum insulin and tissue SOD were dramatically enhanced. *N. sativa* and thymoquinone have been shown to be effective in the treatment of diabetics and the preservation of -cells from oxidative stress [69].

A placebo was given to 99 diabetic patients in an experimental randomized controlled study, while two treatment groups received oral black seed oil. Black seed oil at 1.5 and 3 mL/day for 20 days resulted in significant reductions in glycated hemoglobin A1c and random blood sugar levels [70].

2.3.1.5 Antihypertensive activity

According to a nonrandomized controlled trial, 57 patients who were given 2 g daily supplements of black cumin for one year showed a significant reduction in systolic, diastolic, and mean arterial BP, heart rate, TC, LDL-c, the fractions of TC/HDL-c, and LDL-c/HDL-c, while serum HDL-c was suggestively raised when compared to baseline values and the control group. It was also used to assess the blood pressure-lowering capability and possible processes of *N. sativa* in a rat model, and it was discovered that the seed oil and nicardipine-treated groups had significantly lower blood pressure [71].

3. Conclusions

Medicinal plants are great sources of phytochemicals, which are abundant in a variety of plants and have few negative effects. They include active chemicals that help the body recover itself and re-establish its natural equilibrium. Traditional Islamic natural products are important sources of therapeutic medications with innovative structures and modes of action for the treatment of a variety of ailments as well as the drug discovery process. The recently reported pharmacologically and therapeutically based medicinal plants and their products that are mentioned in Islamic scriptures are presented in this chapter. The current study also emphasizes recent *in vitro*, *in vivo*, and clinical investigations of medicinal plants and their natural compounds. According to these reports, dates palm fruits, figs, and black seeds can be used for a variety of therapeutic applications, and these plant products may hold substantial promise for the development of novel therapeutic strategies for a variety of human diseases.

Acknowledgements

This work was supported by Cell and Tissue Culture Lab, Department of Biotechnology and Department of Biochemistry, Era University, Lucknow, India.

Conflict of interest

The authors declare no conflict of interest.

Author details

Sahabjada Siddiqui[1]*, Afsana Khatoon[2], Khursheed Ahmad[1], Shivbrat Upadhyay[1], Aditi Srivastava[3], Anchal Trivedi[3], Ishrat Husain[3], Rumana Ahmad[3], Mohsin Ali Khan[4] and Md Arshad[5]

1 Deparment of Biotechnology, Era's Lucknow Medical College and Hospital, Era University, Lucknow, India

2 Faculty of Arts, Arab Culture, Karamat Husain Muslim Girls' P.G. College, Lucknow, India

3 Department of Biochemistry, Era's Lucknow Medical College and Hospital, Era University, Lucknow, India

4 Chancellor, Era University, Lucknow, India

5 Department of Zoology, Aligarh Muslim University, Aligarh, India

*Address all correspondence to: sahabjada@erauniversity.in; sahabjadabiotech04@gmail.com

References

[1] Del Rio D, Rodriguez-Mateos A, Spencer JP, Tognolini M, Borges G, Crozier A. Dietary (poly) phenolics in human health: Structures, bioavailability, and evidence of protective effects against chronic diseases. Antioxidants & Redox Signaling. 2013;**18**(14):1818-1892. DOI: 10.1089/ars.2012.4581

[2] Milanizadeh S, Reza Bigdeli M. Pro-apoptotic and anti-angiogenesis effects of olive leaf extract on spontaneous mouse mammary tumor model by balancing vascular endothelial growth factor and endostatin levels. Nutrition and Cancer. 2019;**71**(8):1374-1381. DOI: 10.1080/01635581.2019.1609054

[3] Butler MS, Robertson AA, Cooper MA. Natural product and natural product derived drugs in clinical trials. Natural Product Reports. 2014;**31**(11):1612-1661. DOI: 10.1039/C4NP00064A

[4] Seca AM, Pinto DC. Plant secondary metabolites as anticancer agents: Successes in clinical trials and therapeutic application. International Journal of Molecular Sciences. 2018; **19**(1):263. DOI: 10.3390/ijms19010263

[5] Mehmood A, Khan S, Khan S, Ahmed S, Ali A, Xue M, et al. In silico analysis of quranic and prophetic medicinals plants for the treatment of infectious viral diseases including corona virus. Saudi Journal of Biological Science. 2021;**28**(5):3137-3151. DOI: 10.1016/j.sjbs.2021.02.058

[6] El-Seedi HR, Khalifa SA, Yosri N, Khatib A, Chen L, Saeed A, et al. Plants mentioned in the Islamic Scriptures (Holy Qur'ân and Ahadith): Traditional uses and medicinal importance in contemporary times. Journal of Ethnopharmacology. 2019;**243**:112007. DOI: 10.1016/j.jep.2019.112007

[7] Tungmunnithum D, Thongboonyou A, Pholboon A, Yangsabai A. Flavonoids and other phenolic compounds from medicinal plants for pharmaceutical and medical aspects: An overview. Medicine. 2018;**5**(3):93. DOI: 10.3390/medicines 5030093

[8] Sofowora A, Ogunbodede E, Onayade A. The role and place of medicinal plants in the strategies for disease prevention. African Journal of Traditional, Complementary and Alternative Medicines. 2013;**10**(5): 210-229. DOI: 10.4314/ajtcam.v10i5.2

[9] Baykara O. Current therapies and latest developments in cancer treatment. Horizons in Cancer Research. 2015; **57**:105-156

[10] Al-Alawi RA, Al-Mashiqri JH, Al-Nadabi JS, Al-Shihi BI, Baqi Y. Date palm tree (*Phoenix dactylifera* L.): Natural products and therapeutic options. Frontiers in Plant Science. 2017;**8**:845. DOI: 10.3389/fpls.2017.00845

[11] Alharbi KL, Raman J, Shin HJ. Date fruit and seed in nutricosmetics. Cosmetics. 2021;**8**(3):59. DOI: 0.3390/cosmetics8030059

[12] Hussain Mallhi T, Qadir MI, Ali M, Ahmad B, Khan YH. Ajwa date (*Phoenix dactylifera*): An emerging plant in pharmacological research. Pakistan Journal of Pharmaceutical Sciences. 2014;**27**(3):607-616

[13] Al-Farsi MA, Lee CY. Nutritional and functional properties of dates: A review. Critical Reviews in Food Science and Nutrition. 2008;**48**(10):877-887. DOI: 10.1080/10408390701724264

[14] Nasir MU, Hussain S, Jabbar S, Rashid F, Khalid N, Mehmood A. A review on the nutritional content,

functional properties and medicinal potential of dates. Science Letters. 2015;**3**(1):17-22

[15] Taleb H, Maddocks SE, Morris RK, Kanekanian AD. Chemical characterisation and the anti-inflammatory, anti-angiogenic and antibacterial properties of date fruit (*Phoenix dactylifera* L.). Journal of Ethnopharmacology. 2016;**194**:457-468. DOI: 10.1016/j.jep.2016.10.032

[16] Martín-Sánchez AM, Cherif S, Ben-Abda J, Barber-Vallés X, Pérez-Álvarez JÁ, Sayas-Barberá E. Phytochemicals in date co-products and their antioxidant activity. Food Chemistry. 2014;**158**:513-520. DOI: 10.1016/j.foodchem.2014.02.172

[17] Mirza MB, Elkady AI, Al-Attar AM, Syed FQ, Mohammed FA, Hakeem KR. Induction of apoptosis and cell cycle arrest by ethyl acetate fraction of *Phoenix dactylifera* L.(Ajwa dates) in prostate cancer cells. Journal of Ethnopharmacology. 2018;**218**:35-44. DOI: 10.1016/j.jep.2018.02.030

[18] Siddiqui S, Ahmad R, Khan MA, Upadhyay S, Husain I, Srivastava AN. Cytostatic and anti-tumor potential of Ajwa date pulp against human hepatocellular carcinoma HepG2 cells. Scientific Reports. 2019;**9**(1):1-2. DOI: 10.1038/s41598-018-36475-0

[19] Khan MA, Siddiqui S, Ahmad I, Singh R, Mishra DP, Srivastava AN, et al. Phytochemicals from Ajwa dates pulp extract induce apoptosis in human triple-negative breast cancer by inhibiting AKT/mTOR pathway and modulating Bcl-2 family proteins. Scientific Reports. 2021;**11**(1):10322. DOI: 10.1038/s41598-021-89420-z

[20] Khan F, Ahmed F, Pushparaj PN, Abuzenadah A, Kumosani T, Barbour E, et al. Ajwa date (*Phoenix dactylifera* L.) extract inhibits human breast adenocarcinoma (MCF7) cells *in vitro* by inducing apoptosis and cell cycle arrest. PloS One. 2016;**11**(7):e0158963. DOI: 10.1371/journal.pone.0158963

[21] Khan F, Khan TJ, Kalamegam G, Pushparaj PN, Chaudhary A, Abuzenadah A, et al. Anti-cancer effects of Ajwa dates (*Phoenix dactylifera* L.) in diethylnitrosamine induced hepatocellular carcinoma in Wistar rats. BMC Complementary and Alternative Medicine. 2017;**17**(1):1-0. DOI: 10.1186/s12906-017-1926-6

[22] Al Jaouni SK, Hussein A, Alghamdi N, Qari M, El Hossary D, Almuhayawi MS, et al. Effects of *Phoenix dactylifera* Ajwa on infection, hospitalization, and survival among pediatric cancer patients in a university hospital: A nonrandomized controlled trial. Integrative Cancer Therapies. 2019;**18**:1534735419828834. DOI: 10.1177/1534735419828834

[23] Miller CJ, Dunn EV, Hashim IB. The glycaemic index of dates and date/yoghurt mixed meals. Are dates 'the candy that grows on trees'? European Journal of Clinical Nutrition. 2003;**57**(3):427-430. DOI: 10.1038/sj.ejcn.1601565

[24] Ajiboye BO, Oloyede HO, Salawu MO. *Phoenix dactylifera* Linn fruit based-diets palliate hyperglycemia in alloxan-induced diabetic rats. Journal of Basic and Clinical Physiology and Pharmacology. 2020. DOI: 10.1515/jbcpp-2019-0185. Epub ahead of print. PMID: 32678802

[25] Ahmed S, Alam Khan R, Jamil S. Anti hyperlipidemic and hepatoprotective effects of native date fruit variety "Aseel" (*Phoenix dactylifera*). Pakistan Journal of Pharmaceutical Sciences. 2016;**29**(6):1945-1950

[26] Michael HN, Salib JY, Eskander EF. Bioactivity of diosmetin glycosides isolated from the epicarp of date fruits, *Phoenix dactylifera*, on the biochemical

profile of alloxan diabetic male rats. Phytotherapy Research. 2013;**27**(5): 699-704. DOI: 10.1002/ptr.4777

[27] Al-Shwyeh HA. Date palm (*Phoenix dactylifera* L.) fruit as potential antioxidant and antimicrobial agents. Journal of Pharmacy & Bioallied Sciences. 2019;**11**(1):1. DOI: 10.4103/jpbs.JPBS_168_18

[28] Saafi EB, Louedi M, Elfeki A, Zakhama A, Najjar MF, Hammami M, et al. Protective effect of date palm fruit extract (*Phoenix dactylifera* L.) on dimethoate induced-oxidative stress in rat liver. Experimental and Toxicologic Pathology. 2011;**63**(5):433-441. DOI: 10.1016/j.etp.2010.03.002

[29] Ahmed S, Khan RA, Jamil S, Afroz S. Antidiabetic effects of native date fruit Aseel (*Phoenix dactylifera* L.) in normal and hyperglycemic rats. Pakistan Journal of Pharmaceutical Sciences. 2017;**30**(5):1797-1802

[30] El-Mougy SA, Abdel-Aziz SA, Al-Shanawany M, Omar A. The gonadotropic activity of Palmae in mature male rats. Alexandria Journal of Pharmaceutical Sciences. 1991;**5**:156-159

[31] Singh D, Singh B, Goel RK. Traditional uses, phytochemistry and pharmacology of *Ficus religiosa*: A review. Journal of Ethnopharmacology. 2011;**134**(3):565-583. DOI: 10.1016/j.jep.2011.01.046

[32] Frodin DG. History and concepts of big plant genera. Taxon. 2004;**53**(3):753-776. DOI: 10.2307/4135449

[33] Vinson JA. The functional food properties of figs. Cereal Foods World. 1999;**44**(2):82-87. DOI: 10.1016/B978-0-12-407849-9.00056-7

[34] Barolo MI, Mostacero NR, López SN. *Ficus carica* L. (Moraceae): An ancient source of food and health. Food Chemistry. 2014;**164**:119-127. DOI: 10.1016/j.foodchem.2014.04.112

[35] Jellin JM, Gregory P, Batz F, Hichens K. Pharmacist's Letter/Prescriber's Letter Natural Medicines Comprehensive Database, 3rd Edition. Stockton, CA: Therapeutic Research Faculty, 2000. 1530 pp

[36] Buchman DD. Herbal Medicine. New York, NY: Wings Books; 1996

[37] Duke JA. The Green Pharmacy. New York, NY: Rodale Inc; 1997. p. 453

[38] Goor A. The history of the fig in the Holy Land from ancient times to the present day. Economic Botany. 1965;**19**(2):124-135. DOI: 10.1007/BF02862824

[39] Prasad PV, Subhaktha PK, Narayana A, Rao MM. Medico-historical study of "aśvattha" (sacred fig tree). Bulletin of the Indian Institute of History of Medicine (Hyderabad). 2006;**36**(1):1-20

[40] Badgujar SB, Patel VV, Bandivdekar AH, Mahajan RT. Traditional uses, phytochemistry and pharmacology of *Ficus carica*: A review. Pharmaceutical Biology. 2014;**52**(11):1487-1503. DOI: 10.3109/13880209.2014.892515

[41] Jeong WS, Lachance PA. Phytosterols and fatty acids in fig (*Ficus carica*, var. Mission) fruit and tree components. Journal of Food Science. 2001;**66**(2):278-281. DOI: 10.1111/j.1365-2621.2001.tb11332.x

[42] Veberic R, Jakopic J, Stampar F. Internal fruit quality of figs (*Ficus carica* L.) in the Northern Mediterranean Region. Italian Journal of Food Science. 2008;**20**(2):255-262

[43] Gibernau M, Buser HR, Frey JE, Hossaert-McKey M. Volatile compounds from extracts of figs of *Ficus carica*.

Phytochemistry. 1997;**46**(2):241-244. DOI: 10.1016/S0031-9422(97)00292-6

[44] Oliveira AP, Silva LR, de Pinho PG, Gil-Izquierdo A, Valentão P, Silva BM, et al. Volatile profiling of *Ficus carica* varieties by HS-SPME and GC–IT-MS. Food Chemistry. 2010;**123**(2):548-557. DOI: 10.1016/j.foodchem.2010.04.064

[45] Yancheva SD, Golubowicz S, Yablowicz Z, Perl A, Flaishman MA. Efficient Agrobacterium-mediated transformation and recovery of transgenic fig (*Ficus carica* L.) plants. Plant Science. 2005;**168**(6):1433-1441. DOI: 10.1016/j.plantsci.2004.12.007

[46] Alamgeer IS, Asif H, Saleem M. Evaluation of antihypertensive potential of *Ficus carica* fruit. Pharmaceutical Biology. 2017;**55**(1):1047-1053. DOI: 10.1080/13880209.2017.1278611

[47] Purnamasari R, Winarni D, Permanasari AA, Agustina E, Hayaza S, Darmanto W. Anticancer activity of methanol extract of *Ficus carica* leaves and fruits against proliferation, apoptosis, and necrosis in Huh7it cells. Cancer Informatics. 2019;**18**:117693511 9842576. DOI: 10.1177/11769351198 42576

[48] Gurung AB, Ali MA, Lee J, Farah MA, Al-Anazi KM. Molecular docking and dynamics simulation study of bioactive compounds from *Ficus carica* L. with important anticancer drug targets. Plos One. 2021;**16**(7): e0254035. DOI: 10.1371/journal.pone.0254035

[49] Belguith-Hadriche O, Ammar S, del Mar CM, Turki M, Segura-Carretero A, El Feki A, et al. Antihyperlipidemic and antioxidant activities of edible Tunisian *Ficus carica* L. fruits in high fat diet-induced hyperlipidemic rats. Plant Foods for Human Nutrition. 2016;**71**(2): 183-189. DOI: 10.1007/s11130-016-0541-x

[50] Atkinson FS, Villar A, Mulà A, Zangara A, Risco E, Smidt CR, et al. Abscisic acid standardized fig (*Ficus carica*) extracts ameliorate postprandial glycemic and insulinemic responses in healthy adults. Nutrients. 2019;**11**(8): 1757. DOI: 10.3390/nu11081757

[51] Gilani AH, Mehmood MH, Janbaz KH, Khan AU, Saeed SA. Ethnopharmacological studies on antispasmodic and antiplatelet activities of *Ficus carica*. Journal of Ethnopharmacology. 2008;**119**(1):1-5. DOI: 10.1016/j.jep.2008.05.040

[52] Ahmad A, Husain A, Mujeeb M, Khan SA, Najmi AK, Siddique NA, et al. A review on therapeutic potential of *Nigella sativa*: A miracle herb. Asian Pacific Journal of Tropical Biomedicine. 2013;**3**(5):337-352

[53] Tavakkoli A, Mahdian V, Razavi BM, Hosseinzadeh H. Review on clinical trials of black seed (*Nigella sativa*) and its active constituent, thymoquinone. Journal of Pharmacopuncture. 2017;**20**(3):179. DOI: 10.3831/KPI.2017.20.021

[54] Darakhshan S, Pour AB, Colagar AH, Sisakhtnezhad S. Thymoquinone and its therapeutic potentials. Pharmacological Research. 2015;**95**:138-158. DOI: 10.1016/j.phrs.2015.03.011

[55] Goreja WG. Black Seed: Nature's Miracle Remedy. New York: Amazing Herbs Press; 2003

[56] Abdel-Zaher AO, Abdel-Rahman MS, ELwasei FM. Protective effect of *Nigella sativa* oil against tramadol-induced tolerance and dependence in mice: Role of nitric oxide and oxidative stress. Neurotoxicology. 2011;**32**(6):725-733. DOI: 10.1016/j.neuro.2011.08.001

[57] Yarnell E, Abascal K. *Nigella sativa*: Holy herb of the middle East.

Alternative and Complementary Therapies. 2011;**17**(2):99-105. DOI: 10.1089/act.2011.17203

[58] Hammad Shafiq AA, Masud T, Kaleem M. Cardio-protective and anti-cancer therapeutic potential of *Nigella sativa*. Iranian Journal of Basic Medical Sciences. 2014;**17**(12):967

[59] Amin B, Hosseinzadeh H. Black cumin (*Nigella sativa*) and its active constituent, thymoquinone: An overview on the analgesic and anti-inflammatory effects. Planta Medica. 2016;**82**(01/02):8-16. DOI: 10.1055/s-0035-1557838

[60] Hosseinzadeh H, Taiari S, Nassiri-Asl M. Effect of thymoquinone, a constituent of *Nigella sativa* L., on ischemia–reperfusion in rat skeletal muscle. Naunyn-Schmiedeberg's Archives of Pharmacology. 2012; **385**(5):503-508. DOI: 10.1007/s00210-012-0726-2

[61] Khan A, Chen HC, Tania M, Zhang DZ. Anticancer activities of *Nigella sativa* (black cumin). African Journal of Traditional, Complementary and Alternative Medicines. 2011;**8**(5S):226-232. DOI: 10.4314/ajtcam.v8i5S.10

[62] Atta-UR-Rahman AU, Malik S, Hasan SS, Choudhary MI, Ni CZ, Clardy J. Nigellidine—A new indazole alkaloid from the seeds of *Nigella sativa*. ChemInform. 1995;**26**(30):1993-1996. DOI: 10.1016/0040-4039(95)00210-4

[63] Mahmoud SS, Torchilin VP. Hormetic/cytotoxic effects of *Nigella sativa* seed alcoholic and aqueous extracts on MCF-7 breast cancer cells alone or in combination with doxorubicin. Cell Biochemistry and Biophysics. 2013;**66**(3):451-460. DOI: 10.1007/s12013-012-9493-4

[64] Peng L, Liu A, Shen Y, Xu HZ, Yang SZ, Ying XZ, et al. Antitumor and anti-angiogenesis effects of thymoquinone on osteosarcoma through the NF-κB pathway. Oncology Reports. 2013;**29**(2):571-578. DOI: 10.3892/or.2012.2165

[65] Yimer EM, Tuem KB, Karim A, Ur-Rehman N, Anwar F. *Nigella sativa* L. (black cumin): A promising natural remedy for wide range of illnesses. Evidence-Based Complementary and Alternative Medicine. 2019;**2019**:1528635. DOI: 10.1155/2019/1528635. PMID: 31214267

[66] Onifade AA, Jewell AP, Adedeji WA. *Nigella sativa* concoction induced sustained seroreversion in HIV patient. African Journal of Traditional, Complementary and Alternative Medicines. 2013;**10**(5):332-335

[67] Ozdemir N, Kantekin-Erdogan MN, Tat T, Tekin A. Effect of black cumin oil on the oxidative stability and sensory characteristics of mayonnaise. Journal of Food Science and Technology. 2018;**55**(4):1562-1568. DOI: 10.1007/s13197-018-3075-4

[68] Mostafa RM, Moustafa YM, Mirghani Z, AlKusayer GM, Moustafa KM. Antioxidant effect of garlic (*Allium sativum*) and black seeds (*Nigella sativa*) in healthy postmenopausal women. SAGE Open Medicine. 2013;**1**:2050312113517501. DOI: 10.1177/2050312113517501

[69] Abdelmeguid NE, Fakhoury R, Kamal SM, Al Wafai RJ. Effects of *Nigella sativa* and thymoquinone on biochemical and subcellular changes in pancreatic β-cells of streptozotocin-induced diabetic rats. Journal of Diabetes. 2010;**2**(4):256-266. DOI: 10.1111/j.1753-0407.2010.00091.x

[70] Rachman PN, Darmawan E. The efficacy of black cumin seed (*Nigella sativa*) oil and hypoglycemic drug combination to reduce HbA1c level in

patients with metabolic syndrome risk. In: IOP Conference Series: Materials Science and Engineering. Vol. 259(1). Yogyakarta, Indonesia: IOP Publishing; 2017. p. 012018. DOI: 10.1088/1757-899X/259/1/012018

[71] Badar A, Kaatabi H, Bamosa A, Al-Elq A, Abou-Hozaifa B, Lebda F, et al. Effect of *Nigella sativa* supplementation over a one-year period on lipid levels, blood pressure and heart rate in type-2 diabetic patients receiving oral hypoglycemic agents: Nonrandomized clinical trial. Annals of Saudi Medicine. 2017;**37**(1):56-63. DOI: 10.5144/0256-4947.2017.56

Chapter 2

African Traditional and Complementary Therapies

Josephine Ozioma Ezekwesili-Ofili and Anthony Okechukwu Ogbonna

Abstract

Complementary therapies describe a wide range of healthcare practices that can be used alongside conventional treatments to deal with chronic health problems, treat symptoms, or simply to stay healthy. Examples include herbalism, bloodletting, purgation, prayers and incantations, hydrotherapy, diet, exercise, massage, etc. The basis for these practices stems from core beliefs: imbalance of body functions causes illness, the body can self-heal under the right conditions, and treatment should be of the whole body and not just symptoms; religion, spirituality, and culture are very strong underlying factors. The reasons for using complementary therapies are primarily to maintain good health, dissatisfaction with conventional medicines, taking charge of one's own health, ready availability, and notions of safety. In rural Africa, complementary therapies have been used solely as alternative therapies due to inadequate healthcare. This chapter deals with the African traditional complementary therapies that coexist with conventional medical practices and their advantages and disadvantages.

Keywords: traditional, complementary, alternative integrative, therapies, medicine, African

1. Introduction

The term "complementary therapies or medicine" refers to a broad spectrum of therapeutic and diagnostic practices that exist largely outside conventional medicine and are not fully integrated into the dominant healthcare system [1]. It is often used interchangeable with both alternative medicine and traditional medicine in some countries [2] or collectively called traditional, complementary, and alternative medicine (TCAM). Stricter definitions describe "indigenous traditional medicine" also known as ethno-medicine as the sum total of knowledge and practices, whether explicable or not, used in diagnosing, preventing, or eliminating physical, mental, and social diseases, administered by a trained practitioner or as self-care [3]. This knowledge or practice may rely exclusively on past experience and observation handed down orally or in writing from generation to generation. These practices are native to the country in which they are practiced. The majority of indigenous traditional medicine has been practiced at the primary healthcare level [4]. Complementary medicine (CM), on the other hand, is defined as a broad set of healthcare practices that are neither part of a country's own tradition nor part of conventional medicine and are not fully integrated into the dominant healthcare system. CM practices are used interchangeably with TCAM practices in some countries [5], while alternative medicine refers to practices used in place of conventional practice. Integrative medicine refers to conventional medicine combined with TCAM that are safe and show evidence of efficacy. TCAM is a focus on biological, psychological, social, and spiritual influences to pathology. It is characterized by a belief in the supernatural cause of illness, divination being a diagnostic tool, and the use of a wide variety of agents and techniques in its treatment [6, 7]. In the modern African setting, it may encompass local herbal medicines or products, indigenous healthcare practices [6, 8], and imported complementary and alternative medicine products and practices (e.g., acupuncture or chiropractic, etc.). Sub-Saharan Africa (SSA) is one region of the world in which TCAM has long been held to be widespread, with a considerable number of its population relying on it to maintain their health or prevent and treat communicable and noncommunicable diseases [9, 10]. However, some peculiar practices of TCAM, which include voodooism, incantations, chants and mysticism, etc., generate controversies and reduce the scientific credibility. The traditional healers'/attendants' rituals/incantations and other peculiar practices appear to be more important than the pharmacological effects of herbs and other practices. The traditional medical practitioner is usually a well-known and trusted person in his community, with competence to provide healthcare by using plant, animal, and mineral substances and other methods based on and religious practices. He makes use of indigenous social, cultural, and knowledge, beliefs, and/or experiences to treat disease and promote health. Healing power is passed down through generations via oral transmission and apprenticeship or through knowledge imbued by the "gods." Its powers and skills are generally reserved for the members of certain families by inheritance or the members of regional or cultural communities [8, 11].

TCAM is an important and often underestimated health resource with many applications, especially in the prevention and management of lifestyle-related chronic diseases and in meeting the health needs of indigenous populations, especially in Sub-Saharan Africa, where conventional healthcare systems are largely inadequate. Other terminologies that have been used include natural medicine, nonconventional medicine, or holistic medicine [2]. Common to most TCAM systems is a focus on individualizing treatment [1]. TCAM encompasses products, practices, and practitioners. TCAM has evolved over millennia by drawing on the religious beliefs and social structures of indigenous people and by exploiting natural products in their environment and more recently by developing and validating therapeutic and preventive approaches through scientific methods [12]. Despite the promise of contemporary medical practice, large segments of humanity either cannot access its benefits or cannot afford; rather, people opt for practices based on their culture, proof of efficacy, and accessibility. TCAM use is indeed very common in Africa but varies among different populations based on their beliefs and sociocultural practices [13, 14]. At least 4 out of 10 adults have used some form of TCAM.

In Africa, TCAM is interwoven with religious practices involving body and soul, hence the name holistic. This spiritual aspect of healing encompasses belief and worship to God and reverence and acknowledgement of ancestors. Ancestors are compassionate spirits of departed blood relatives of an individual and may involve a whole lineage spanning generations. They are revered but not worshipped as one would pray to God but serve to mediate between the living and God to bring healing and luck to them. They are regarded as custodians of the lives of future generations and, therefore, occupy a position of dignity and respect among their descendants [15]. According to [9], a considerable number of people in Sub-Saharan Africa (SSA) rely on traditional, complementary, and alternative medicine (TCAM) to meet their primary healthcare needs; yet, there remains a dearth of research evidence on the overall picture of TCAM utilization in the region. There have been reports of varied prevalence of the use of TCAM in Africa. In comparison, the use of TCAM products was found to be higher than that of practitioner services, especially for self-care and over-the-counter use among the general population. TCAM may be used alone or in combination with orthodox medicine, in both general population and specific health conditions.

2. Types of complementary therapies

The National Institutes of Health has grouped TCAM into five overlapping domains, namely, biologically based therapies, manipulative and body-based approaches, mind-body medicine, alternative medical systems, and energy medicine [1, 12]. Some complimentary therapies are discussed as follows:

- *Biologically based practices:* Nutritional excess and deficiency have been problems in today's society, both leading to certain chronic diseases. Thus, many dietary and herbal approaches are used to balance the body's nutritional well-being, e.g., vitamins and mineral supplements, unconventional diets (such as low-carbohydrate and keto diets), and natural products [16]. A dietary supplement could be intended to supplement the diet and will contain, for instance, a vitamin, a mineral, an herb, a botanical, or an amino acid. A dietary supplement might also be intended to supplement the diet by increasing the total daily intake of a concentrate, a metabolite, a constituent, an extract, or a combination of these ingredients. Health foods, including functional foods, are any natural food popularly believed to promote or sustain good health by containing vital nutrients. Functional foods also include any foodstuff enhanced by additives and marketed as beneficial to health or longevity. Examples include cereals, breads, or beverages, which are fortified with vitamins and herbs. Health foods and/or functional foods may be advertised or marketed with specific health claims and may, therefore, be regulated differently than other foods [4]. Eating nutritious foods help patients get important nutrients, such as protein, vitamins, and minerals. Depending on the ailment, patients may experience appetite loss, weight loss, or weight gain. Eating well helps to maintain a healthy body weight during and after treatment. Natural products are substances produced by living organisms and built by cells from biomolecule, e.g., botanicals, minerals, herbs and herbal preparations, and probiotics. Animal fats, cartilage, bones, and other parts are also part of natural products. Herbal medicines include herbs, herbal materials, herbal preparations, and finished herbal products that contain phytochemicals (alkaloids, tannins, glycosides, flavonoids, etc.) as active ingredients, parts of plants (leaves, seeds, roots, flowers, and bark) are used for medicinal purposes, other plant materials, or combinations thereof. In some countries, herbal medicines may contain, by tradition, natural organic or inorganic active ingredients that are not of plant origin (e.g., animal and mineral material) [4].

- *Manipulative and body-based approaches:* These focus primarily on the structures and systems of the body. They include massage, chiropractic (spinal manipulation), osteopathy, and traditional bone setting. Womb manipulation and alignment is also an important aspect of preconception therapy. Spinal manipulation is used to treat an array of conditions that arise as a result of abnormal alignment or stress on the vertebrae, often due to musculoskeletal complaints. Traditional bone setting is the traditional form of osteopathy.

Though appearing crude because of the lack of the use of X-ray, it has recorded tremendous success. The bonesetter may often make used of herbs to relieve pain and promote healing and may use primitive forms of straps and wooden splints to hold the bone in place.

- *Mind-body medicine:* This is based on the fact that the mind exerts powerful influences on bodily functions and *vice versa*. They include an array of approaches that incorporate spiritual, meditative, and relaxation techniques, including hypnosis, yoga, acupuncture, Tai chi, Qi gong, and breathing exercises. Appropriate psychotherapy was found to reduce depression and anxiety and improved coping skills.

- *Alternative medical systems:* Health is based on the balance and flow of vital energies through the body. For example, in acupuncture, vital energy flow is restored by placing needles at critical body points.

- *Energy medicine:* This involves the use of energy either biofield- or bioelectromagnetic-based interventions, e.g., reiki, purging, bleeding/bloodletting, and treatment with heavy metals.

Based on literature, biological therapies, such as the use of herbal and animal products, are the most common forms of TCAM used in Sub-Saharan Africa, followed by faith-based healing methods, such as prayer/spirituality [17, 18], and mind and body therapies (traditional bone setting, meditation and yoga, massage, relaxation, and music and art therapy). Others include acupuncture, Tai chi and Qi gong, massage, hydrotherapy, physical activity, and diet and nutrition [19]. Some of these health practices, though not originally African, have been adopted overtime and are included in complementary therapies practiced today in modern Africa, especially Chinese medicine due to the recently increased influx of the Chinese into Africa.

Acupuncture is a form of complementary medicine and a component of traditional Chinese medicine and is one of the imported complementary therapies in Africa [20, 21]. It involves the use of very thin needles or pressure to stimulate specific points on the body. Acupuncture causes changes in the fascia, which is the connective tissue that covers the muscles and bones. This can lead to changes in the brain, such as the release of chemicals like serotonin or changes in electrical activity. These changes are thought to explain, in part, how acupuncture works to treat different symptoms. Acupuncture has been used for the alleviation of pain [22], nausea, vomiting [23], fertility, childbirth chronic asthma, epilepsy, and addiction, among others. The efficacy of acupuncture is considered to be due to the release of endorphins and the stimulation of the peripheral nervous system when the skin is punctured [24]. The safety of acupuncture is assured when administered by well-trained practitioners using sterile needles. However, being an invasive procedure, adverse effects have been reported, such as hemorrhage, hematoma and bacterial infection, nerve injuries, hepatitis, kidney damage, etc. [25].

Homeopathy: According to the principles of homoeopathy, certain remedies, when given in high concentrations, tend to mimic the symptoms presented by the patient, and that upon dilution and vigorous shaking releases the curative "essence." Dilution continues until no more of the original substance remains, but the water molecules are believed to retain a "memory" of the original substance [26]. While no scientific evidence has been found to support the theories of homeopathy, some successes have been reported. Randomized clinical trials have suggested that it might be effective for treating influenza, allergies, and postoperative ileum [12]. Some schools of thought consider it to be a little more effective than placebo [27].

Yoga is another important aspect of complementary therapies. Yoga promotes slow breathing techniques used to relax mind and body, as well as to increase oxygenation [28]. It reduces stress and anxiety by using breathing exercises, meditation, relaxation techniques, and poses to stretch and flex different muscle groups. Yoga also calms the mind and connects mind and body. Studies have shown that yoga increases the activities of the parasympathetic nervous system by releasing γ-amino butyric acid, GABA [29].

The benefits of yoga include improved overall quality of life, increased physical functioning, and increased ability to conduct the activities of daily living. Yoga also improves mood and physical well-being, improves nausea, reduces pain and fatigue, improves sleep problems, and helps regulate stress hormones. It also decreases inflammation and increases immune function.

Tai chi and Qi gong are part of traditional Chinese medicine that combine a series of fluid movements, which are slow and deliberate, meditation, regulated breathing, and calming of the mind, thus enhancing physical health and emotional well-being. Derived from martial art, Tai chi and Qi gong can improve the quality of life, reduce sleep problems, and decrease inflammation. Tai chi is based on spiritual and philosophical ideas that advocate for a need for balance in the body, mind, and spirit, with the notion that life energy or "*chi*" needs to flow freely for good health to occur. Qi gong, also derived from martial art, on the other hand, trains both body and soul and focuses on the relationship between the individual and the cosmic environment [30, 31].

Meditation is the practice of focusing your attention to calm the mind and relax the body. Sometimes, a calming word or chant is silently repeated. Other times, there is only focus on breathing or just being aware of thoughts and feelings with no judgment, attachment, or interpretation. Meditation can be self-taught or guided by others. There are many different types, including focused meditation, open awareness and mindfulness, and compassion or loving-kindness meditation, with or without religious undertone. Studies show that meditation can decrease chronic pain, improve mood and many other aspects of quality of life, lower stress hormones, and improve immune function [32].

Music therapy involves the use of musical and rhythm-based interventions to support and develop physical, mental, social, and spiritual well-being. It is a non-invasive, nonpharmaceutical, relatively inexpensive but effective therapy, which targets improvements in cognitive function and physical rehabilitation. Music has been shown to have psychosocial, behavioral, and motor benefits as treatment for neurological dysfunctions. Music induces changes by linking brain regions within multisensory and motor networks, thereby having effects on emotion and reward systems. Evidence suggests that music-based therapy improves balance and functional mobility in patients with Parkinson's disease and positive benefits in dementia as well as mitigating pain, improving blood flow and joint flexion required for a more rapid healing process during the rehabilitation phase after stroke [33, 34].

Art therapy is a form of complementary psychotherapy that uses artistic materials (visual art, painting, and drawing) as palliative care focused on relieving suffering patient with serious illness to ameliorate symptom burden and adapt to the stressful life experiences associated with life-limiting diagnosis. It utilizes the expressive qualities of art to improve physical, mental, and emotional well-being. It also improves cognitive and semimotor functions, fosters self-esteem and self-awareness, cultivates emotional resilience, promotes insight, enhances social skills, reduces and resolves conflict and distress, and advances societal and ecological changes. Art therapy is used mainly for cancer, depression, anxiety, autism, dementia, and cognitive impairment, especially in situations when verbal interaction becomes difficult and provides a safe and indirect way to connect oneself to others [35, 36].

Massage can help promote relaxation, ease tension, increase comfort, and reduce pain, especially in musculoskeletal conditions. People with cancer may especially benefit from massage and its subspecialty called oncology massage. In addition to receiving massage from a massage therapist, a caregiver can do simple massage to help relax. It is also possible to do a self-massage [32].

Research shows that massage can reduce pain, decrease tension and stress, help with recover after surgery, ease anxiety and depression, and help with sleep problems and fatigue [32].

Regular exercise: A growing amount of research shows that exercise can greatly improve different aspects of patients' physical and mental health during every phase of treatment. An exercise program can rejuvenate a patient, if used appropriately [37].

3. Factors affecting and reasons for TCAM use

A number of factors were identified as being promoters of TCAM use. Generally, the use of TCAM could simply be for health promotion and maintenance, but could equally be dependent on the type of illness and severity. Favorites among diseases include mental illness, impotence, infertility in females, and chronic disorders. Key factors that affect its use include relatively low cost and flexibility of payment of products and services, accessibility, availability affordability, compatibility, and suitability for the treatment of various diseases particularly certain chronic ones that orthodox medicine has not been able to cure, and the perception that because these products are natural, they must be safe with fewer side effects [38]. It was observed that patients that use TCAM also access conventional medicine, which more common in developing countries [39]. The fact that TCAM is in alignment with sociocultural, religious, and spiritual values is also a strong factor. Trust and confidence in traditional medicine practitioners and the perceived privacy as well as recommendation by elders, relatives, and friends also contributed to the choice to patronize TCAM products and facilities. Furthermore, recent increase in scientific research and validation of traditional medicines and aggressive advertisement of products and services are enhancing factors.

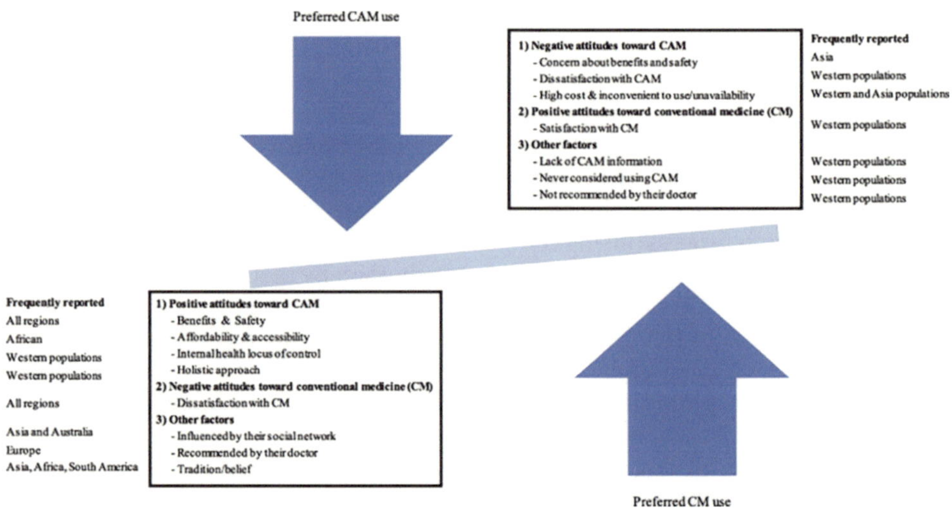

Figure 1.
Factors related to reasons for TCAM use and nonuse [41].

Dissatisfaction with conventional medicine, inadequate health facilities, unavailability of drugs, difficulty in accessing healthcare, negative attitudes of health workers, lengthy procedures, and long waiting time are other push factors to patronizing TCAM. Furthermore, TCAM is sought for: i) health conditions that had failed to respond to initial treatment, ii) health conditions stigmatized at communities of origin, and iii) health conditions thought to have resulted from supernatural causes [40]. Some of the benefits of complementary therapies are the holistic approach, which is more or less according to the philosophies and beliefs of a people, and the individualized approach to patients' care, involving them as active participants in their own health, portraying a high degree of physical, psychological, and spiritual contribution to treatment with a sense of self-satisfaction. There is also a strong emphasis on use as preventive medicine [41, 42] (**Figure 1**).

4. Barriers to the use of TCAM

Limiting factors to the use of TCAM in Africa include absence of scientific evidence supporting TCAM practices, lack of belief in safety and efficacy, lack of appropriate dose, unhygienic preparations [43], unregulated TCAM practitioner practice, and lack of education and proper training of practitioners. There are also no standard regulations as in orthodox medicine such that fake, ineffective substances and practices may be commonplace. The World Health Organization (WHO) further advocates that for future existence and integration of TCAM into conventional healthcare, attention ought to be paid to overcome the following hurdles: lack of research data, lack of mechanisms to monitor the safety of products, lack of expertise within national health authorities and control against appropriate mechanisms to monitor and regulate practitioners and products, lack of cooperative channels between national health authorities to share information about TCAM mechanisms to monitor the safety of products, and lack of mechanisms to control and regulate TCAM advertising and claims [4]. In addition, the lack of control of overharvesting and the conservation of endangered species and dwindling biodiversity due to climate change, thereby resulting possibly in extinction, are of great concern [44]. All these present major challenges to any effort to optimize TCAM.

5. Safety of TCAM

TCAM is still very much in use in modern-day Africa after hundreds of years of its existence without much reported cases of adverse effects [40]. Limited correlation between research and scientific evidence on safety and efficacy of most TCAM treatments has made them potential risks. Although practices such as acupuncture, homeopathy, and medication are low risks, adverse effects due to TCAM alone or in combination with conventional medicines have been reported [45]. These may be due to the side effects of TCAM products or drug interaction with conventional medicine. Herbs have been found to be toxic and produce herb-drug interactions due to their content of substances that have powerful pharmacological effects. Commonly observed effects include allergies, nausea, vomiting, diarrhea, abdominal pains, as well as dizziness, headache, and general malaise, and even death may ensue [46]. Liver and kidney problems have been observed among the chronic users of TCAM products [47]. However, the results of many evidence-based clinical trials have equally promoted credibility in TCAM.

6. Economic factors affecting the use of TCAM

Although social, medical, and cultural reasons account for why people in any given country prefer TCAM to conventional medicines, economic factors play a vital role in influencing TCAM use. The cost of TCAM, which is much cheaper than the cost of accessing conventional medical services, is the primary factor. Others include choosing a trusted traditional healer in whom much confidence is reposed, ease of access, and convenience. The poor are more likely to use TCAM, although people with high income are also likely to use TCAM for different reasons [48]. The method of payment is flexible, often on credit, in exchange for labor or contingent on outcome.

7. Prevalence of TCAM in Sub-Saharan Africa

Africa African traditional medicine is said to be one of the oldest and most diverse of all medicine systems, even though the medicines are poorly recorded. In developing countries, TCAM use is driven mostly by tradition and lack of resources. Over the years, the use of TCAM in both rural and urban areas across Africa has increased, but there is a great concern for its safety [45], efficacy, and control, and this poses a great challenge for health authorities and the general public [14]. There have been reports that there is varied prevalence but substantial use of TCAM, more of products (either for self-care and over-the-counter) than practitioner services, among the general population and specific clinical populations [19]. At least 80% of populations in Africa use TCAM [4].

The prevalence of TCAM during pregnancy, childbirth, and pregnancy termination is between 12% and 90.3% [49], but fewer patronage of TCM services during pregnancy but high use in the case of infertility, enhancing libido, general gynaecological conditions, and sexually transmitted diseases [50, 51].

TCAM products are highly used by patients with diabetes: Tanzania (77.1%), Nigeria (43%), Guinea (33%), and Kenya (12.4%) [52]. A higher rate was reported for cancer: Nigeria (65%), Ethiopia (79%), and Ghana (73.5%) [53]. Psychosis in some African countries (Nigeria, Ethiopia, Ghana, and Malawi) was also high (73%) [54]. The elusive COVID-19 was not left out in TCAM use. Massage and steam inhalation with various African herbs and spices were highly used and were believed to be effective for prevention and treatment.

Other reports revealed the following prevalence for noncommunicable diseases (61%), asthma (50%), epilepsy (65.5%), and schizophrenia (76%) [19, 38]. Musculosketetal problems, osteoarthritis, and bone fracture showed high patronage for bonesetters. All other health conditions, such as diarrhea, infantile colic, oral health, etc., were reported with varying prevalence.

In terms of different categories of people, a higher TCAM utilization rate was observed among outpatients than inpatients (72% versus 18.5%) [55]. Among student population, a higher utilization rate of products was found with high school than undergraduates, and much less for medical and paramedical students in both Ghana and Nigeria [56, 57]. Among healthcare professionals, TCAM use was much lower in Nigeria (20.777%) and South Africa (23.5%) [58, 59].

Sociodemographic studies indicated that TCAM users compared with non-TCAM users are more likely to be of low socioeconomic and educational status, unemployed and unskilled, while there were inconsistencies in age, sex, spatial location, and religious affiliation between TCAM users and non-TCAM users. Some reports, however, indicated that urban and semiurban dwellers were found to be younger (20–50 years) than rural dwellers (>58 years). Users were also found to be higher among married than not married [60] and women more likely than men [13].

The mean prevalence of concurrent use of TCAM products and conventional medicine within the general population and for specific health conditions in SSA was reported to be high but lower among patients with HIV/AIDS, and least with noncommunicable diseases such as diabetes [19].

Most TCAM users (55.8–100%) in SSA fail to disclose TCAM use to their healthcare providers, with the main reasons for nondisclosure being fear of receiving improper care, healthcare providers' negative attitude and a lack of enquiry about TCAM use from healthcare providers.

Evidence suggests that Africans in diaspora still maintain their use of TCAM overseas, and it is commonplace to find them transporting medicines from Africa to their country of abode [61].

The increasing uptake of TCAM services across the continent in recent decades has attracted the attention of policy makers, researchers, and healthcare professionals. In the past 20 years, the WHO regional office for Africa spearheaded the implementation of a regional strategy endorsed by African Heads of State in Lusaka, Zambia to promote the role of TCAM in health systems in the African region [62]. The gains experienced since the adoption of the regional plan include policy formation in 36 countries and research promotion, including the establishment of TCAM research centers in some countries such as Nigeria, Ghana, and South Africa. The regional plan has also promoted the inclusion of TCAM courses into the curricula of healthcare training institutions in countries across the continent. For instance, such plan has seen the inclusion of TCAM courses in some South African and Nigerian universities at both undergraduate and postgraduate levels. In Ghana, universities offer a BSc in herbal medicine. In Guinea, Sierra Leone, and Tanzania, Master's degree in herbal medicine has been made compulsory for pharmacists [62]. It has also promoted the training of TCAM practitioners and the local production and cultivation of medicinal plants, as well as the establishment of intellectual property rights for traditional medicine knowledge in few nations [55]. Despite such progress, most African countries continue to grapple with an absence of TCAM policy or its implementation, inadequate TCAM research infrastructure, and insufficient regulation of TCAM products and practices [15, 62]. For instance, by 2005, only 32% and 27% of the African countries who responded to the WHO global survey had a national policy and law or regulation on TCAM [63].

8. Conclusion

The pattern of disease is changing in developing countries of Africa as a result of globalization, mostly due to contributing factors such as lifestyle, diet, obesity, lack of exercise, stress, etc. A steady rise in the prevalence of chronic noncommunicable diseases is significantly contributing to Africa's disease burden and is adding to healthcare systems already strained due to the high incidence of infectious diseases. It is, therefore, postulated that TCAM will continue to play an integral role in the health and well-being of people suffering from chronic diseases in Africa as it is part and parcel of African heritage.

Although the use of TCAM is increasing in both developed and developing countries, while this may be substantial, it continues to exist only at the periphery of conventional medicine. It is noteworthy that Western religion, education, modernization, and globalization in Africa have not affected the continuous existence of TCAM, as practiced both in urban and rural areas. This is because it is affordable, dependable, and culture oriented, taking care of healthcare needs of the people. The continued use and future of TCAM is to a great extent hinged on its coexistence with conventional medicine. The extent to which this integration will occur in future as well as the nature of this integration will be greatly influenced by the attitude of physicians, which is mostly negative. For futuristic purposes, the medical students' attitude toward TCAM is, therefore, important in assessing the possibility that this may change. Students' attitudes and beliefs may have a strong impact on the way they will ultimately practice this type of integrative medicine in future. A proper policy and practice response to increasing TCAM use requires an in-depth insight into the nature of TCAM use, including the profile of TCAM users as well as the drivers and barriers that facilitate and limit the use of TCAM. It is, therefore, important for health departments and governments across Africa to put forward policy designs and implementations regarding TCAM, its current role and future possibilities in healthcare systems in general and promoting TCAM training, research and development, as well as integration into mainstream healthcare systems and educational systems as a means of advancing TCAM use.

The WHO, in spite of the challenges of uplifting the role of TCAM in Africa, has noted quite a number of achievements, namely, formation of national policies and regulatory framework in some African member countries, promotion of research by the production of scientific evidence on the safety, efficacy, and quality of TCAM products and services, the development of inventories and monographs on medicinal plants and herbal pharmacopoeia, and capacity building by the inclusion of TCAM in training curricula of health professionals, educating, training, and integration of traditional health practitioners for primary healthcare. However, some challenges yet to be addressed in many African countries exist. There are limited data on safety, efficacy, and quality, limited resources for clinical trials, integrating TCAM to tertiary institutions healthcare systems, and inadequate protection of indigenous knowledge and intellectual proprietary rights. The way forward would, therefore, be to tackle these challenges. No doubt, there are differences between the degrees of organization and integration of TCAM into the mainstream health systems. While some countries may have no structure in place, others have considerable structures in place.

Overall, there is definitely hope for growth and future of TCAM in Africa.

Author details

Josephine Ozioma Ezekwesili-Ofili[1]* and Anthony Okechukwu Ogbonna[2]

1 Department of Applied Biochemistry, Nnamdi Azikiwe University, Awka, Nigeria

2 Department of Medicine, Enugu State University Teaching Hospital, Enugu, Nigeria

*Address all correspondence to: ezekjossie@gmail.com

References

[1] Pace O. Complementary and alternative medicine facts and figures. The Journal of Malta Collee of Family Doctors. 2012;**1**(1):18-24

[2] Mothibe ME, Sibanda M. African Traditional Medicine: South African Perspective. London, UK: IntechOpen Publishers; 2019

[3] Sirios FM, Salamousen A, Kristofferson AE. Reasons for continuing use of complementary and alternative medicine in students: A consumer commitment model. BMC Complementary and Alternative Medicine. 2016;**16**:75-84

[4] WHO. WHO Global Report on Traditional and Complementary Medicine. Geneva: World Health Organization; 2019; License: CC BY-NC-SA 3.0 IGO [Accessed July 10, 2021]

[5] WHO. Traditional, Complementary and Integrative Medicine. Geneva: WHO; 2013 [Accessed July 5, 2021]

[6] WHO. Traditional Medicine Strategy. 2014-2023. Geneva: World Health Organization (WHO); 2013 Available from: https://www.who.int/medicines/publications/traditional/trm_strategy14_23/en/ [Accessed 20 August, 2021]

[7] Rasamiravaka T, Kahumba J, Okusa PN, Bakari A, Bizumukama L, Kalonji JN, et al. Traditional African Medicine: From ancestral Knowledge to a modern integrated future. Science. 2015;**350**(6262):S61-S63

[8] Sofowora A. Medicinal Plants and Traditional medicine in Africa. 2nd ed. Ibadan, Nigeria: Spectrum Books Limited, Sunshine House; 1993, 1993. p. 289

[9] World Health Organization. Promoting the role of traditional medicine in health systems: A strategy for the African region. 2000

[10] Bannerman RH. The role of traditional medicine in primary health care. In: Burton J, Editor. Traditional Medicine and Healthcare Coverage: A Reader for Health Administrators and Practitioners. Geneva: WHO; 1983. pp. 318-327

[11] Ezekwesili-Ofili JO, Okaka ANC. Herbal medicines in African traditional medicine. In: Herbal Medicines. London, UK: IntechOpen Publishers; 2019

[12] Debas HT, Laxminarayan R, Straus SE. Complementary and Alternative Medicine In: Jamison DT, Breman JG, Measham AR, et al., editors. Disease Control Priorities in Developing Countries. 2nd edition. Washington (DC): The International Bank for Reconstruction and Development/The World Bank, Co-published bu Oxford University Press, New York; 2006. Chapter 69

[13] OnyiaPat E, Okoronkwo I, Ogbonnaya N. Complementary and alternative medicine use among adults in Enugu, Nigeria. BMC Complementary and Alternative Medicine. 2011;**11**(1):19

[14] Chukwuma EC, Soladoye MO, Feyisola RT. Traditional medicine and the future of medicinal plants in Nigeria. Journal of Medicinal Plants Studies. 2015;**3**(4):23-29

[15] Abdullahi A. Trends and challenges of traditional medicine in Africa. African Journal of Traditional, Complementary and Alternative Medicine. 2011;**8**(Suppl. 5):115-123

[16] Obu RN. Herbal/Alternative Medicine: The New Frontier West Africa All Herbal/Alternative Medicine

Conference Awards. Accra, Ghana: Holiday Inn; 2019 [Accessed 20 July, 2021]

[17] Bearon LB, Koenig HG. Religious cognition and use of prayer in health and illness. The Gerontologists. 1990;**30**(2):249-253

[18] Obu RN, Aggrey-Bluwey. Naturopathic Doctors qualitative study of prayer in Ghana: How much do we know? Ghana Alternative Medicine Journal. 2021;**2**(1):17-20

[19] James PB, Wardle J, Steel A, Adams J. Traditional, complementary and alternative medicine use in Sub-Saharan Africa: A Systematic review. British Medical Journal Global Health. 2018;**3**(5):e000895

[20] Adams D, Cheng F, Jou H, Aubg S, Yasui Y, Vohra S. The safety of paediatric acupuncture: A systematic review. Pediatrics. 2011, 2011;**128**(6):1575-1587

[21] Kantai C. Chinese Medicine is China's Fastest Growing Export in Africa?. Available form: https://pandaily.com/whytraditional [Accessed 26 December 2021]

[22] MPatil S, Sen S, Bral M, Reddy S, Bradley KK, Cornett EM, et al. The role of Acupuncture in Pain Management. Current Pain and Headache Reports. 2016;**20**(4):22

[23] Lee A, Fan LT. Stimulation of the wrist acupuncture point P6 for prevention of postpartum nausea and vomiting. Cochrane Database of Systematic reviews. 2009;**2**:CD003281

[24] Sun Y, Gan TJ. Acupuncture for the management of chronic headache: A systematic review. Anesthesia and Analgesia. 2008;**107**(6):2038-2047

[25] Ernst E. Death after acupuncture: A systematic review. The International Journal of Risk and Safety in Medicine. 2010;**22**(3):131-136

[26] Teixeira J. Can water possibly have a memory: A skeptical view. Homeopathy. 2007;**96**(3):158-163

[27] Shang A. Are the clinical effects of homeopathy placebo effects? Comparative study of placebo-controlled trials of homeopathy and allopathy. The Lancet. 2005;**366**(948):726-732

[28] Sharma M, Haider T. Yoga as an alternative and complementary therapy for patients suffering from anxiety: A systematic review. Journal of Evidence-Based Complementary and Alternative Medicine. 2013;**20**(2):143-153

[29] Rocha KK, Ribeiro AM, Rocha KC, et al. Improvement in physiological and psychological parameters after 6 months of yoga practice. Conscious Cognition. 2012;**21**:843-850

[30] Sharma M, Haider T. Tai chi as an alternative and complementary therapy for anxiety: A systematic review. Journal of Evidence-Based Integrative Medicine. 2015;**20**:143-153

[31] Siu JY. The use of qigong and tai chi as complementary alternative medicine (CAM) among chronically ill patients in Hong Kong. In: A Compendium of Essays on Alternative Therapies. 2012. pp. 175-192

[32] American Society of Clinical Psychology (ASCO). Types of Complementary Therapies. Available from: https://www.cancer.net/types of complimentary therapies [Accessed 6 December 2021]

[33] Machado Sotomayor MJ, Arufe-Giráldez V, Ruíz-Rico G, Navarro-Patón R. Music therapy and Parkinson's Disease: A systematic review from 2015-2020. International Journal of Environmental Research Public Health. 2021;**18**(21):11618. doi: 10.3390/ijerph182111618. PMID: 34770129; PMCID: PMC8582661

[34] Daniel A, Koumans H, Ganti L. Impact of music therapy on gait after stroke. Cureus. 2021;**13**(10):e18441. DOI: 10.7759/cureus.18441

[35] Hu J, Zhang J, Hu L, Yu H, Xu J. Art therapy: A complementary treatment for mental disorders. Frontiers in Psychology. 2021;**12**:686005

[36] Iguina MM, Kashan S. Art Therapy. Treasure Island (FL): StatPearls Publishing; 2021

[37] The Well Project, Complementary Therapies. 2020. Available from: https://www.thewellproject.org/complementary therapies. 2020 [Accessed June 18, 2021]

[38] Adeyeye OO, Onadeko BO, Ogunleye O, Bamisele RT, Olubisi A. The use of complementary and alternative medicine by asthma patients receiving care in an urban tertiary center in Nigeria. International Journal of Medical Research. 2011;**2**(4): 1026-1030

[39] Thomas K, Coleman P. Use of complementary or alternative medicine in a general population in Great Britain. Results from the National Omnibus Survey. Journal of Public Health. 2004;**26**(2):152-157

[40] Okigbo RN, Mmeka EC. An Appraisal of Phytomedicine in Africa. KMITL Science and Technology Journal. 2006;**6**(2):83-94

[41] Abbott RB, Hui K, Hays RD, Mandel J, Goldstein M, Winegarden B, et al. Medical students' attitude toads. Complementary, Alternative and Integrative Medicine. 2011; Article ID 985243:1-14

[42] Tangtjiakumjai M, Boardman H, Walker DM. Potential factors that influence usage of complementary and alternative medicine worldwide: A systematic review. BMC Complementary Medicine and Therapies. 2020;**20**(1):363

[43] Ezekwesili-Ofili JO, Onyemelukwe NF, Agwaga P, Orji J. The bioload and Aflatoxin content of herbal medicines from selected states in Nigeria. African Journal of Traditional, Complementary and Alternative Medicine. 2014;**11**(3):143-147

[44] Ottuh JA, Ottuh PO. Herbal medicine in Nigeria (Ezekiel, 47:12): Towards a synergy between the African medical practice and Western medicine in Urhobo land. Saudi Journal of Humanities. 2012;**1**(1):179-200

[45] Adewumi CO, Ojewole JAO. Safety of traditional medicines, complementary and alternative medicines in Africa. African Journal of Complementary and Alternative Medicine. 2004;**1**(1):1-3

[46] Okaiyeto K, Oguntibeju OO. African herbal medicines: Adverse effects and cytotoxic potentials with different therapy applications. International Journal of Environmental Research and Public Health. 2021;**18**:5988

[47] Ezekwesili-Ofili JO, Udensi JA, Okwara J. Liver and Kidney function in medicinal plant users in South-East, Nigeria: A pointer to herbal toxicity? Journal of Applied Science. 2012;**15**(1): 100638-110649

[48] Winston CM, Patel. Use of traditional and Orthodox Health Services in Urban Zimbabwe. International Journal of Epidemiology. 1995;**24**(5):1006-1012

[49] Mureyi DD, Morena-Penduka TG, Maponga CC. Prevalence and patterns of prenatal use of traditional medicine among women at selected Harare clinics: A cross-sectional study. BMC Complementary and Alternative\ Medicine. 2012;**12**(1):164

[50] Nelms LW, Gorski J. The role of African traditional healer in women's health. Journal of Transcultural Nursing. 2006;**17**(2):184-189

[51] Kaadaaga HF, Ajeani J, Ononge S, Alele PE, Nakasuijja N, Manabe YC, et al. Prevalence and factors associated with use of herbal medicine among women attending an infertility clinical in Uganda. BMC Complementary and Alternative Medicine. 2014;**14**:27

[52] Ogbera AO, Dada O, Adeyeye F, Jewo PI. Complementary and alternative medicine use in diabetes mellitus. West African Journal of Medicine. 2010;**29**(3):158-162

[53] Ezeome ER, Anarado AN. Use of complementary and alternative medicine by cancer patients at the University of Nigeria Teaching Hospital, Enugu, Nigeria. BMC Complementary and Alternative Medicine. 2007;**7**:28-35

[54] Girma E, Sefaye M. Patters of treatment seeking behavior for mental illness in southwest Ethiopia: A hospital based study. BMC Psychiatry. 2011;**11**(1):138

[55] Adinma E, Azuike E, Okafor-Udah C. Pattern and practice of complementary and alternative medication among patients in a tertiary hospital in Nigeria. European Journal of Preventive Medicine. 2015;**3**:44-48

[56] Alade GO, Kpako E, Ajibesin KK. Indigenous Knowledge of herbal medicines among adolescents in Amassoma, Bayelsa State, Nigeria. Global Journal of Health Science. 2016;**8**:217

[57] Nworu CS, Udeogaranya PO, Okafor CK, Adikwu AO, Akah PA. Perception, usage and knowledge of herbal medicines by students and academic staff of University of Nigeria: A survey. European Journal of Integrative Medicine. 2015;**7**:218-227

[58] Awodele O, Agbaje EO, Abiola OO, et al. Doctors' attitude towards the use of herbal medicines in Lagos Nigeria. Journal of Herbal Medicine. 2012;**2**:16-22

[59] Mbutho NP, Gqaleni N, Korporaal CM. Traditional, complementary and alternative medicine: Knowledge, attitudes and practices of health care workers in HIV and AIDS clinics in Durban hospitals. African Traditional, Complementary and Alternative Medicine. 2012;**9** (Suppl. 3):64-72

[60] Okoronkwo I, OnyiaPat J-L, Okpala P, Agbo M. Patterns of complementary and alternative medicine use, perceived and adverse effects among users in Enugu Urban, South-Eastern Nigeria. Evidence-Based Complementary and Alternative Medicine. 2014;**2014**:1-6

[61] Shewamene Z, Dune T, Smith CA. The use of Traditional medicine in maternal care among women in Africa and in the diaspora: A systematic review. BMC Complementary, Alternative and Alternative Medicine. 2017;**17**(1):382

[62] Kasilo OM, Trapsida JM, Mwikisa CN, Lusamba-Dikassra PS. An overview of the traditional medicine situation in the African Region. African Health Monitor. 2010;**14**:7-15

[63] WHO. National Policy on Traditional Medicine and Regulation of Herbal Medicines: Report of a WHO Global Survey. Geneva: World Health Organization; 2005

Chapter 3

Mibyou Care is A Key for Healthy Life Elongation: The Role of Mibyou-Care Functional Foods

Tetsuya Konishi

Abstract

Mibyou was originally defined in the traditional Chinese Medicine as the certain physiological state being not perfectly well but not ill and was recognized that the treatment of Mibyou is more important than treating diagnosable diseases. As the life span of human is getting sufficiently elongated, the demand for the healthy life expenditure increased, and the Mibyou is recognized to be the target for securing the healthy aging and wellness in the longevity society. Consequently, the concept of Mibyou is currently reevaluated, especially, in the preventive medicine. However, as sub-healthy condition is alternatively used for the Mibyou, the Mibyou was rather obscure concept, and thus, a new concept and definition of Mibyou was proposed by the Japan Mibyou Association (e.g., Japanese Society of Mibyou System) in 2006. According to the definition, the Mibyou is the specific physiological and disease condition distinct from the terminal diseases, which needs hospitalization and medical treatments, and includes such conditions that the individuals are able to enjoy normal life activity and well-being even if the clinical inspections show some abnormality. This made clear the targets of Mibyou care practices including dietary approach. For the beneficial use of functional foods in the Mibyou care practices, it is worthy to categorize the currently distributed functional foods into newly defined Mibyou-Care functional foods.

Keywords: Mibyou, Mibyou care, Mibyou-care functional food, preventive and integrative medicine

1. Introduction

The life span of human is getting elongated especially in developed countries, although the maximum life span is expected no longer than 135 years [1]. Under this situation, the needs for elongation of healthy life span are social concern [2]. The healthy life span is the life period in that individuals can actively enjoy their life activities and wellness without hospitalization or with fewer assistance by others, even if they carry any manageable disorders. In the longevity society, the life style and age-related diseases such as diabetes, dementia, and cancer are disincentive for the healthy life span [3]. They are the complex diseases with multiple pathogenic factors and symptoms, and thus, the treating strategy of modern western medicine to remove specific pathogen is often useless. Therefore, the prevention and control of these disorders are recognized more important rather than the treatment of serious endpoint diseases lead by these disorders. The importance of preventive medicine has been discussed in the traditional oriental medicines using the term Mibyou [4]. The Mibyou was defined as a certain pathogenic condition being not healthy but not ill, and the treatment of Mibyou was considered more important than treating the diagnosed diseases since Mibyou is an entrance for the serious endpoint diseases. Mibyou that is also often described as sub-healthy condition in the present day [5] is thus an important concept that should be renovated in the current preventive medicine as a target for attaining healthy life expenditure.

2. Mibyou, traditional, and current concepts

Mibyou concept was established in ancient China more than 2000 year ago. The term was first appeared in one of the oldest Chinese medicine literature called "*Huangdi Neijing*" as a physiological condition that is not ill but not healthy [4]. It is important to treat the Mibyou before it progresses to diagnose endpoint diseases. Although this idea is quite valuable in today's preventive medicine, the Mibyou condition is hardly diagnosed by the routine clinical test to give specific disease name. The pathological definition of Mibyou was left obscure and has not been well accepted in the modern medicine, although the term Mibyou was reconfirmed and approved at the 7th Asian-Oceanian International Aging symposium in 2003. There are several efforts to identify the Mibyou condition, which are now progressed. For example, the group of Toyama University observed progressive change of gene expression in adipocyte for 3 months using genetically defined spontaneous metabolic syndrome model rat and found 147 genes showed characteristic change of expression pattern before metabolic syndromes developed [6].

On the other hand, recent development of clinical examination technologies such as biochemical assay-detecting disease markers in blood and also physical methods for imaging nidus such as MRI (magnetic resonance imaging), CT (computed tomography), and ultrasound echo allow us to detect diseases, even cancers at very early stage. In such stages of disorder, the patients can behave and enjoy the life activity as normal without hospitalization. The Japan Mibyou Association currently distinguished these early stages of diseases from the diseases that need medical care with hospitalization and defined them as modern Mibyou [7]. According to the newly proposed definition, there are two types of Mibyou, the western medicine Mibyou (Modern Mibyou) and the traditional oriental medicine Mibyou (Classical Mibyou), and the Modern Mibyou is further classified into two conditions, Mibyou I and Mibyou II as shown in **Figure 1**. The Mibyou I is such conditions that individuals feel uneasy or ill but clinical examinations including blood biochemical markers

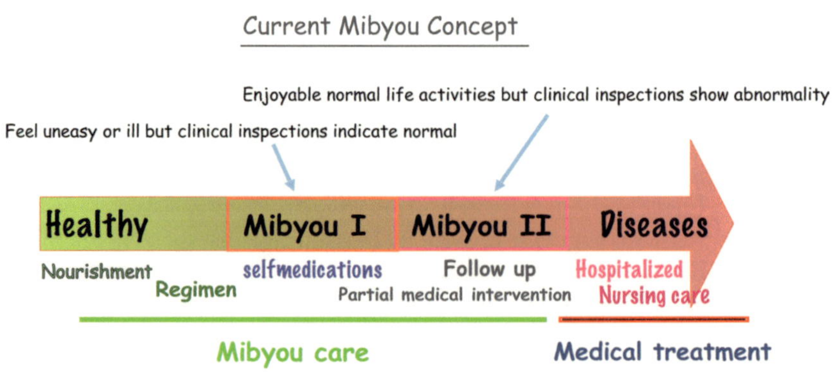

Figure 1.
Current Mibyou concept and Mibyou-Care for healthy life expenditure.

or imaging check do not show detectable abnormality. On the other hand, Mibyou II is defined as the condition where individuals do not feel abnormality or ill and can spend regular daily life by keeping wellness but clinical examinations show some abnormal level of disease markers or the presence of some abnormal images.

According to this new definition of Mibyou, the Mibyou I covers the condition related to classical Mibyou and several uneasy symptoms such as anxiety, sleep defect, physical pains, overweigh, fatigue, and frail. The Mibyou II on the other hand covers many familiar disorders including obesity, hypertension, hyperglycemia, hyperlipidemia, diabetes, hyperuricemia, tiny stroke, latent cardiac failures, liver fat diseases, hepatitis virus B carrier, sarcopenia, and even early stage of cancers. By this categorization, such diseases as life style diseases and metabolic syndromes are covered by Mibyou II. This new definition of Mibyou provides more clear targets for Mibyou care practices.

3. Mibyou care practices

The health care targeting Mibyou (Mibyou-care practices) will be a reliable strategy to approach the healthy life span and to improve QOL (Quality of Life). The Mibyou I care, such as the daily behavioral habits carried out by normal healthy individuals for sustaining health, is especially important in the preventive medicine.

It is said that meal, physical excise, and brain activity (both mental and psychological) are the three factors sustaining health and wellness. Indeed, the Mibyou-care practices such as diet, exercises, acupuncture, Yoga, meditation, mental stimulation, and others are more or less related to or are targeting these factors.

The Mibyou II conditions are reflected in the disease markers such as blood sugar level, and thus are controllable by certain medical and nutritional intervention targeting these markers in collaboration with clinical stuffs. For example, diabetic condition could be managed by observing blood HBA1c level regularly as a diagnosed marker [8]. The Mibyou II-care practices for diseases prevention, amelioration, and stimulation of recovery include the actions such as remedy, nourishment, self-medication, and the medications assisted by co-medical stuffs such as physician, pharmacist, and nutritionist.

In these Mibyou care practices, the diet plays the most basic and essential part.

4. Food functions

Currently, the food functions are discussed by the following three categories. Those are 1: Nutritional, 2: Sensory, and 3: pharmacological functions [9]. The nutritional function is the basic property of foods functioning as the source of the building block for constructing body architecture (structures) and also the energy required for functioning the structure (activities). Foods usually accompany such sensory properties as taste, flavor, and color as well to stimulate appetite so that the nutrients are smoothly taken. The third category of food function is currently attracting extensive attention since a book of knowledge is getting accumulated that certain components existing in food ingredients often show pharmacological activity and they are called food factors [10]. The food factors are implicated as the very molecules taking part in the observed pharmacological functions of foods, especially of the foods traditionally used as folk medicine and the food for nourishing and astringent purpose [11].

Obviously, the nutritional and sensory roles of foods are playing essential roles in the Mibyou care, especially in Mibyou I care. On the other hand, the third role of foods contributing to the medicinal functions of foods will take pivotal part in Mibyou II care.

The pharmacological function of foods is historically attracting much attention. "Foods are medicine" is well accepted in both oriental and western countries from ancient. One example is the oldest literature of herbs called "*Shennong bencaojing*" in China, in that 365 natural resources including botanicals, minerals, and animals were collected and classified into three categories according to their nutritional and pharmacological health benefits [12]. The listed first group is edible as food and suggested to eat routinely in the daily meals because of having potentials not only of nourishing and tonic functions but also elongating life span. The second group is not recommended to eat every day because of having a weak pharmacological activity, but is useful to ameliorate certain physiologically distorted conditions. The third group is toxic and is unable to eat, but often used as medicine to treat specific diseases.

These classifications of natural resources are interesting as reflected on the current category of the so called functional foods. The first group is the same as the dietary or nutritional supplements and the second group is overlapped to the so-called functional foods such as HOSHU, nutraceuticals, and pharmafoods. The third group is the medicine, and the resources in this group have been the target for developing clinical medicines or their prototypes [13].

From the view of the Mibyou care, the botanicals listed in the first and second categories of *Shennong bencaojing* are especially interesting, because they will be useful in functional application such as in the form of supplement and functional food.

5. Functional foods

The functional food is denoted as the food with certain health beneficial function given by the pharmacologically active ingredient named "food factor." The food factors are essentially not nutrient as exemplified by polyphenols and dietary fibers, [14] but some nutrient molecules show pharmacological functions and are thus food factors [15]. For example, vitamin D [16] and omega-3 fatty acids [17] that are nutrients required as structural component of bone and cellular membranes, respectively, have other physiological functions such as immune modulation [18].

There are many types of functional foods currently in the market, which target certain abnormal physiology and disorder such as hyperglycemia, obesity, and even dementia and immune, and the forms are also variable such as fresh fruit and vegetables, processed foods, and even tablet and capsule.

In Japan, FOSHU (foods for specialized health uses) was legally approved that can claim certain health benefit such that the product is recommended to the individuals who have the signs of hyperglycemia and want to manipulate the blood sugar level [19]. FOSHU provided one model of the government regulation for developing functional foods, but there are many types of functional foods that are globally in the market such as the dietary supplements established in US, and other commonly named functional foods such as pharmafoods, nutraceuticals, and fortified foods [20].

Those functional foods distributed in the current society are contributing certain extent to the human health; however, due to the complexity such as found in above-mentioned naming and also in the usage, the social benefits of functional foods are not fully satisfied or often mislead. There are also some discussions left whether the medicinal functions of foods are simply explained by the ligand-receptor theory applied for drug action [21]. It is worthy to renovate the classification of functional foods from the view of Mibyou care.

6. Mibyou-care functional food

Whatever the types or appearances of functional food products, the functional foods can be classified into following four groups according to the objectives of usage. (1) The first group is used for sustaining health and preventing diseases; thus, individuals who are not ill and healthy will intake. (2) The second is used by the individuals who feel ill or uneasiness but clinical test does not show significant change or abnormality in disease markers (Mibyou I). (3) The third group is used by the individuals who shows certain abnormal level in disease markers or physical inspections such as CT but can spend normal daily life (Mibyou II). (4) The fourth group is used by the hospitalized patients to ameliorate or to help recovery of diseases under medication, or to assist the therapy as an adjuvant such as in cancer therapy, and thus used in the integrate medicine. Except this 4th group, all other functional foods are able to define as the Mibyou-Care functional food.

These Mibyou-Care functional foods are basically grouped into two types as shown in **Figure 2**. One is the Mibyou-Care functional food-1 that is used mainly for sustaining health and preventing diseases. Therefore, the foods in the groups 1 and 2 of above classification of usage are included. Another group of functional foods denoted as Mibyou-Care functional food-2 is used for keeping well-being, and amelioration and recovery of the Mibyou condition assessed by diseases markers. Therefore, the Mibyou-Care functional foods-2 essentially have certain pharmacological function, which can manipulate the Mibyou condition evaluated by the changes of respective diseases marker.

6.1 Targets of Mibyou-Care functional food-1

Oxidative stress and inflammation are the commonly encountered cell-damaging factors during normal life activity. It is known that the system or the respective component devices working in the metabolism as life process are damaged even under normal condition by the oxidative stress [22] and the associated inflammation [23]. It is implicated that the accumulation of such damages is the major cause of aging [24]. Therefore, the protection against these abuses is exclusively important to maintain the health and also prevent the diseases.

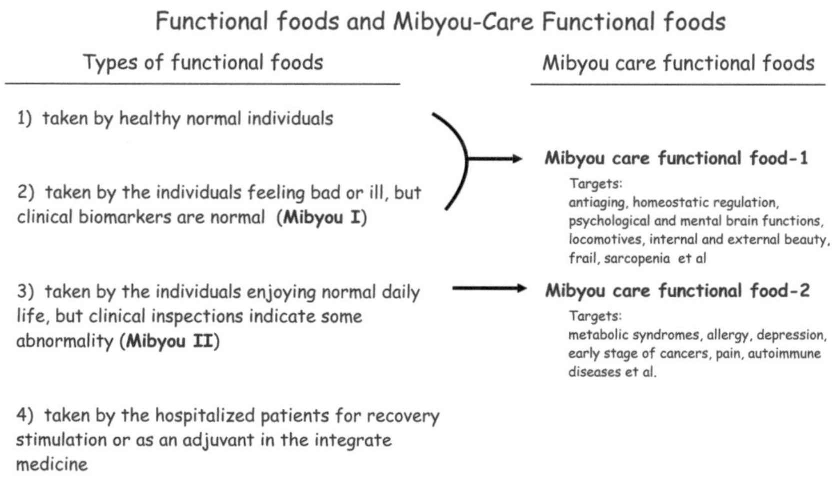

Figure 2.
Targets of functional foods and Mibyou-Care functional foods

On the other hand, healthy condition is often described by the potential to maintain the homeostatic balance that is reflected in the ability how extent the system can tolerate against the stimuli that distort the dynamic equilibrium of metabolism. The Mibyou was often described as the condition that the homeostatic potential is decreased or is hardly sustainable. It is known that neural, endocrine, and immune functions are the physiological factors controlling the homeostasis, and nutritions are exclusively necessary to support these systems to function [25], both the major nutrients (protein, lipid, and sugar) that are essentially needed for the maintenance of the system and also micronutrients that are the catalyst for driving the system. Therefore, it is evident that appropriate daily meals are essential to supply these necessary nutrients. Moreover, it became apparent that certain non-nutrient-edible molecules including food factors and also natural products as xenobiotics are playing a pivotal role in manipulating homeostatic factors, especially immune system [26, 27].

Natural products, especially botanical ingredients, are the treasure source of antioxidant and anti-inflammatory functions [28, 29] and thus used as attractive resources to develop the Mibyou-Care functional food-1. Currently, the vegetables and fruits with enriched health beneficial ingredients are in the market; therefore, there are many types and appearances of functional foods are possible from such fortified fresh vegetables and fruits, processed foods, restaurant menus, take-out menus such as Bento (take-out pack), and even tablet or capsule. The Mibyou-Care functional food-1 will cover the target area related to anti-aging, homeostatic regulation, *Qi* modulation, locomotive functions, internal and external beauty, mental and pscychological brain activities including stress tolerance, and some area of age-related symptoms such as frail and sarcopenia.

6.2 Targets of Mibyou-Care functional food-2

On the other hand, the second group of Mibyou-Care functional foods (Mibyou-Care functional food-2) targets the specific disorders or abnormality assigned by the biochemical or physical examinations from the respective disease markers or nidus imaged, for example, blood sugar for diabetics, transaminases for liver damage, and echo image for fatty liver. Therefore, the presently distributed functional foods such as FOSHU are included in this category. The Mibyou-Care functional foods-2 carry medicinal functions mediated by the food factors in addition to the basic functions usually associated with foods such as nutritional, antioxidant, and anti-inflammation activities, with which the amelioration of distorted conditions or the prevention of disease progression is anticipated. They are used to manage the variety of distorted physiological states such as related to the metabolic syndromes (hyperglycemia, hypertension, and hyperlipidemia), early stage of cancer, depression, allergy, and pains, so as to prevent the progression of early stage of disorders into the serious diseases such as heart attack, stroke, cancer, and dementia. The functional food application in integrative medicine will be another promised field and is also covered by the Mibyou-Care functional food-2 category. Specially designed foods for adjuvant use are such example to enhance the efficacy of medication such as in cancer chemo- and radiotherapies.

These functional foods are usually taken as tablet- or capsule-type supplements but many other forms of food products are also possible such as granule, drink, gel, candy, other processed and fortified foods, and served or ready-to eat foods such as restaurant menus and Bentou (take-out pack), so that they are beneficially used in the self-medication strategy.

New category of functional foods proposed from the view of Mibyou care not only helps the effective usage of functional foods in the Mibyou care practices but also stimulates further basic studies such as the search of appropriate Mibyou markers and functional food design and development.

7. Conclusion

Current development of functional foods is obviously contributing to the human health. Elongation of life span reminds us the importance of healthy life expenditure and well-being demands. Western medicines are not sufficiently effective against the age-related complex diseases in the longevity society, so that the disease prevention becomes primary concern. Mibyou was a classical concept but is recognized more important in the current preventive medicine and thus renovated. In the newly defined Mibyou concept, the condition where individuals are able to spend normal daily life even if clinical inspection indicates certain ills was distinguished from the diseases which need medications in the hospital, and is covered by the newly defined Mibyou.

As the term Mibyou was defined more clearly, the Mibyou care became a target for the healthy life expenditure. Mibyou care practices will be important daily routines such as exercise, diet, and mental and psychological activities of the brain. Among them, the diet shares the most basic and essential part. The functional foods are thus one of the beneficial tools playing a pivotal role in the Mibyou care practices. The new definition of Mibyou care functional foods category will be helpful to use and develop the functional foods in Mibyou care.

Conflict of interest

There is no conflict of interest.

Author details

Tetsuya Konishi[1,2]

1 Niigata University of Pharmacy and Applied Life Sciences (NUPALS), Japan

2 Office HALD Food Function Research, Japan

*Address all correspondence to: janja.zupan@ffa.uni-lj.si

References

[1] Pearce M, Raftery AE. Probabilistic forecasting of maximum human life span by 2100 using Bayesian population projections. Demographic Research. 2021;**44**:1271-1294

[2] Lindgren B. The Rise in Life Expectancy, Health Trends among the Elderly, and the Demand for Health and Social Care. Working paper no.142, March 2016 published by the National Institute of Economic Research (NIER) https://www.konj.se

[3] Jaul E, Barron J. Age-related diseases and clinical and public health implications for the 85 years old and over population. Frontiers in Public Health. 2017;**5**:335. DOI: 10.3389/fpubh.2017.00335

[4] Memory of the world register Nuang Di Nei Jing. Available from: http://www.unesco.org/new/fileadmin/MULTIMEDIA/HQ/CI/CI/pdf/mow/nomination_forms/China%20Huan%20di%20Nei.pdf

[5] Chan RYP, Chien WT. Concepts of body constitution, health and sub-health from traditional Chinese medicine perspective. World Journal of Translational Medicine. 2013;**2**:56-66

[6] Koizumi K, Oku M, Hayashi S, et al. Identifying pre-disease signals before metabolic syndrome in mice by dynamical network biomarkers. Scientific Reports. 2019;**9**;8767 DOI:10.1038/s41598-019-45119-w

[7] Japanese Guideline of Mibyou for the Prevention of Cardiovascular diseases and Long-time Care ed by Japan Mibyou Society. 2016

[8] Hussain N. Implications of using HBA1c as a diagnostic marker for diabetes. Diabetology International. 2016;**7**:18-24

[9] Arai S. Physiological functions of foods. Developments in Food Engineering. Boston, MA: Springer; 1994. pp. 48-53. DOI:10.1007/978-1-4615-2674-2_9

[10] Terao J. A perspective of the research on food factors in human health: A return to the mechanistic approach Journal of Nutritional Science and Vitaminology. 2015; **61**(Supplement):S98-S99

[11] Andrew R, Izzo AA. Principles of pharmacological research of nutraceuticals. British Journal of Pharmacology. 2017;**174**:1177-1194

[12] An Encyclopedia on Chinese History, Literature an Art. Available from: http://www.chinaknowledge.de/Literature/Science/shennongbencaojing.html

[13] Mand al. SC, Mandal V, Konishi T. eds, Natural products and drug discovery: An integrated approach. Amsterdam, Netherland: Elsevier; 2018

[14] Abuajah CI, Ogbonna AC, Osuji CM. Functional components and medicinal properties of food: A review. Journal of Food Science and Technology. 2015;**52**(5):2522-2529. DOI: 10.1007/s13197-014-1396-5

[15] Rucker RB, Keen CL, Steinberg FM. Vitamins and food-derived biofactors. Encycloped Agricul Food Systems. Vol 5, San Diego, CA: Elsevier; 2014. pp. 356-377

[16] Aranow C. Vitamin D and the immune system. Journal of Investigative Medicine. 2011;**59**:881-886

[17] Gutierrez S, Svahn S, Johansson M. Effects of omega-3 fatty acids on immune cells. International Journal of Molecular Science. 2019;**20**:5028. DOI: 10.3390/ijms2020502Onega

[18] Thurnham D. Micronutrients and immune function: Some recent developments. Journal of Clinical Pathology. 1997;**50**:887-891

[19] Food for Specialized Health Uses (FOSHU) Ministry of Health, Labour and Welfare Japan. Available from: https://www.mhlw.go.jp/english/topics/foodsafety/fhc/02.html

[20] Bagchi D. ed, Nutraceutical and Functional food Regulations in the United States and Around the World. Third edition. NY: Academic Press; 2019

[21] Konishi T. Weak Direct and Strong Indirect Interactions are the Mode of Action of Food Factors. Functional Food Health Disease. 2014;4(6). DOI:10. 31989/ffhd.v4i6.7

[22] Dalle-Donne I, Rossi R, Colombo R, et al. Biomarkers of oxidative damage in human disease. Clinical Chemistry. 2006;**52**:601-623

[23] Hunter P. The inflammation theory of disease. *EMBO Reports*. 2012; **13**:968-970

[24] Liguori I, Russo G, Curcio F, et al. Oxidative stress, aging, and diseases. Clinical Interventions in Aging. 2018;**13**:757-772

[25] Childs CE, Calder PC, Miles EA. Diet and immune function. Nutrients. 2019;**11**:1933. DOI:10.3390/nu11081933

[26] Detopoulou P, Demopoulos CA, Antonopoulos S. Micronutrients, phytochemicals and mediterranean diet: A potential protective role against COVID-19 through modulation of PAF actions and metabolism. Nutrients. 2021;**13**:462. https://doi.org/10.3390/nu13020462

[27] Behl T, Kumar K, Brisc C, et al. Exploring the multifocal role of phytochemicals as immunomodulators. Biomedicine & Pharmcotherapy. 2021;**133**:110959

[28] Allegra M. Antioxidant and anti-inflammatory properties of plants extract. *Antioxidants* (Basel). 2019;**8**:549. DOI: 103390/antiox8110549

[29] Arulselvan P. Role of antioxidants and natural products in inflammation. Oxidative Medicine and Cellular Longevity. 2016;**2016**. Article ID 5276130/ 15pages, http://dx.doi.org/10.1155/2016/5276130

Section 2

Complementary Therapies and mental disorders

Chapter 4

Cognitive Hypnotherapy and EMDR: Two Effective Psychodynamic Therapies for the Rapid Reduction of Cognitive Anxiety

Elizabeth Brooker

Abstract

In the main research into cognitive anxiety has focused on the conscious mind. The aim of this chapter is to review two psychodynamic psychotherapies, cognitive hypnotherapy (CH) and eye movement desensitisation and reprocessing (EMDR). Both therapies focus on implicit or unconscious processes for the rapid relief of cognitive anxiety. The objective is to give credence to CH and EMDR both in the scientific and medical domains. The philosophy is concerned with changing negative cognitions and dysfunctional feelings through a process of desensitisation and reprocessing, utilising positive imagery. CH and EMDR were investigated in an intervention study with advanced pianists (n = 46). Participants were of mixed gender aged 18–26 and were randomly assigned to a therapy or control group. The therapy groups received two therapies of either CH or EMDR during a two week period between two concerts. Quantitative data were collected through the Spielberger State-Trait Anxiety Inventory. Results showed that both therapy groups (but not the control) experienced a significant reduction in state anxiety post-therapy and trait anxiety decreased significantly below baseline levels in the EMDR group. This chapter further reviews research into CH and EMDR documented through a case study allowing for qualitative assessment of the therapies where two sessions only were required to effect positive change.

Keywords: cognitive anxiety, implicit processes, explicit processes, CH, EMDR, psychodynamic therapy

1. Introduction

Cognitive anxiety is a widespread problem. It exerts a negative effect on human behaviour with individuals experiencing a gamut of mental, emotional and physical feelings. It has psychological and physiological effects which can be devastating. A plethora of research documents the outcomes of complementary therapies for the reduction of cognitive anxiety; however in the main the therapies focus on the conscious mind (explicit processes that are in conscious awareness) and these therapies can be both time consuming and costly. Both CH and EMDR focus on implicit or unconscious processes (thoughts and actions no longer consciously perceived) as well as explicit processes. By this means the therapies target the root cause of the condition which allows for rapid alleviation of anxiety and effects long-lasting change. EMDR and CH, both hypnotically-based therapies, offer positive healing in a short space of time in comparison with other psychotherapies. As a therapeutic treatment each focuses on implicit processes and addresses the contemporary stimuli that might independently trigger the person's fear. Each offers relief of symptoms for small or 't' trauma; however EMDR is also used as a leading therapy for significant trauma, for subjects deemed to have experienced life-threatening situations.

The chapter first discusses cognitive anxiety looking at both trait and state anxiety, how anxiety arises and manifests itself before looking at the complexity and components of this debilitating condition. The cognitive/emotional connection is discussed and the role and importance of implicit memories, thoughts and emotions in the exacerbation and maintenance of cognitive anxiety. The use of alternative therapies for the reduction of cognitive anxiety is reviewed looking at their effectiveness and outcomes and the number of sessions required to effect positive change.

To enable the reader to understand the genesis and development of CH an overview of hypnosis is given followed by a synopsis of cognitive behaviour therapy (CBT). The assimilation of the two therapies has become known as CH and the rationale for this integration is discussed. The background, techniques and procedures of CH are outlined and current research critiqued where CH has been the intervention for a variety of dysfunctional conditions. The chapter continues with a review of EMDR looking at the theory, protocols and practice of this psychotherapeutic treatment and documents research conducted in a number of different domains for traumatic and debilitating conditions where EMDR has been used.

The remainder of the chapter documents the quantitative and qualitative research into CH and EMDR and gives scientific evidence for the effectiveness and rapid results of both therapies. In conclusion, the future direction and importance of CH and EMDR are considered in the light of current knowledge, their effectiveness as psychodynamic therapies for the treatment of cognitive anxiety, and their relevance to current research as well as the medical practice.

2. Cognitive anxiety

Cognitive anxiety is a complex (learned) emotion where fear is combined with other emotions such as anger, guilt, shame and embarrassment; all of these can be extremely disruptive to human behaviour [1]. Research informs us that there are two types of anxiety: trait and state. Trait anxiety is an individual's normal level of anxiety when in a non-threatening situation and it has been suggested that it is influenced by genetics and as such remains roughly at the same level throughout the life-span [2]. However more recent research has shown that it is also influenced by an individual's experiences and in fact is mutable and can be lowered positively through desensitisation of traumatic memories and negative cognitions [3]. State anxiety is a temporary condition which can be heightened according to environmental situations. It is the anxiety felt for instance when individuals feel they are in the spotlight or 'on show' and are under pressure to do their best. However it returns to its generic level when the situation has passed [4].

It has been found that there is a relationship between trait and state anxiety and that individuals with high trait levels of anxiety will experience correspondingly high state levels of anxiety in what is deemed to be a threatening situation [4, 5].

Evidence from the literature emphasises the multi-dimensional aspects of anxiety, and the affective role that experiences have on primary emotions such as fear and apprehension. This can affect the degree to which cognitive processes influence assumptions, expectations, physiological symptoms and behaviour [6–11].

2.1 The components of anxiety

A complexity of components that have an impact on anxiety have been found, including affective, cognitive, physiological and behavioural factors [12], and this investigative research corroborates the findings of previous work in this field:

- affective subjective experiences generate arousal of pleasure or displeasure [13].

- cognitive processes are generated in a situational state and have effects which lead to either negative or positive appraisal [14].

- physiological adjustments to cognitive processes activate arousal causing uncomfortable somatic symptoms which are unhelpful in a performance state [15].

- behaviour which is not goal-directed can have a negative outcome on the experience [16].

Table 1 shows four interrelated components of anxiety [12].

During the application of both CH and EMDR the principles of affect, cognition, physiology and behaviour as documented in this table are broadly addressed.

affective experience/trauma of situational states is targeted by accessing both explicit and implicit memories

leads to

↓

cognitive appraisals and reviewing of negative/positive experiences allowing for changed perceptions

activating

↓

physiological adjustments and emotional reprocessing

leading to

↓

changed behaviour that is both goal directed and adaptive

Table 1.
Components of anxiety.

2.2 The role of memories and emotions in generating anxiety

In the 1890s Sigmund Freud observed that memories of negative experiences or events could be changed over time having a new meaning. In conducting his analysis of patients both during and after treatment, he found that subjective memory of events could be re-transcribed years after they had occurred. To be changed however, he argued that memories had to be consciously perceived and those memories in the unconscious mind should be relived rather than just remembered [17].

Research into the phenomenology of memory found that when meaningful material is encoded, associated information such as thoughts and feelings are also encoded; this allows activation of the recollection process which leads to a 'remember' response. This triggers an interaction of latent patterns of negative thoughts, emotions and behaviours, causing both psychological and physiological symptoms [18]. Further research has shown that new experiences are assimilated into existing memory networks, and that pathology results when unprocessed experiences are stored in their own neural network, unable to link up with anything more adaptive. Recall invokes content and affect, and the implicit thoughts and feelings, although no longer in conscious awareness, will impact on present day experiences [19]. In fact it is argued that cognitive disorders can be thought of as mal-connections between the various synaptic regions of the brain, and that mal-adaptive experiences or memories disassemble the connections; however these can be reassembled by positive experiences that bring about change [20].

Implicit processes, sometimes referred to as automated processes, produce an automatic response [21]. This has important implications for the recall of implicit memory and emotions and for the effectiveness of CH and EMDR. Both therapies focus on these processes and are specifically designed to desensitise and reprocess dysfunctional cognitions and memories, giving the individual the opportunity to revisit and change the maladaptive memory from a safe environment [5].

3. Complementary therapies currently adopted for the treatment of cognitive anxiety

A variety of treatment therapies are presently adopted for the reduction of stress and cognitive anxiety, however the main interventions adopted are listed below and fall into several categories:

- Cognitive behavioural interventions: focus is on dysfunctional thoughts, how these may have been generated, coping skills, positive imagery, attentional focus and goal setting.

- Physiological and physically-based interventions: Alexander technique, biofeedback, muscle relaxation and music-enhanced relaxation.

- Meditative interventions: meditation, yoga and autogenic training.

- Psychodynamic interventions: cognitive hypnotherapy, eye movement desensitisation and reprocessing.

In discussing the above interventions positive effects have been reported in the literature in the cognitive therapies; however a large number of sessions are required [3, 22]. Further to this, core problems are insufficiently focused upon and the relapse rate for individuals who have undergone symptom-based CBT is cause for concern [23]. The physiological and physically-based therapies and assertiveness training demonstrate little beneficial effect; however more promising results have been found in the reduction of cognitive anxiety in meditation and yoga [23]. It has been found however that it takes time to acquire these skills and as with the cognitive therapies the drawback is the length of time taken to effect positive change [3, 23]. More details of the above interventions can be found in the author's doctorate [3].

This chapter now reviews CH and EMDR, two psychodynamic therapies that target implicit processes, thoughts and actions no longer in conscious awareness, for the alleviation of cognitive anxiety. The rationale is that by focusing on the role that these processes exert on anxiety both therapies have the potential to reduce cognitive anxiety quickly and effectively.

4. Cognitive Hypnotherapy

CH is the integration of two disciplines, hypnosis and CBT; therefore to enable the reader to understand the genesis of CH this section of the chapter first reviews hypnosis. This is followed by a brief synopsis of the background of CBT including the protocols and procedures adopted in this therapy. The rationale is given and discussed for the assimilation of these two disciplines before documenting the roots, development and theory of CH. This section concludes with the findings from research in various domains where CH has been adopted for the reduction of cognitive anxiety.

4.1 Hypnosis

Hypnosis dates back over 220 years as an area of scientific research and clinical practice and has been adopted to bring about positive change in diverse psychological conditions [24]. However there are different approaches to hypnosis. Traditional hypnosis, which is believed to be the earliest form of hypnosis, is more authoritative, using direct commands and orders to bring about positive changes, and has been shown to be less effective than the modern hypnosis [25]. Modern hypnosis was developed by the psychologist Dr. Milton Erikson in the 1930s and was known as Eriksonian Hypnosis. Eriksonian philosophy revolutionised the process of hypnotherapy by recognising that individuals are able to access their own inner resources to improve their quality of life. It adopts a holistic approach to each client, understanding their needs and their individual situation and is the form of hypnosis used by the author when conducting cognitive hypnotherapy. This approach uses metaphors by comparing and contrasting experiences and situations, rather than commands and suggestions. Working in this way it enables the brain to think more creatively, and the suggestions become more acceptable to the unconscious mind [26]. It has been suggested that during hypnosis the memory and meaning of negative experiences and the effect of fear can be changed through emotional processing [27, 28]. It is further suggested that when hypnosis is added to therapy such as cognitive behavioural therapy (CBT) the hypnotic relationship enhances the efficacy of the treatment effects [29].

4.2 Cognitive behavioural therapy

CBT, which has been adopted for anxiety and diverse disparate conditions since the 1980s, uses a combination of behavioural and cognitive interventions aimed at changing dysfunctional thoughts and memories. Individuals are helped in the pursuit of goals, and emotional problems by directing cognitions towards memories, images, thoughts and attention [30]. Through its development over the last 40 years CBT has adopted treatments for diverse anxiety conditions and emotional disorders [31]. There are a number of protocols and procedures adopted in CBT which allow clients to re-access early negative experiences and enable more understanding of how the negative thoughts, emotions and behaviours have been generated. However for the purpose of this review the formulation by Persons is illustrated as this is most usually associated with CBT [32].

Persons' Formulation 1989

Early Experience: Negative experience either from teacher, parents or peers.

↓

Schemas: Become maladjusted and lead to mistrust. Mistrusts ability to do things.

Core Beliefs: Negative cognitions result in anxiety leading to behavioural and physiological problems.

↓

Assumptions: I know I will feel anxious because it always happens and then I will ………… (becomes a self-fulfilling prophecy).

↓

Trigger: Thought of an impending event.

↓

Vicious Cycle:

Negative Automatic Thought (NAT): Negative thoughts of dread, apprehension, failure.

↑ ↓

Consequence: The conceptualised belief regarding the event is realised.

Feeling: Hopelessness, worthlessness, depression, shame, withdrawal.

↑ ↓

Behaviour: Decision not to (put themselves in that situation again).

By following the guidelines of the above model CBT helps to redress negative cognitions, and encourages the association of positive thoughts, changing the negativity into positive outcomes. In fact it is argued that suppositions are reiterated with corrected thoughts, enabling positive visualisation of present and past experiences, giving the client confidence in their ability to handle situations so that a positive outcome can be achieved [33].

However, the literature reports that no theory/therapeutic action is without flaws, and a number of issues have been identified with the CBT approach: the effective role that cognition plays on physiological symptoms in the body; the failure to recognise the role of the unconscious mind in overt behaviour; and the failure to recognise that human thought and action are socially embedded [34]. Further to this, evidence from the literature indicates that one of the main drawbacks with CBT is the number of sessions required to effect positive change (10 or more sessions in the majority of cases) [3]. New cognitive models are being developed considering the role of cognitions and emotions in generating anxiety, including a meta-cognitive model (MCM) [35], and an emotion dysregulation model (EDM) [36]. However neither of these models takes into account the role of the unconscious mind in the way that anxiety develops.

4.3 The rationale for the integration of hypnosis with CBT

It has been proposed that hypnosis is based on the affect theory of human emotion and that cognitions locked to unpleasant emotions can become disturbingly resistant to change until hypnosis alters the affective perceptions of the individual [37]. Intransigent symptoms of dysfunctional cognitions and emotions can be approached and treated through a sequence of interactions as thoughts previously locked to negative affect are processed and changed positively [37]. Indeed It is argued that as a result of incorporating techniques from two disciplines the core ideas of each are integrated changing both and resulting in a new assimilative model [38]. The rationale for the integration of the two disciplines is well documented in the literature. It has been suggested that by combining the treatment of two disciplines gives a quicker resolution of the dysfunctional condition [39]. Further to this it is argued that hypnosis combined with CBT offers a powerful form of treatment approach with rapid effects and has been shown that this treatment approach offers a template for the guidance of treatment strategies for cognitive and emotional conditions [40].

CH uses a model first adopted in the 1990s, not dissimilar to cognitive behavioural therapy (CBT). However the fusion of hypnotic techniques with CBT first proposed in 1994 strengthens the therapeutic outcome, offering an addition to therapy by facilitating the resolution of resistant symptoms [41]. By focusing on the unconscious mind cognitive hypnotherapy targets implicit memories and cognitions no longer in conscious awareness. The impact and added strength of integrating two disciplines maximise therapeutic effect [39].

4.4 Protocols and procedures of CH

CH uses an integrative and holistic approach in the treatment of disparate conditions and focuses on both explicit and implicit processes. Case formulation is guided by case history and the therapist's interpretation of this and a treatment plan is then outlined to the patient. An explanation of hypnosis is given making sure that the patient feels comfortable with this. Whilst in trance the therapist attempts to address the unconscious mind, as during this state the critical part of the mind is bypassed allowing the establishment of positive thoughts, substituting former judgemental cognitions with helpful ones [33]. During the process of hypnotherapy implicit processes which appear to be causing negative cognitions, emotions and behaviours are targeted whist the patient is in a state of deep relaxation or a trance-like state. In this state the unconscious mind is receptive to positive ideas and behaviours, hypnotic relaxation, positive mood induction, ego strengthening and post-hypnotic suggestions [33].

4.5 Findings from research using cognitive CH as an intervention

The research documented below gives evidence for the effectiveness of CH in various domains and documents the beneficial effects of integration. In fact a meta-analysis was conducted looking at comparative studies of CBT and CH and gave evidence that patients receiving CH as opposed to CBT showed a 70% improvement in their mean scores in comparison with the CBT group [42].

Significant benefits have been found for the following conditions using CH:

Anxiety disorders [43], general anxiety disorder [44], anxiety in cancer patients [45], PTSD [46], cognitive anxiety/trauma [47], pain relief [48], sleep disorders [49], diabetes [50], anxiety in public speaking [51], music performance anxiety [5, 52]. For more information on these studies see Brooker [3].

The above research testifies to the effectiveness of CH for the above conditions. Eye movement desensitisation and reprocessing (EMDR), another psychodynamic therapy used widely for anxiety conditions, is now reviewed.

5. Eye Movement Desensitisation and Reprocessing

EMDR has evolved from a simple technique into an integrative psychotherapy that addresses both the cognitive perception of trauma and the resultant physiological condition, an interaction of mind and body. Psychological problems are addressed and successful treatment outcome is achieved in a short space of time, as negative cognitions and emotions are replaced with positive thoughts and memories, body sensations are changed, and new behaviours emerge [53]. Changes in anxiety and fear are only by-products of a comprehensive reprocessing of the whole experience. The conceptualisation of the transformation of stored disparate experiences and the accompanying memories through a rapid learning process is the key to understanding the basis and application of EMDR [53].

5.1 Background

Initially EMDR was called Eye Movement Desensitisation, beginning with a behavioural orientation similar to the roots of CBT [54, 55], as it was thought that eye movements were unique in causing an effective desensitisation. Subsequently it was discovered that other forms of bilateral stimulation (tactile and auditory) also resulted in positive effects [56]. The word 'reprocessing' was added when it was realised that through a process of desensitisation the treatment achieved positive changes in traumatic memories, as well as a reduction in anxiety. EMDR is a relatively new psychotherapy first used in the treatment of post-traumatic stress disorder (PTSD) [57]. However since its inception it has expanded widely now treating a wide range of pathologies including treatment of trauma, anxiety disorders and associative conditions as well as phobias. The treatment protocols have evolved enabling treatment of diverse forms of trauma responsible for psychological and physiological disorders, particularly those that are anxiety-based. The philosophy underlying this hypnotically-based approach to treatment is that individual conditions that are emotionally-based can be healed quickly, effectively and profoundly; dissociative disorders and phobias, and the consequences of these and other past negative-rooted traumas can be changed using EMDR [58]. In 2004 it was placed in the "A" category as strongly recommended for the treatment of trauma and anxiety-related conditions in both the American Psychiatric Association and the American Department of Defence. Through a process of desensitisation it was found that dissociative disorders and past negative-rooted experiences can be changed effectively and quickly, allowing for the emergence of new positive behaviours [58].

5.2 Theory

EMDR is based on the premise that earlier life experiences can elicit a continued pattern of similar affect, behaviour and cognition (the three main constituents of anxiety [59], and that present-day stimuli can elicit similar affective behavioural memories of earlier experiences. The theory of EMDR adopts a model that emphasises cognitive information processing of past negative experiences and memories, the bilateral movements adopted inducing a light hypnotic trance. Both physical and emotional memories of subjective trauma can be reprocessed resulting in a state of positive mental and emotional wellbeing [56]. A putative neurobiological mechanism for the efficacy of EMDR has been offered [60], which presents a complete model of how EMDR could lead to specific improvements in PTSD and related conditions. It suggests that during EMDR the flow of information from the hippocampus (which stores information) to the neo-cortex (which analyses information) is directionally reversed in EMDR similar to REM sleep cycles. This allows for cognitive re-evaluation of previously maladjusted/negative encoded information. The theory is that, through guided eye movements or other sources of bilateral brain stimulation such as hand taps or alternating sounds, traumatic information held in neurological networks is changed and connected to more positive cognitions stored in subjective memory [56, 61].

5.3 Disparate memories and EMDR practice

EMDR targets memories directed at the negative/traumatic experience and deals specifically with reprocessing these memories as quickly as possible. It is aimed at the pivotal event that caused the initial fear/reaction and addresses all the contemporary stimuli that might independently trigger the subjective fear [62]. It is believed that traumatic information of disparate memories cause dysfunctional cognitive and emotional behaviour [63], and that this information, held in neurological networks in the brain, is changed during the process of EMDR [61].

It is argued that through assimilation negative memory adds to subjective knowledge regarding expectations and potential warning signs and suggests that when a distressing experience results in persistent anxiety the information processing system has stored the experience without adequately processing it to an adaptive resolution. The event is 'frozen in time' in the moment of fear and pain and this lays the foundation for future inappropriate dysfunctional responses to similar events [62].

When subjective implicit memories have not been processed this may be at the root of a variety of psychological issues in the present [20, 64]. Emotions, sensations and perspectives of earlier events colour the perceived view of similar present-day events; a current situation similar to an earlier event will automatically link into the memory network in which the earlier event is stored [53].

The procedures have been developed to identify, access and target dysfunctionally stored experiences and to stimulate the innate processing system. This allows adaptive resolution of the information and shifts the information to the appropriate memory systems [60, 63]; pinpointing the target (the traumatic experience) and reprocessing the disparate memory is crucial in the initial stages of treatment.

5.4 Protocols and procedure in therapy

During therapy a dual-attention approach is used to facilitate the processing of the cognitive, affective and sensory elements of a recalled disturbing event [64]. An eight-phase psychotherapeutic treatment approach has been adopted with standardised procedures and protocols to address the full range of clinical conditions caused or exacerbated by previous negative experiences [64]. Subsequently this developed into an adaptive information process (AIP) model, the premise of which is that every person has both an innate tendency to move towards health and wholeness and the inner capacity to achieve it [64].

The AIP model has been adopted for experiences for the highest level of trauma, 'A' category, as well as for small trauma designated as 't' trauma. Small trauma is described as experience not rising to the highest level of trauma, but nonetheless causing significant psychological damage to require treatment. The treatment of both 'A' and 't' trauma guides the procedures and protocols of the clinical practice of EMDR [53].

The AIP model: Standardised EMDR protocols and procedure.

1. History taking

   This determines whether the subject is an appropriate candidate for EMDR and includes treatment planning.

2. Preparation

   Preparing the subject for any disturbance that may arise during the session or between sessions.

3. Assessment

   Finding a target or targets and defining its/their components. Memories, physical feelings and negative cognitions.

4. Desensitisation

   Using bilateral movements: eye, tactile or auditory to reprocess targets.

   Use of Subjective Unit of Disturbance Scale (SUD).

5. Installation

   Strengthening the positive cognition throughout the neuro-networks.

   Use of Validation of Cognition Scale (VOC).

6. Body scan

   Identifying physical feelings manifested in any part of the body and reprocessing any target revealed by the identification.

7. Closure

   Returning the subject to emotional equilibrium, discussion of ongoing processing which may cause further disturbances. If this occurs it should be recorded in a diary/log in readiness for the next session. Instruction in the use of relaxation techniques to maintain a state of calm.

8. Re-evaluation

   As the processing proceeds memories may emerge that are linked by similar cues such as beliefs or sensations.

5.5 Clinical studies

The methodology used in EMDR has been extensively validated in the following clinical studies and has provided evidence for the effectiveness of this treatment for category 'A' patients (the highest level of trauma, threat of death, extreme trauma):

Survivors of earthquake [65]; terrorist attack (9/11) [66]; sexually abused girls [67]; railway employees, person under train accident [68]; children with PTSD [69].

Further studies have been conducted into experiences categorised as small or 't' trauma (anxiety conditions contributing to significant psychological distress:

Trauma from life events [70]; distressful experiences [71]; depression and social anxiety [72]; pain reduction [73, 74]; phobias (dental) [75].

EMDR standard protocols have been applied to alleviate anxiety in the following fields:

Dressage [47, 76]; athletics [77, 78]; swimming [79]; test anxiety [80]; music performance anxiety [5, 81, 82]. EMDR has also developed a peak performance protocol used to enhance performance, enabling individuals to overcome subjective negativity and anxiety [83].

For more detailed information on all of the above studies see Brooker [3].

This section of the chapter now gives a very brief overview of the effectiveness of CH and EMDR through the quantitative and qualitative research conducted by the author from her doctoral thesis at the University of Leeds [3] and from her private practice [5].

6. Quantitative research: method

At the start of the study 46 advanced pianists (aged 18–26 years and of mixed gender) from three higher educational institutions were randomly assigned to a therapy or control group. The therapy groups received two interventions of either CH or EMDR during a two-week period between two concerts. A quantitative assessment of the state component of cognitive anxiety of all participants was obtained from the Spielberger State-Trait Anxiety Inventory (STAI-Y1) taken at baseline and prior to both performances. The findings reported here are on state anxiety; for the full findings of the author's research, including trait anxiety, somatic/physiological symptoms of anxiety and the behavioural aspects of performance anxiety see Brooker [3].

6.1 Results

At the end of data collection to establish whether anxiety levels decreased more in the intervention groups than the Control, an ANCOVA was calculated comparing levels of state anxiety across the three groups at the first and second performances (before and after treatment). There was a main effect of condition ($F(2, 42) = 4.92$, $p = .012$) such that participants in the two treatment conditions, CH and EMDR, showed significantly lower cognitive anxiety than the Control group at the second performance, post-intervention and that both treatment groups were significantly effective in achieving this (Helmert contrasts, .005 significance level).

This suggests that the therapies applied between the two performances significantly lowered anxiety in both the CH and EMDR groups prior to the second performance and this required two sessions only. This effect was not demonstrated in the Control group.

Figure 1 below shows the standard error of the mean score of state anxiety at the two performances calculated from the STAI Y-1 questionnaire, where 80 represents the highest level of anxiety and 20 the lowest. It illustrates the decrease in state anxiety at the second performance across the three groups.

7. The qualitative research: case study

Qualitative information on music performance anxiety (MPA) is documented here in the form of a case study, taken from the author's private practice [47]. A personal account of performance experience is given which allows for more detail, sensitivity and insight into the understanding of MPA which could not be obtained from quantitative research alone. It gives insight into the process of therapy by

Error bar graph of the mean score of state anxiety at the two performances

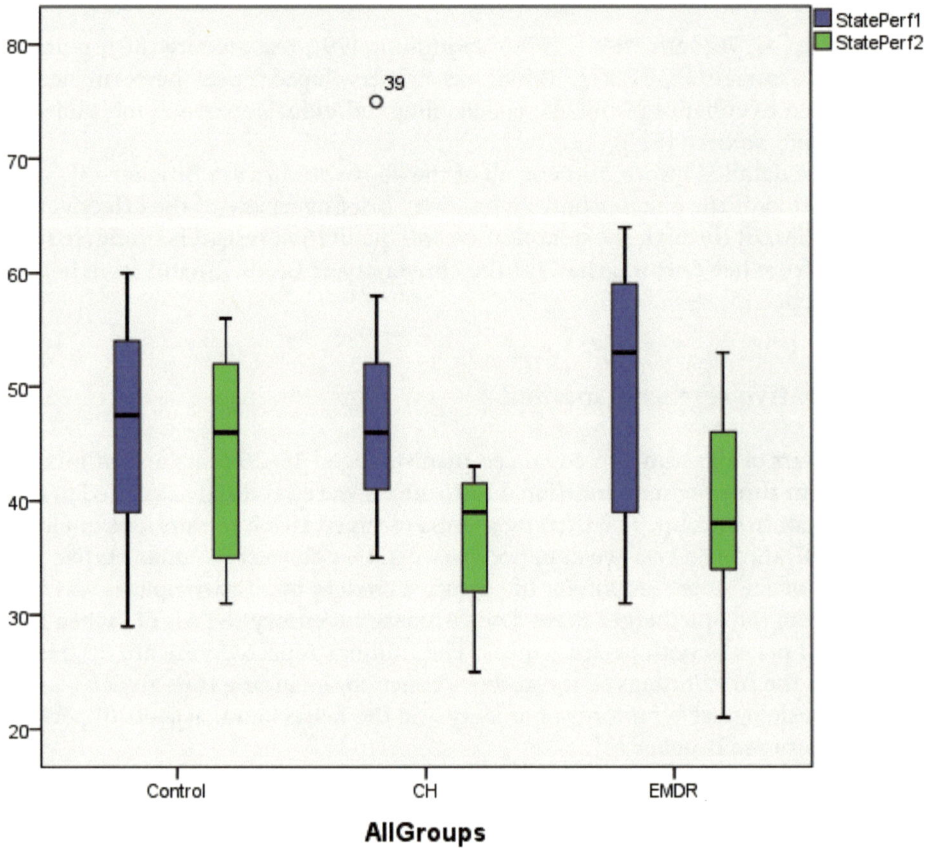

Figure 1.
The standard error of the means of state anxiety from the STAI Y-1 questionnaire taken 15 min prior to performances 1 and 2: error bars show 95% CI of mean.

exploring the internal thoughts, feelings and experience of the individual. This case study begins with the individual's own words (the narrative). It then continues with an abbreviated description of the progression of treatment and documents the therapeutic outcome, as well as reflecting on the suitability of the treatment administered from a research standpoint and comparisons of possible treatment effects of other treatments. It is the documentation of an individual who received one therapy of EMDR and one of CH for the treatment of MPA, (the name is anonymised).

Identifying information
Name: Rebecca.
Music performance anxiety: Voice.
Age: 41.
Occupation: Student with the Open University studying English and Music (first instrument, voice).

7.1 Case history: Rebecca's narrative

I had always felt very nervous when performing and always seemed to have the image of my father in the background; I felt that he was judging and criticising me and that I was letting myself down. I was having singing lessons at this time and giving small informal recitals but I was never happy with the outcome; I always felt I fell short of my true potential. I took Grade 8 ABRSM Singing examination but failed quite badly and this felt like the ultimate disaster. Although I was confident practising on my own, I found singing lessons 'nerve racking' and at the examination I just 'fell apart'.

After I moved here and restarted singing lessons I was very interested in taking part in the Christmas concert as your research was close to my heart as I always get very nervous in performance. I was singing in the second half of the concert but felt nervous in the first half and this got worse, and as soon as I started singing my throat felt tense and I had saliva in my mouth which I had to keep swallowing before the long runs, my heart was beating quickly and I could feel my cheeks flushing. Because of all this I felt that I had not connected with the audience and was disappointed with my performance. I did enjoy taking part however and being part of the research into music performance anxiety and found it somewhat reassuring that others taking part were also feeling nervous, I wasn't the only one.

7.2 Case formulation

Therapist's summary and interpretation of Rebecca's narrative.

Important features in this narrative indicate that the domineering personality and the physically abusive behaviour of her father, who was against her musical ambitions, have had far-reaching consequences on Rebecca's singing performances both as a teenager and as an adult. These emotions are so strong in present-day performances that she imagines the spectre of her father while she is performing. The negative criticism that she experienced from her father has affected her self-esteem and self-worth as a musician in spite of her belief that she has talent as a singer. This was compounded by a boyfriend who had a similar attitude as her father towards her regarding her music. She is confident practising on her own where she perceives that she is not being judged; however she experiences both cognitive anxiety and distressing physiological and somatic symptoms of anxiety in a performance or examination situation where she feels she 'falls apart'.

7.3 Critical analysis: therapist

An analysis of Rebecca's narrative suggests that she is suffering from social phobia in situations where she feels threatened and under scrutiny, such as a singing examination or a live concert performance. Social phobia, rooted in social anxiety, has been summarised [84].

a. Negative cognitions operating in social situations which include fear of negative evaluation, self-consciousness, self-deprecating thoughts and self-blaming attributions for difficulties.

b. Heightened physiological activity.

Rebecca experiences cognitive anxiety as well as physiological and somatic symptoms of anxiety in a performance situation. However, although she experiences destructive and crippling anxiety when performing, this phobic reaction does not occur in other areas of her life. The therapist purports that this is as a result of the criticism and physical abuse that she received from her father during her teenage years regarding her ambitions as a singer ('my father literally tried to knock it out of me') and this I believe has had a profound psychological effect on her self-esteem and confidence in her music performances.

In therapy Rebecca presented with the following negative schemas regarding her anxiety (direct quotes):

'I know I'll screw it up'

'I can't control my thoughts'

'I'm hopeless'

'I can't control my emotions'

'I can't control my body'

'I can't control my nerves'

Physiological and somatic symptoms of anxiety were:

rapid heartbeat;

shaking/trembling;

tension in throat;

an excess of saliva.

7.4 Treatment plan: EMDR and CH

7.4.1 First treatment (EMDR): 30 May 2010

Rebecca's MPA is complex as it is not related to a single incident but the systematic criticism that she received as a teenager, undermining her self-belief in the possibility of her pursuing a professional career in music as an adult. The primary aspect of the overall treatment would be targeting the trauma experienced at this time which in the opinion of the therapist is best addressed initially through EMDR by systematic desensitisation of these experiences.

In therapy the negative criticism and upsetting experiences revealed in Rebecca's narrative regarding her father were the main targets, beginning with the most upsetting incident which she rated as 9/10 on the subjective unit of disturbance scale (SUD) (10 being the highest level of anxiety). This rating indicates that significant trauma had been experienced at this time. The most painful negative emotions when recalling this incident were of fear and anger; the strongest physical sensation was tension throughout her whole body which was accompanied by heightened breathing. After fifty minutes of EMDR her rating on the SUD scale decreased to 0, indicating that the negative memories had been desensitised. The negative schemas that she had presented with at the start of treatment had now changed. Where previously she had six negative self-perceptions (four beginning with 'I can't ...'; see above), post-treatment these had changed into positive perceptions of 'I can ...'). She no longer thought of herself as being hopeless or that she would 'screw it up'.

Her rating on the validity of cognition scale (VOC scale was 6/7 (7 being the highest level of positivity): negative schemas cited earlier had been reprocessed. Her bodily sensations which she had experienced at the start of therapy when recalling the traumatic memories had now gone completely, her breathing had normalised and she had no tension anywhere in her body. Having targeted and desensitised the most traumatic memories first, the lesser memories of trauma regarding performance when reviewed were more difficult to hold, and no longer caused Rebecca the former anguish or physiological/somatic symptoms of anxiety. If the past has been one of negativity or trauma regarding aspects that are important to the individual, the subjective behavioural response to a similar present-day experience will be consistent with the negative affective responses of the past [56]. An adult may experience feelings of fear and being out of control, and will react emotionally and display negative behaviour accordingly.

7.4.2 Second treatment (CH): 6 June 2010

The second treatment session (1 h) was shorter than the first (90 min), the important groundwork having been accomplished in the first session. As the disparate memories had been desensitised and reprocessed in the first session CH should now be beneficial in supporting the reprocessed cognitive perceptions. It should also enhance the positivity achieved in the previous session. Rebecca had experienced hypnotherapy some years previously but it had not been particularly effective. However it was explained that it should enhance the EMDR treatment and the combination of the two therapies would strengthen treatment effects. The most important aspects of her singing performance were discussed; she wanted to feel confident, calm and in control in performance, to connect with her audience and feel eager to do more. Her key words, which were 'anchored' on her dominant wrist during hypnotherapy, were *confident*, *calm* and *in control*; these she felt were the words that would enable her to give her optimum performance. The therapy focused on enhancement of performance and included visualisation of her perfect performance.

On completion of hypnotherapy Rebecca was given the therapist's *Self-Confidence for Musicians* CD and advised to listen to this as often as possible, and especially on the day/evening prior to a performance; this would further relax her and add to her confidence. She left feeling happy and relaxed looking forward to her next singing lesson and her next performance.

7.5 Rebecca's self-assessment of treatment

My singing in front of audiences can be adversely affected by pre-performance nerves, which seem to stem from my first solo concerts when I suffered with acute stage fright. The EMDR treatment brought my worst singing nightmares to the surface and I was initially sceptical that anything could be done to help my anxiety when performing. However I came away from the first treatment feeling unburdened as if a weight that I had been carrying around for years had lifted. It was like coming out from underneath a dark cloud. The CH treatment in the second session focused my mind on enjoying singing so that when I performed I was in control and relaxed. It appeared to reinforce everything so that I am now looking forward to performing instead of dreading it.

(Email message, June 2010)

7.6 Therapist's assessment of treatment and reflections from a research standpoint

This case study supports current research into anxiety which suggests that negative affect and beliefs from the past control the individual in the present; however they can be healed quickly, effectively and profoundly when past negative-rooted traumas are changed [58, 64]. The negative cognitions and previous perceptions of subjective performance that this patient held were successfully desensitised and reprocessed in two treatments.

There can be no doubt that the treatment was effective; however reflecting on this as a researcher there are other possible explanations for the resolution of the problems presented here which need to be explored. These outcomes may be explained by a number of different factors. For instance some individuals improve because they have entered therapy, regardless of the specific treatment: a variant of the placebo effect. Fascinating research has been conducted into the well-known phenomenon of the placebo effect with various medical conditions: headaches, pain reduction and even the visual effects of packaging in headache tablets [85, 86].

It could further be suggested that 'narrative smoothing' plays a part in resolving psychological issues, and many psychotherapists support this view [87–89]. It is believed that the process of reconstruction of the initial narration gives more control over the story and can change the patient's perception into something more positive; this underpins the central goals of therapy [87]. Rebecca's narrative was highly charged with specific negative experiences and relating this allowed a different subjective perception.

CBT might also be effective as a therapy in this instance as it similarly uses narration in therapy but treats the presenting symptoms rather than the cause. CBT has similarities with psychodynamic therapies but there are a number of different elements which are distinctive. CBT focuses on the way individuals think and act in specific circumstances and how emotional and behavioural problems may be overcome [90]. However, although CBT appears to be the preferred treatment for anxiety-based conditions, no theory/therapeutic action is without flaws, and a number of issues have been identified with this approach [34]:

1. The failure to consider experiences in the past in relation to the present in generating anxiety.

2. The effective role that cognition plays on physiological symptoms in the body.

3. The failure to recognise the role of the unconscious mind in overt behaviour.

4. The failure to recognise that human thought and action are socially embedded.

5. Core problems are not treated.

In fact there is increasing concern regarding the relapse rate at follow-up sessions for those patients who have undergone symptom-based CBT [19, 90]. It treats the symptoms rather than the cause and as such this may only provide a short-term solution to the problem [16, 34].

7.7 Longitudinal outcome

Since Rebecca's therapy treatments in 2010 she has completed her Open University degree and now holds a Masters in Professional Voice Practice. She still enjoys performing and has regular engagements. Her dream of becoming a professional musician has been realised.

8. Conclusion

The aim of this chapter was to give more exposure to and greater understanding of two highly effective therapies for the rapid reduction of cognitive anxiety: CH and EMDR. The complexities of cognitive anxiety were discussed and the role that dysfunctional memories, particularly implicit memories no longer consciously perceived, can exert on present-day experiences. The chapter reviewed CBT and the benefits of hypnosis as an adjunct to this therapy, now called CH, as well as comorbid conditions where CH has been an effective treatment. The background and theory of EMDR was documented discussing the role of disparate memories in EMDR practice. The procedures and protocols used in EMDR were highlighted before reviewing the clinical studies that have adopted EMDR as a treatment. The final section of the chapter documented the author's research using CH and EMDR, giving both quantitative and qualitative findings. Both the quantitative and qualitative research documented above (pp. 8–13) gave evidence for the effectiveness and rapid results of CH and EMDR in comparison with other complementary treatments where the main drawback appears to be the length of time required to effect positive change. This chapter further highlighted the important contribution that CH and EMDR have made to current research and in doing so has shown the need for further scientifically-based research into the complexities of anxiety and the role that implicit memories play in maintaining this.

In the UK the treatments of choice being advocated by the National Health Service (NHS) for PTSD and anxiety disorders still tend to be medication or CBT and as such there is no financial cost incurred by the patient. Where individuals experience no positive effects, or are dissatisfied with treatment, they are guided towards private therapists at their own financial cost. The medical profession are aware of CH and EMDR but as yet these treatments are not widely available to the general population, although EMDR is available for PTSD in the military domain. This state of affairs needs to be remedied given the effective and dynamic results which are being seen from both CH and EMDR.

Author details

Elizabeth Brooker
University of Leeds, Leeds, UK

*Address all correspondence to: elizabeth.brooker@hotmail.co.uk

References

[1] Izard CE. Human Emotions. New York, NY: Plenum Press; 1977

[2] Cattell RB. Personality and mood by Questionnaire: A Handbook of Interpretive Theory, Psychometrics, and Practical Procedures. San Francisco: Jossey-Bass; 1973

[3] Brooker E. Music performance anxiety: An investigation into the efficacy of cognitive hypnotherapy and eye movement desensitisation and reprocessing when applied to Grade 8 pianists [doctoral dissertation eThesis]. UK: University of Leeds; 2015. Retrieved from: http://etheses.whiterose.ac.uk/12130

[4] Spielberger CD, Gorsuch RL, Lushene RE. State-trait Anxiety Inventory for Adults. Palo Alto, California: Consulting Psychologists Press; 1977

[5] Brooker E. Brooker E. Music performance anxiety: A clinical outcome study into the effects of cognitive hypnotherapy and eye movement desensitisation and reprocessing in advanced pianists. Psychology of Music. 2018;**46**(1):107-124

[6] Beck AT. Thinking and depression. Part II: Theory and therapy. Archives of General Psychiatry. 1964;**9**:324-333

[7] Beck AT. Cognitive therapy: Nature and relation to behaviour therapy. Behavior Therapy. 1970;**1**(2):184-200

[8] Kenny DT. The role of negative emotions in performance anxiety. In: Juslin PN, Sloboda JA, editors. Handbook of Music and Emotion: Theory, Research, Applications. New York: Oxford University Press; 2010. pp. 425-451

[9] Kirchner JM. A qualitative inquiry into musical performance anxiety. Medical Problems of Performing Artists. 2003;**18**:78-82

[10] McCraty R. Heart-brain Neurodynamics: The Making of Emotions (Publication No. 03-01). Boulder Creek, CA: HeartMath Research Center, Institute of HeartMath; 2003

[11] McCraty R. The Scientific Role of the Heart in Learning and Performance (Publication No. 02-030). Boulder Creek, CA: HeartMath Research Center, Institute of HeartMath; 2003

[12] Miller SR, Chesky K. The multidimensional anxiety theory: An assessment of and relationships between intensity and direction of cognitive anxiety, somatic anxiety, and self-confidence over multiple performance requirements among college music majors. Medical Problems of Performing Artists. 2004;**19**(1):12-20

[13] Oatley K, Jenkins JM. Understanding Emotions. Oxford, UK: Blackwell; 1996

[14] Steptoe A. Negative emotions in music making: The problem of performance anxiety. In: Juslin PN, Sloboda JA, editors. Music and Emotion: Theory and Research. Oxford, UK: Oxford University Press; 2001. pp. 291-307

[15] Fredrikson M, Gunnarsson R. Psychobiology of stage fright. Biological Psychology. 1992;**33**:51-61

[16] Salmon PG. A psychological perspective on musical performance anxiety: A review of the literature. Medical Problems of Performing Artists. 1990;**5**(1):2-11

[17] Freud S. Introductory Lectures on Psycho-analysis. London: George Allen and Unwin Ltd; 1949

[18] Baddeley AD. Essentials of Human Memory. Hove: Psychology Press; 1999

[19] Debiec J, Diaz-Mataix L, Bush DE, Doyere V, LeDoux JE. The amygdala encodes specific sensory features of an aversive reinforce. Nature Neuroscience. 2010;**13**(5):536-537

[20] LeDoux J. The Synaptic Self: How Our Brains Become Who We Are. New York: Viking; 2002

[21] LeDoux J. Cognitive-emotional interactions in the brain. Cognition and Emotion. 1989;**3**:267-289

[22] Tarrant RA, Leatham JM. A CBT-based therapy for music performance anxiety. In: Einstein DA, editor. Innovations and Advances in Cognitive Behavioural Therapy. Bowen Hills, Australia: Australian Academic Press; 2007. pp. 3-17

[23] Kenny DT. The Psychology of Music Performance Anxiety. Oxford: Oxford University Press; 2011

[24] Barnier AJ, Nash MR. Introduction: A roadmap for explanation, a working definition. In: Nash MR, Barnier AJ, editors. The Oxford handbook of hypnosis: Theory, Research and Practice. Oxford, UK: Oxford University Press; 2008. pp. 1-18

[25] Sani I. What Is Traditional Hypnosis?. 2011. Available from: https://EzineArticles.com/expert/Ian_Sani/130890

[26] Moore J. Types of Hypnosis. 2011. Available from: https://www.selfdevelopment.net/hypnosis/hypnosishypnotism/types-of-hypnosis

[27] Bryant R, Moulds ML, Guthrie R, Nixon R. The additive benefit of hypnosis and cognitive-behavioral therapy in treating acute stress disorder. Journal of Consulting and Clinical Psychology. 2005;**73**:334-340

[28] Spiegel D, Classen C. Acute stress disorder. In: Gabbard GO, editor. Treatments of Psychiatric Disorders. Vol. 2. Washington, DC: American Psychiatric Publishing; 1995. pp. 1521-1535

[29] Alladin A. Evidence-based hypnotherapy for depression. International Journal of Clinical and Experimental Hypnosis. 2010;**58**(2):165-185

[30] Cooper P. Introduction: Why cognitive behavior therapy? In: Butler G, editor. Overcoming Social Anxiety and Shyness. London: Robinson Publishing; 1999

[31] Butler G. Overcoming Social Anxiety and Shyness. London: Robinson Publishing; 1999

[32] Persons JB. Cognitive Therapy: A Case Formulation Approach. New York: W. W.Norton; 1989

[33] Rossi EL, Cheek DB. Mind-body Therapy: Methods of Ideodynamic Healing in Hypnosis. New York: W.W. Norton; 1994

[34] Clark A. Supersizing the Mind: Embodiment, Action, and Cognitive Extension. New York, NY: Oxford University Press; 2008

[35] Wells A. Worry, metacognition, and GAD: Nature, consequences, and treatment. Journal of Cognitive Psychotherapy. 2002;**16**(2):179-192

[36] Mennin DS, Heimberg RG, Turk CL, Fresco DM. Applying an emotion regulation framework to integrative approaches to generalized anxiety disorder. Clinical Psychology: Science and Practice. 2002;**9**:85-90

[37] Nathanson DL. Affect and hypnosis: On paying friendly attention to disturbing thoughts. International

Journal of Clinical and Experimental Hypnosis. 2009;**57**(4):319-342

[38] Messer S. A critical examination of belief structures in integrative and eclectic psychotherapy. In: Norcross JC, Goldfried MR, editors. Handbook of Psychotherapy Integration. New York: Basic Books; 1992. pp. 130-168

[39] DePiano FA, Salzberg HC, editors. Clinical Applications of Hypnosis. Norwood, NJ: Ablex; 1986

[40] Alladin A, editor. Special Issue: Evidence-based practice in clinical hypnosis—Part 1. International Journal of Clinical and Experimental Hypnosis. 2007;**55**(2):115-249

[41] Alladin A. Cognitive hypnotherapy with depression. Journal of Cognitive Psychotherapy: An International Quarterly. 1994;**8**(4):275-288

[42] Kirsch I, Montgomery G, Saperstein G. Hypnosis as an adjunct to cognitive-behavioral psychotherapy: A meta-analysis. Journal of Consulting and Clinical Psychology. 1995;**63**:214-220

[43] Wolfe BE. Understanding and Treating Anxiety Disorders: An Integrative Approach to Healing the Wounded Self. Washington: American Psychological Association; 2005

[44] Daitch C. Cognitive behavioral therapy, mindfulness, and hypnosis as treatment methods for generalized anxiety disorder. American Journal of Clinical Hypnosis. 2018;**61**(1):57-69. DOI: 10.1080/00029157.2018.1458594

[45] Chen P-Y, Liu Y-M, Chen M-L. The effect of hypnosis on anxiety in patients with cancer: A meta-analysis. Meta-analysis. 2017;**14**(3):223-236. DOI: 10.1111/wvn.12215

[46] Abramowitz EG, Barak Y, Ben-Avi I, Knobler HY. Hypnotherapy in the treatment of chronic combat-related PTSD patients suffering from insomnia: A randomised, Zolpidem-controlled clinical trial. International Journal of Clinical and Experimental Hypnosis. 2008;**56**(3):270-280

[47] Brooker E. Transforming Performance Anxiety Treatment using Cognitive Hypnotherapy and EMDR. London and New York: Routledge; 2019. p. 2019

[48] Abbasi M, Ghazi F, Barlow-Harrison A, Sheikhvatan M, Mohammadyan F. The effect of hypnosis on pain relief during labor and childbirth in Iranian pregnant women. International Journal of Clinical and Experimental Hypnosis. 2009;**57**(2): 174-183

[49] Graci GM, Hardie JC. Evidence-based hypnotherapy for the management of sleep disorders. International Journal of Clinical and Experimental Hypnosis. 2007;**55**: 288-302

[50] Xu Y, Cardena E. Hypnosis as an adjunct therapy in the management of diabetes. International Journal of Clinical and Experimental Hypnosis. 2008;**56**(1):63-92

[51] Schoenberger NE, Kirsch I, Gearan P, Montgomery G, Pastyrmak S. Hypnotic enhancement of a cognitive-behavioral treatment for public speaking anxiety. Behavior Therapy. 1997;**28**:127-140

[52] Stanton HE. Research note: Alleviation of performance anxiety through hypnotherapy. Psychology of Music. 1993;**21**:78-82

[53] Shapiro F. EMDR and case conceptualization from an adaptive information processing perspective. In: Shapiro F, Kaslow FW, Maxfield L, editors. Handbook of EMDR and Family Therapy Processes. Hoboken, NJ: John Wiley and Sons; 2007. pp. 3-34

[54] Orman EK. Effect of virtual reality graded exposure on heart rate and self-reported anxiety levels of performing saxophonists. Journal of Research in Music Education. 2003;**51**(4):302-315

[55] Orman EK. Effect of virtual reality graded exposure on anxiety levels of performing musicians: A case study. Journal of Music Therapy. 2004;**41**(1): 70-78

[56] Shapiro F. Alternative stimuli in the use of EMDR. Journal of Behavior Therapy and Experimental Psychiatry. 1994;**25**:89

[57] Shapiro F. Efficacy of the eye movement desensitization procedure in the treatment of traumatic memories. Journal of Traumatic Stress. 1989;**2**: 199-223

[58] Shapiro F. Paradigms, processing, and personality development. In: Shapiro F, editor. EMDR As an Integrative Psychotherapy Approach: Experts of Diverse Orientations Explore the Paradigm Prism. Washington, DC: American Psychological Association; 2002. pp. 3-26

[59] Aigen K. Thoughts on Nordoff-Robbins music therapy, music psychotherapy and psychotherapy—Stimulated by 'Music for Life'. Newsletter of the International Association of Nordoff-Robbins Music Therapists. 1996;**1**:8-12

[60] Stickgold R. EMDR: A putative neurobiological mechanism of action. Journal of Clinical Psychology. 2002; **58**(1):61-75

[61] Grand D. Emotional Healing at Warp Speed: The Power of EMDR. New York: Present Tents Publishing; 2003

[62] Shapiro F. Eye movement desensitization and reprocessing procedure: From EMD to EMDR: A new treatment model for anxiety and related traumata. The Behavior Therapist. 1991; **14**:133-135

[63] Siegel DJ. The developing mind and the resolution of trauma: Some ideas about information processing and an interpersonal neurobiology of psychotherapy. In: Shapiro F, editor. EMDR As an Integrative Psychotherapy Approach: Experts of Diverse Orientations Explore the Paradigm Prism. Washington, DC: American Psychological Association; 2002. pp. 85-122

[64] Shapiro F. Eye Movement Desensitization and Reprocessing: Basic Principles, Protocols and Procedures. 2nd ed. New York: Guilford Press; 2001

[65] Konuk E, Knipe J, Eke I, Yusek H, Yurtsever A, Ostep S. Effects of EMDR therapy on post-traumatic stress disorder in survivors of the 1999 Marmara, Turkey earthquake. International Journal of Stress Management. 2006;**13**:291-308

[66] Silver SM, Rogers S, Knipe J, Colelli G. EMDR therapy following the 9/11 terrorist attacks: A community-based intervention project in New York City. International Journal of Stress Management. 2005;**12**:29-42

[67] Jaberghaderi N, Greenwald R, Rubin A, Zand SO, Dolatabali S. A comparison of CBT and EMDR for sexually abused Iranian girls. Clinical Psychology and Psychotherapy. 2004; **11**:358-368

[68] Hogberg G, Pagani M, Sundin O, Soares J, Aberg-Wistedt A, Tarnell B, et al. On treatment with eye movement desensitization and reprocessing of chronic post-traumatic stress disorder in public transportation workers: A randomized controlled study. Nordic Journal of Psychiatry. 2007;**61**(1):54-61

[69] Kemp M, Drummond P, McDermott B. A wait-list controlled

study of eye movement desensitization and reprocessing (EMDR) for children with post-traumatic stress disorder (PTSD) symptoms from motor vehicle accidents. Clinical Child Psychology and Psychiatry. 2010;**15**:5-25

[70] Mol SSL, Arntz A, Metsemakers JFM, Dinant G, Vilters-Van Montfort PAP, Knottnerus A. Symptoms of post-traumatic stress disorder after non-traumatic events: Evidence from an open population study. British Journal of Psychiatry. 2005;**186**:494-499

[71] Cvetek R. EMDR treatment of distressful experiences that fail to meet the criteria for PTSD. Journal of EMDR Practice and Research. 2008;**2**:2-14

[72] Power KG, McGoldrick T, Brown K, Buchanan R, Sharp D, Swanson V, et al. A controlled comparison of eye movement desensitization and reprocessing versus exposure plus cognitive restructuring, versus waiting list in the treatment of post-traumatic stress disorder. Journal of Clinical Psychology and Psychotherapy. 2002;**9**:299-318

[73] Ray AL, Zbik A. Cognitive behavioural therapies and beyond. In: Tollison CD, Satterhwaite JR, Tollison JW, editors. Practical Pain Management. 3rd ed. Philadephia: Lippincott; 2001. pp. 189-208

[74] Schneider J, Hofmann A, Rost C, Shapiro F. EMDR in the treatment of chronic phantom limb pain. Pain Medicine. 2008;**9**(1):76-82

[75] De Jongh A, van den Oord HJM, Ten Broeke E. Efficacy of eye movement desensitization and reprocessing in the treatment of specific phobias: Four single-case studies on dental phobia. Journal of Clinical Psychology. 2002; **58**(12):1489-1503

[76] Crabbe B. Can Eye-Movement Improve Your Riding. November: Dressage Today; 1996. pp. 28-33

[77] Foster S, Lendl J. Eye movement desensitization and reprocessing: Initial applications for enhancing performance in athletes. Journal of Applied Sport Psychology. 1995;**7**(Suppl):63

[78] Gracheck KA. Evaluating the Efficacy of EMDR as an athletic performance enhancement intervention [unpublished dissertation]. Colorado: The University of the Rockies; 2011

[79] Graham L. Traumatic swimming events reprocessing with EMDR. The Sport Journal. 2004;**7**(1):1-5

[80] Maxfield L, Melynyk WT. Single session treatment of test anxiety with Eye Movement Desensitization and Reprocessing (EMDR). International Journal of Stress Management. 2000;**7**: 87-101

[81] Feener RS. EMDR: Eye movement desensitization and reprocessing: A new method in the treatment of performance anxiety for singers [unpublished DM thesis]. Florida State University; 2005

[82] Plummer CD. Performance enhancement for brass musicians using eye movement desensitization and reprocessing [unpublished DM thesis]. University of Cincinatti; 2007

[83] Lendl J, Foster S. EMDR performance enhancement psychology protocol. In: Luber M, editor. EMDR Scripted Protocols: Basics and Special Situations. New York: Springer Publishing; 2009. pp. 377-396

[84] Turner SM, Beidel DC, Townsley RM. Social phobia: Relationship to shyness. Behaviour Research and Therapy. 1990;**2**:497-505

[85] Blackwell B, Bloomfield SS, Buncher CR. Demonstration to medical students of placebo responses and non-drug factors. Lancet. 1972;**1**(7763): 1279-1282

[86] Montgomery GH, Kirsch I. Mechanisms of placebo pain reduction: An empirical investigation. Psychological Science. 1996;7:174-176

[87] Brandchaft B. Systems of pathological accommodation and change in analysis. Psychoanalytic Psychology. 2007;**24**(4):667-687

[88] Sroufe LA, Waters E. Attachment as an organizational construct. Child Development. 1977;**48**:1184-1199

[89] Stolorow RD. Anxiety, authenticity and trauma: The relevance of Heidegger's existential analytic for psychoanalysis. Psychoanalytic Psychology. 2007;**24**(2):373-383

[90] Alladin A. Cognitive Hypnotherapy: An Integrated Approach to the Treatment of Emotional Disorders. Chichester: John Wiley & Sons; 2008

Chapter 5

Intervention of Yoga in Stress, Anxiety and Depression

Chandra Nanthakumar

Abstract

Yoga is not only an art but also an ancient science that evolved more than 5000 years ago. It is practised by people from all walks of life in almost every part of the world. In the past, the practice, which was seen to be spiritual and divine, used to be confined to smaller groups of individuals who were seeking moksha or liberation; however, the trend has transformed over the decades. Today, there are so many yoga studios worldwide, and this has made it easy for yoga enthusiasts. This chapter investigates the effectiveness of yoga not only as a complementary therapy but also as a viable option in the management of stress, anxiety and depression. Articles were retrieved using PubMed, MEDLINE and PsychInfo databases. The findings reveal that the practice of yoga as a complementary therapy and stand-alone therapy is effective in managing stress, anxiety and depression. However, further research is needed as all the studies reviewed were limited in terms of heterogeneity, sample size, intervention styles, frequency and duration of practice, and also teaching methods. The chapter concludes with suggestions for home practice.

Keywords: intervention of yoga, stress, anxiety, depression

1. Introduction

Amongst all the mental health disorders, anxiety, depression and stress appear to be the most common ones inflicting the human society. These diseases are disorders of the biochemical and neurophysiological systems which have an impact on not only the release of mood-regulating chemicals such as serotonin, dopamine and noradrenaline, but also on the cortisol and gamma amino-butyric acid (GABA) levels [1]. More than 264 million of people regardless of age, gender or creed suffer from depression [2]. Compared to men, women are more prone to this disorder, but the worrying trend is that depression leads to suicide. Evidence shows that approximately 700,000 people worldwide take their own lives annually, and what is more shocking is that suicide is deemed the fourth cause of death amongst 15 to 19-year-olds [3].

Not only depression, but also anxiety and stress are interrelated with physical well-being. For instance, cardiovascular diseases can lead to depression and vice versa. On a same note, the deadly Covid-19 pandemic which took the entire world by a storm in 2020 has had a significant undesirable impact on mental health. As the pandemic continues to ravage lives of innocent people in every nook and corner of the globe, a wide range of psychological outcomes have been observed at different layers of the society – individual, community, national and international levels. At the individual level, people are still apprehensive of falling ill or experiencing a painful death due the virus or being stigmatized by the society [4]. Health care workers and families with infected patients are completely fatigued. School and college-going students are not only totally demotivated, but also displeased as they have had to switch to virtual learning which in turn has impacted not only their eyesight, but also their physical health due to prolonged hours of being glued to the computer screen, and their social life. Family bread winners in various sectors who have lost jobs, and those in dire need of financial aid are totally dejected and devastated. Findings also reveal that those who have been quarantined or isolated, experienced quite a significant amount of stress, anxiety, mood swings, depression, and insomnia [5–7]. Frequent exposure to media appears to be another detrimental contributing factor to stress and anxiety [8]. It appears that patients with depression more often than not show symptoms of anxiety disorders, while those with anxiety disorders exhibit signs of depression [9]. Nonetheless, it is evident that both disorders tend to co-exist [10]. There are still so many people out there who are anxious and stressed out that they or their loved ones may contract the disease and not survive.

As anxiety and depression are affiliated with morbidity and mortality, it is imperative that these illnesses be identified and treated. Common treatments for these mental health disorders are available. Besides psychosocial treatments, psychological treatments such as cognitive behavioral therapy and pharmacotherapy such as selective serotonin reuptake inhibitors (SSRIs) and tricyclic antidepressants (TCAs) are usually used as the first line of treatment in moderate to severely depressed individuals [11]. Antidepressants augmented with antipsychotics have shown positive results in treating anxiety. It is noteworthy that some of the drug-based treatments for anxiety have been reported to produce a sharp decline in depressive symptoms [12, 13]; however, the strategy involved in preventing depression by treating anxiety successfully warrants further clinical investigation. Benzodiazepine, a common drug-based medication that enhances the effects of GABA at its receptor, on the other hand, is only effective in treating anxiety and not depression [9].

While treatments are readily available, some of the victims do not seek help because of financial issues, fear of being stigmatized for visiting a mental health counsellor, ignorance or for no rationale at all. Furthermore, there could be concerns about the adverse outcomes and compliance of these drugs [14].

In many parts of the world today, complementary and alternative medicine treatments are gaining popularity by all and sundry. Mindfulness-based interventions such as meditation and yoga are widely used in the therapy of both psychological and also physical ailments as research has shown a link between these practices, and physical and psychological health changes [15]. Findings seem to reveal that the practice of yoga can positively affect the biochemical and neurophysiological systems by regulating the autonomic nervous system and stress response, hence lowering the stress, anxiety and depression levels [16]. There is evidence that patients favour these conventional methods of treatment compared to mainstream approaches such as psychotherapy or psychotropic medications [17].

This chapter will look at the philosophy and benefits of yoga, review some recent research that have been done on the intervention of yoga as an adjunct or stand-alone therapy for stress, anxiety and depression, the effectiveness of this mind-body regime and its implications for the sufferers of the current society.

2. Background

2.1 The philosophy of yoga

Yoga, an ancient mind-body movement practice, originated in India more than five millenniums ago. Also commonly referred to as a meditative movement practice, it involves movement, a meditative state of mind, breath focus and deep relaxation for purposes of enhancing or healing the physical, mental and emotional well-being [18].

Yoga appears to be a form of alternative medicine [19], and its philosophy is based on the eight limbs schematised by Maharishi Patanjali, one of the main pillars of classical yoga. These eight limbs comprise yama (universal moral ethics), niyama (internal attitudes for personal discipline), asana (yoga posture), pranayama (expansion of life force), prathyahara (withdrawal of senses), dharana (contemplation of one's true nature), dhyana (meditation) and samadhi (liberation) [20].

The first three limbs or stages – yama, niyama and asana, are considered the outward quests (bahiranga sadhana). With the practice of yama and niyama, the practitioner works towards keeping his passions and emotions under control, while the asana component, if practised diligently, keeps the body strong and healthy, and in harmony with nature. Breath regulation and mind control take place in the next two stages, that is, pranayama and prathyahara. Since these stages work at the inner level, they are known as inner quests or antaranga sadhana in Sanskrit. The last three stages – dharana, dhyana and samadhi, elevate the practitioner into the deeper recesses of the soul [21].

As yoga is not a religion or a cult, anyone regardless of age, creed or gender can learn and practise it. For the genuine seeker, whose desire is to experience the universal self within, the practice of yoga is an unbroken journey. Nevertheless, this ancient practice can be simplified and performed in a number of ways to suit the practitioner [22].

The practice of yoga is so flexible that the practitioner can simply utilize some, if not all, of the limbs to their own comfort. In a conventional 1 h yoga session, it is not uncommon to have the asanas integrated with practices of pranayama, prathyahara, dharana and dhyana. Having said that, there are many styles of yoga; precision and alignment, asthanga yoga, flow yoga, asana yoga, gentle yoga and hot yoga are some of the common styles [23].

2.2 Benefits of yoga

The practice of yoga brings about tremendous benefits to the body and mind. In the past nine decades, empirical research has been carried out on the techniques of yoga to test its credibility. Pioneer experiments conducted by Swami Kuvalayananda in 1924 focused on parameters like heart rate, blood pressure fluctuations, and intra-esophageal air pressure during the performance and also after the practice of asanas and pranayama [24].

Due to promising results, yoga has since been classified by the National Institute of Health as a form of complementary and alternative medicine, and people from all walks of life have incorporated this scientific practice into their lifestyles [25].

Unlike other forms of exercise, yoga focuses on being present in the moment. Hence, the practitioner needs to be mindful regardless of whether they have assumed a static position while holding an asana for a couple of breaths, or in motion especially during the performance of an asana. Preliminary research has advocated that yoga may increase levels of mindfulness in the practitioner [26, 27]. The asanas when performed steadily and joyfully, are useful in preventing and correcting structural imbalances in the body [28].

As this ancient science also appears to be a form of moving meditation, there have been suggestions that practitioners are more likely to be engaged in the movement aspect of yoga as it stimulates the cognitive processes related to mindfulness [29]. In addition, the meditative movement, which coordinates each movement with the breath systematically, increases physical endurance in the practitioner over time. As the muscles recurrently contract with more force while performing a particular movement, their strength eventually increases. An example would be in the classical cobra pose (bhujangasana). In this pose, the practitioner starts of by lying flat facing downward on the mat. As the upper torso and head are lifted of the mat upon inhalation, the back extensors are engaged and contracted strongly. Hence, if the position is held long enough (while breathing normally), and if the movement is repeated a couple of times in each practice, the back muscles will be strengthened [30].

Muscles and connective tissues are stretched in asanas to increase flexibility. Regardless of whether the stretch is with or against gravity, the body will experience a stretch, thus increasing flexibility [30]. Unfortunately, in the current situation today where many, who work from home, pay little attention to their sitting position, the structural alignment is greatly compromised. Certain sporting activities like tennis and football, which require strenuous use of one side of the body, are equally to be blamed too. Asanas taught in yoga have been known to prevent and correct structural misalignments in the body.

Having said that, existing research unveils that the benefits of yoga are not limited to only correcting structural misalignments, enhancing stretching and improving flexibility; yoga also enhances emotional and psychosocial health and brings about an increase in proprioceptive and interoceptive awareness [31, 32]. There have been propositions that if yoga is practised consistently, it has the ability to induce neuroplasticity i.e., changes in the neural pathways of the brain, thus improving psychological skills [33]. This augurs well for the yoga practitioner as it suggests that the brain can be rewired just like a muscle in the physical body.

3. Intervention of yoga in stress, anxiety and depression

Yoga as therapy or therapeutic yoga has been defined as application of yoga postures and practice to the treatment of health conditions [34]. Evidence from a growing body of research supports the notion that yoga may bring about positive effects not only in one's physical but also mental health through the downregulation of the hypothalamo–pituitary adrenal (HPA) axis and the sympathetic nervous system (SNS) [35].

3.1 Methodology of yoga intervention

Since the aim of this review is to look into the impact of yoga specifically on stress, anxiety and depression in this contemporary society, only findings from articles that were published from 2014 to 2021 were reviewed and included. A combination of databases including PubMed, MEDLINE and PsychInfo were used to identify these articles with the help of keywords and phrases such as "intervention of yoga," "anxiety," "stress," and "depression." The search was streamlined to include only studies that were conducted with adults as participants, irrespective of gender or creed. Those that were conducted with children or teenagers below the age of 18 were excluded completely. In addition, studies that included adults suffering from multiple diseases and/or mental health issues, such as psychosis, obsessive – compulsive disorder and health-related aspects of physical fitness were not included in the discussion here. Studies that included pregnant and post-partum participants were also omitted as it is not unusual for this category of participants to undergo depression and anxiety during that period. In terms of the intervention, only studies that integrated classical yoga were included. Hence, the discussion is substantiated with findings from nine studies conducted between 2014 and 2021.

Authors	Description of Intervention	Findings
Kinser et al. [40]	RCT; YG: 75 min of hatha yoga (asanas, breathing techniques, relaxation, guided meditation) per week over 8 weeks; CG: health education activities (lectures, videos, discussions) Both groups continued with prescribed medication and maintained their lifestyle activities.	YG experienced multiple benefits of yoga including a boost of confidence; Gained new skills to be used in daily life to manage depression and stress;
Doria et al. [39]	Pre-test post-test; Grp 1: medication+SKY+self-help group weekly; Grp 2: SKY+self-help group weekly but no medication 6 months prior to study Intervention: 10 sessions of 2 h SKY in 2 weeks followed by weekly SKY for 6 months (asanas, pranayama, chanting, prathyhara, dharana)	A reduction in anxiety and depression levels in both groups No significant differences in scores between both groups
Falsafi and Leopard [37]	Quasi-experimental (repeated measures with one group); Intervention: 90 min yoga per week for 8 weeks (asanas, pranayama and mindfulness practice)	Significant decrease ($p < 0.05$) in depressive symptoms
De Manincor et al. [41]	RCT; YG: A 6 week yoga program; 30 min of vini yoga practice (asanas, pranayama, relaxation, mindfulness, meditation) for 4.8 days per week + TAU; CG: TAU – yoga was given after waitlist period.	A significant reduction in depression and anxiety scores; YG showed greater reduction compared to CG.
Falsafi [36]	RCT (stratified- randomised controlled repeated measures); YG: 8 weeks hatha yoga; 75 min session once a week; 20 min daily home practice. CG: absence of yoga MIG: mindfulness practice	YG and MIG showed significant reduction in depression, stress and anxiety compared to CG; no significant change in CG; No difference between YG and MIG, but self-compassion scores significant in MIG.
Prathikanti et al. [42]	RCT (stratified-randomised controlled); YG: A 8 week yoga program (asana, pranayama, dharana, prathyahara); 90 min per session, two sessions a week; props used; TAU. CG: 90 min of Yoga history workshop twice a week for 8 weeks, TAU. No medication for both groups.	YG showed a significant decrease in depression compared to CG ($p = 0.034$). YG more likely to achieve remission. YG requested for more sessions per week and also permission to attend yoga history workshop.
Uebelacker et al. [44]	RCT (stratified-randomised controlled); YG: A 10 week yoga program (asana, pranayama, dharana, dhyana, prathyahara); 80 min per session; one or two sessions per week; TAU. CG: A 10 week healthy-living workshop; 60 min per session; one or two sessions per week; TAU.	Insignificant difference between YG and CG; YG demonstrated lower levels of depressive symptoms, better social and role functioning, and general health perceptions when compared to CG.
Shohani et al. [43]	Quasi-experimental (pre/post -test); YG: 60–70 min hatha yoga, three times a week for 4 weeks	A significant, decrease in depression, stress and anxiety in the YG ($p < 0.001$).
Simon et al. [38]	RCT (three-arm controlled single blind); YG: A 12 week program (asana, pranayama, dharana, prathyahara dharana, dhyana) 120 min per session CBT: evidence-based GAD protocol CG: stress education	YG and CBT showed efficacy for treatment of GAD; CBT remains first-line treatment.

CG: control group; CBT: cognitive behavioral therapy; GAD: generalized anxiety disorder; MIG: mindfulness intervention group; RCT: randomized controlled trial; TAU: treatment as usual; and YG: yoga group.

Table 1.
Summary of the intervention and findings of the selected studies.

The design of all the studies varied considerably from pre-test/post-test to quasi-experimental and randomised controlled trials (RCTs). One of the RCTs was a stratified-randomised controlled with repeated measures [36]. The sample size incorporated in all these studies was relatively small, ranging from 18 [37] to a maximum of 226 [38]. While this review is not limited to qualitative and quantitative studies, the instruments used in each study varied rather significantly. In all these studies, the intervention of yoga was heterogeneous. Studies that had incorporated transcendental meditation or mindfulness meditation (or any other forms of meditation) or pranayama as stand-alone practices are not included in this discussion.

Only studies that assimilated aspects of classical hatha yoga specifically asana, pranayama, prathyahara, dharana and dhyana were included, though the duration of each class and frequency of sessions varied considerably. One study had administered Kundalini yoga; however, it had incorporated all the aspects of classical hatha yoga, hence the findings of that study were included in this review [38]. It is interesting to note that another study had incorporated chanting as part of the intervention [39].

3.2 Outcomes

On a positive note, most of the studies reviewed (2014–2021), if not all, exhibited appreciable outcomes; intervention of yoga, with or without pharmacotherapy, appeared to be effectual in reducing the symptoms of these mental health disorders [36–44]. A summary of the intervention and findings is provided in **Table 1**. Even though the duration of each and every study reviewed in this chapter varied considerably, that is, from 4 weeks to 6 months, there are implications that the practice of yoga advocates changes in the neural pathways of the human brain, resulting in favorable effects to the brain activity. Evidence has shown that, when compared to controls, there is less activation in the dorsolateral prefrontal cortex of yoga practitioners [45]. It appears that if there is consistency in the practice of yoga, the alpha, beta and theta brainwaves are activated; these have been linked to improvement in not only memory, but also mood and anxiety.

4. Discussion

All the studies reviewed in this chapter incorporated the fundamental limbs of Patanjali yoga, that is, asanas, pranayama, prathyahara, dharana and dhyana. The first two limbs in yoga, that is, yama and niyama, are therapeutic in nature as both entail code of ethics that work at not only intrapersonal (yama), but also interpersonal (niyama) levels [46]. Yama includes practices such as ahimsa (non-violence), satya (non-stealing), asteya (non-lying), brahmacharya (non-excessiveness) and aparigraha (non-greediness). Niyama, on the other hand, encompasses traits such as saucha (cleanliness), santosha (contentment), tapas (sacrifice), swadyaya (self-study) and Ishwara pranidana (surrendering to the higher power). It is imperative to note that while none of these studies reported the inclusion of yamas and niyamas as part of the intervention, it is believed that these two limbs may have been interleaved into the yoga sessions in an informal manner [47].

It is common to prompt students in a timely manner specifically during the asana session to practise ahimsa, for example. While mindfully challenging oneself to perform a strenuous or a dynamic pose is encouraged, using unwarranted force recklessly to get into the pose is not. For obvious reasons, just like in any sporting activities, adding excessive pressure at certain joints in the body can and will bring about unforeseen injury to the practitioner. More importantly, while the pose is being held (being in the pose), students are persistently reminded to bring their awareness to the deep joy and pleasurable feelings that they are experiencing at that moment regardless of whether they are in the full pose or in a modified version. This act of experiencing joy while being in a particular position brings us to one of the niyamas, that is santosha. Hence, in this manner, the other yamas and niyamas are introduced and expounded during a yoga session at the academy where classes are conducted.

In the studies that have been reviewed in this chapter, the instructors assigned to the yoga sessions may have implicitly incorporated the yamas and niyamas but may have inadvertently failed to report the minutiae and hence, the details of the latter were not highlighted in the papers published. Just like in any study, implicit details are imperative for informed choices to be made. If the specifics of the yoga intervention for each study had been reported, it would have been instrumental not only to the researcher and the reader, but also to the participant who may be keen on exploring the philosophical roots of the yogic practice [47].

It is noteworthy that despite the insignificant sample size, heterogeneity in the sample population, varied duration of the intervention and wide-ranging styles of yoga taught, all studies reviewed demonstrated positive results in reducing the scores in depression, anxiety, and also stress.

In one study, where both the yoga group (YG) and the control group (CG) underwent pharmacotherapy during the intervention, the YG not only experienced a significant decrease in ruminations, but also found solace in the practice; participants used yoga as a strategy to help cope with ill-thoughts and other symptoms of depression in daily life [40]. This could be due to the impact of one of the components in the yoga practice, i.e., yoga nidra (guided meditation) that may have enhanced the self-regulatory capacities in the participants. On the hindsight, participants of this study acknowledged that the practice of yoga had intensified their confidence and that the practice had become an internal motivator for continued participation.

Similar results were seen in another study that engaged sudharshan kriya yoga (SKY) [39]. There was hardly any difference in the scores between the two groups (one group did SKY with pharmacotherapy, while the other group did SKY sans pharmacotherapy), purely suggesting that SKY may be effective not only as a stand-alone therapy, but also as an adjunct therapy for patients undergoing medical treatment. This study was exceptional as it had incorporated chanting in the yoga session. Chanting appears to have a healing effect not only on the physical and emotional, but also on the mental and spiritual body. It provides the drifting mind with a focal point. Though the chanting aspect was brief in this study, previous research has revealed that chanting has the potential to bring about deactivation in the amygdala, parahippocampal and hippocampal brain regions [46]. By stimulating the auricular branches of the vagal nerves, chanting creates vibrations at the cellular level. It is these vibrations that create neuro-linguistic effects which induce tranquility in the body and mind. Those suffering from depression tend to have a noisy mind – one that is cluttered with heaps of unnecessary thoughts. It is believed that the sounds of the mantra have the ability to mask the negative voices in the brain. Only when these ruinous thoughts are eradicated, can the mind have room for positive contemplations.

Similarly, the eight-week yoga intervention study which was conducted on 18 patients diagnosed with anxiety in the US showed a significant reduction in depressive symptoms ($p < 0.05$) [37]. However, in the stratified RCT study that engaged college students in the USA, yoga and mindfulness practices were seen to be equally effective in reducing not only depression and anxiety, but also stress, even though the self-compassion scores were more significant for the mindfulness practice group [36]. The intervention in the study also lasted 8 weeks.

In a study conducted amongst a subsyndromal population in Australia, a six-week yoga intervention was found to be effective in reducing depressive and anxiety symptoms in both groups of participants, the YG and the CG [41]. There was reduction in psychological stress and rumination, an increase in resilience, and an improvement in mental well-being. It is interesting to note that findings of this study revealed that the yoga participants, on their own accord, had reduced medication dosage and frequency of visiting the counsellor. Though the reasons for these actions are indistinct and warrants deeper investigation, the yoga intervention mode appeared effective in managing the issue at hand of these participants. Pharmacological interventions for depression and anxiety usually produce a delay of approximately 4 weeks before exerting significant mood effects over placebo; it may take up to 12 weeks to achieve full anti-depression effects with medication [48]. Hence, time is definitely a parameter for consideration in yoga intervention. However, in this Australian study, it was suggested that a 30 min yoga practice over 5 days per week should suffice for all and sundry.

Similar positive outcomes of practicing yoga were observed in a depressive and withdrawn community who participated in a randomized controlled trial in San Francisco [42]. Unlike other studies, participants in the YG in this study not only asked for more yoga sessions, but also sought permission to attend the theoretical sessions on yoga history that were specifically held for the CG. It appears that these participants were definitely eager to do yoga for the benefit of their own mind-body health, but at the same time, interested in understanding the physiology behind this ancient science. Specific asanas such as dhanurasana (bow pose), ardhakati chakrasana (half waist wheel pose), ardha chakrasana (half wheel pose), Bhujangasana (cobra pose), setu bandhasana (bridge pose), sarvangasana (shoulder stand) and matsyasana (fish pose) employed in this study were found to be effectual in helping the participants manage their depressive moods and anxiety. It is interesting to note that most of these asanas are heart/chest openers. It appears that in the process of expanding the chest and rib cage to oxygenate the lungs efficiently, these asanas have helped in managing symptoms of depression such as grief, anger and frustration.

The findings from an Iranian study which was carried amongst 52 women suffering from some form of mental health disorders albeit free from pharmacotherapy, was equally positive; the intervention of yoga as a stand-alone therapy brought upon a reduction in anxiety, depression and also stress levels ($p = 0.001$) in the participants who did 12 sessions of yoga over a four-week period [43].

While most studies showed promising outcomes, one study hardly showed any significant statistical difference between the YG and the CG even though there was evidence of a reduction in depressive symptoms and better social functioning in the YG [44]. These positive effects could have been merely an after effect due to the relaxation techniques included in the yogic regime. Relaxation techniques in yoga are known to downplay the sympathetic activity and balance the autonomic nervous system responses.

Finally, in one recent three-arm controlled single blind clinical trial, where participants were randomized over a period of 12 weeks to either the kundalini yoga (KY) or cognitive behavioral therapy (CBT) while the CG was subjected to stress education, it was found that the KY group and the CBT group had shown significant reduction in generalized anxiety disorder symptoms. That said, the findings also revealed that CBT appears to be more effective than yoga, and it was concluded that the former shall remain the first line of treatment for anxiety disorders [38].

However, in most, if not all, of the studies reviewed in this chapter, they were subjected to limitations. For example, a few of the studies were predominantly a female sample [40, 43]. While there is a greater tendency for women to suffer from depression compared to men [49], the sample size in these studies was disproportionately represented. Also, most of the studies were limited by the insignificant sample population and heterogeneity. Due to the absence of controls in certain studies, it was challenging to establish whether the results obtained were due intervention of yoga or another factor. RCTs are known to be intervention research of high standards, but most of the studies reviewed here were challenged due to several reasons. Either the randomization was inappropriate, yoga styles in terms of postures, breathing and meditative techniques were too varied and/or incongruence in teaching methods.

Despite the limitations, it appears that participants who have benefitted from these yoga sessions may now have an extra tool at hand to help them manage stress, anxiety and depression. Since there were no adverse effects reported in any of the studies, yoga appears to be a safe practice.

5. Conclusion

All studies that have been reviewed in this chapter incorporated the fundamental limbs of Patanjali yoga that is, asanas, pranayama, prathyahara, dharana and dhyana. Despite the limitations such as heterogeneity in the sample population, insignificant sample size, varied durations of intervention and styles of yoga taught, most studies, if not all, demonstrated substantial positive outcomes in reducing the scores in depression, anxiety and stress. Previous studies have shown that the practice of asana, pranayama, dharana and dhyana have the ability to still not only the mind, but also the body, thus lowering anxiety levels, and these effects were seen in the studies reviewed in this chapter.

Having said that, another factor to delve into is the time (duration) required for participants to master the yoga asanas, especially for those whose flexibility is compromised, and the breathing techniques. The duration for the psycho-physiological factors mediating specific mood benefits of yoga to develop and exert a quantifiable effect in the participant is equally important. While factors such as duration of a yoga session, frequency and duration of each limb in a yoga session warrant further investigation, selection of asanas in a yoga intervention should not be neglected.

At the Malaysian Yoga Academy, students, regardless of their mental or physical health conditions, are encouraged to practise yoga daily for at least 45 min. This is not only to ensure there is sufficient time to practise most, if not all the limbs, but also to sustain a healthy mind and body, and keep diseases at bay; this step is crucial as studies have indicated that many people suffer from some form of anxiety and/or mood disorder at some point in their life.

6. Suggestions for home practice

Here are some simple postures (asanas) and breathing practices one can do two to three times daily. All practices should be done on an empty stomach. A suggestion would be to practice before sunrise, and/or at sunset and/or before bedtime. If food has been consumed, allow 2 h for digestion before the practice. It is imperative to note that these practices do not replace any form of prescribed medication. They are merely suggested complementary practices towards better mental and physical health, and tools that can be used to manage a sudden onslaught of stress, anxiety and/or a depressive mood.

6.1 Postures

i. *Swaying palm tree pose*: Stand with the legs 2 feet apart. Upon inhalation, the hands are raised vertically upwards. Upon exhalation, the torso is stretched sideways to the right. This position is held for 2–3 s. Upon inhalation, the torso is brought to the center. Then upon exhalation, the torso is stretched sideways to the left. This right and left movement is considered one set. Depending on one's capacity, one may perform up to five sets of this asana.

ii. *Double angle pose*: Standing with the legs 2–3 feet apart, interlace the fingers at the back of the body. In this starting position, inhale slowly and deeply. Upon exhaling, stretch the torso forward. If the body allows a greater stretch, bring the torso a horizontal position while gently lifting the hands away from the body. While breathing normally, hold this position for approximately 5 s before inhaling to bring the torso up to a vertical position. Depending on one's capacity, one may repeat this stretch three times, increasing the 'holding duration' from 5 to 10 s in the second and third repetition.

iii. *Half wheel pose*: Stand with the legs hip width apart. Place palms at the back of the waist with all fingers pointing downward. This is the starting position. Upon inhalation, bend the torso backwards from the lumbar region. Then exhale and continue with normal breathing while holding this position for 10 s. Inhale and bring the torso up the original position. Depending on one's capacity, this posture may be repeated three to five times.

6.2 Breathing techniques

i. *Deep breathing with hand movement*: In a comfortable sitting position (on the floor or on the chair), stretch the hands out to the front parallel to floor. The palms are in contact with each other. This is the starting position. Upon inhalation, bring the hands away from each other and stretch it to the back without any exertion. Hold for 2 s. Upon exhalation, bring the palms together to the starting position. This is one set, and one may do up to 10 sets in a nice and slow manner with breath awareness.

ii. *Alternate nostril breathing*: Sit in a comfortable position (on the floor or on the chair). If one is seated on the floor cross-legged, they may lean against the wall for support. Place the left palm facing upward on the left knee and allow the tip of the index finger to be in contact with the tip of the thumb throughout the practice. The remaining three fingers are stretched out without strain. Close the right nostril with the right thumb. For convenience, the index and the middle finger may be folded towards the palm, while keeping the ring and little fingers stretched out. This is the starting position. Inhale deeply through the left nostril. Then close the left nostril with the ring and index fingers. Subsequently, release the right thumb and exhale completely through the right nostril. Next, inhale through the right nostril. At the end of the inhalation, close the right nostril with the thumb and open the left nostril to exhale. This complete cycle is one round of alternate nostril breathing. One may practice up to 10 rounds at one sitting, bearing in mind that the inhalation and the exhalation should not only be slow and steady, but also silent and controlled.

iii. *Humming bee's breath*: Sit in a comfortable position (on the floor or on the chair). Back of the palms are rested on the knees – right palm on the right knee and left palm on the left knee. This is the starting position. Inhale deeply through both the nostrils. Allow the breath to stop effortlessly. Then exhale slowly while producing a humming sound like a bee. This is one round. One may practise up to 10 rounds at one sitting and increase the number of repetitions gradually.

All these postures and breathing techniques induce relaxation for the body and mind. One may practice all the postures and breathing techniques given here at any one sitting; alternatively, one may practice a few.

Acknowledgements

The author is grateful to Malaysian Association of Yoga Instructors (MAYI) Yoga Academy and the Malaysian Yoga Society for all the trainings and certifications she has received over the years.

Conflict of interest

The author declares no conflict of interest.

Notes

As a yoga instructor and therapist, the author has shared lots of personal experiences and provided home practice for the benefit of those who need it. Thank you.

Author details

Chandra Nanthakumar
HELP University, Kuala Lumpur, Malaysia

*Address all correspondence to: nankumar60@yahoo.com; chandratk@help.edu.my

References

[1] Cramer H, Lauche R, Langhorst J, Dobos G. Yoga for depression: A systematic review and meta-analysis. Depression and Anxiety. 2013;**30**(11): 1068-1083. DOI: 10.1002/da.22166

[2] World Health Organisation. Depression [Internet]. 2020. Available from: https://www.who.int/news-room/fact-sheets/detail/depression [Accessed: June 10, 2021]

[3] World Health Organisation. Suicide [Internet]. 2021. Available from: https://www.who.int/news-room/fact-sheets/detail/suicide [Accessed: June 20, 2021]

[4] Salari N, Khazaie H, Hosseinian-Far A, Khaledi-Paveh B, Kazeminia M, Mohammadi M, et al. The prevalence of stress, anxiety and depression within front-line healthcare workers caring for COVID-19 patients: A systematic review and meta-regression. Human Resources for Health. 2020;**18**(100):1-14. DOI: 10.1186/s12960-020-00544-1

[5] Brooks SK, Webster RK, Smith LE, Woodland L, Wessely S, Greenberg N, et al. The psychological impact of quarantine and how to reduce it: Rapid review of the evidence. Lancet. 2020;**395**(10227):912-920. DOI: 10.1016/S0140-6736(20)30460-8

[6] Wang Y, Xu B, Zhao G, Cao R, He X, Fu S. Is quarantine related to immediate negative psychological consequences during the 2009 H1N1 epidemic? General Hospital Psychiatry. 2011;**33**(1):75-77. DOI: 10.1016/j.genhosppsych.2010.11.001

[7] Rubin GJ, Wessely S. The psychological effects of quarantining a city. BMJ. 2020;**368**:m313. DOI: 10.1136/bmj.m313

[8] Neria Y, Sullivan GM. Understanding the mental health effects of indirect exposure to mass trauma through the media. Journal of the American Medical Association. 2011;**306**(12):1374-1375. DOI: 10.1001/jama.2011.1358

[9] Tiller JWG. Depression and anxiety. The Medical Journal of Australia. 2013;**199**(6):S28-S31. DOI: 10.5694/mja12.10628

[10] Garber J, Weersing VR. Comorbidity of anxiety and depression in youth: Implications for treatment and prevention. Journal of Clinical Psychology. 2010;**17**(4):293-306. DOI: 10.1111/j.1468-2850.2010.01221.x

[11] Gautam S, Jain A, Gautam M, Vahia VN, Grover S. Clinical practice guidelines for the management of depression. Indian Journal of Psychiatry. 2017;**59**(1):S34-S50. DOI: 10.4103/0019-5545.196973

[12] Kendall PC, Safford S, Flannery-Schroeder E, Webb A. Child anxiety treatment: Outcomes in adolescence and impact on substance use and depression at 7.4-year follow-up. Journal of Consulting and Clinical Psychology. 2004;**72**(2):276-287. DOI: 10.1037/0022-006X.72.2.276

[13] Manassis K, Mendlowitz SL, Scapillato D, Avery D, Fiksenbaum L, Freire M, et al. Group and individual cognitive-behavioral therapy for childhood anxiety disorders: A randomized trial. Journal of the American Academy of Child and Adolescent Psychiatry. 2002;**41**(12): 1423-1430. DOI: 10.1097/00004583-200212000-00013

[14] de Manincor M, Bensoussan A, Smith C, Fahey P, Bourchier S. Establishing key components of yoga interventions for reducing depression and anxiety, and improving well-being: A Delphi method study. BMC Complementary and Alternative Medicine. 2015;**15**(1):1-10. DOI: 10.1186/s12906-015-0614-7

[15] Cuijpers P, Smit F, Bohlmeijer E, Hollon SD, Andersson G. Efficacy of cognitive-behavioural therapy and other psychological treatments for adult depression: Meta-analytic study of publication bias. The British Journal of Psychiatry. 2010;**196**(3):173-178. DOI: 10.1192/bjp.bp.109.066001

[16] Salmon P, Lush E, Jablonski M, Sephton SE. Yoga and mindfulness: Clinical aspects of an ancient mind/body practice. Cognitive and Behavioral Practice. 2009;**16**(1):59-72. DOI: 10.1016/j.cbpra.2008.07.002

[17] Kessler RC, Soukup J, Davis RB, Foster DF, Wilkey SA, Van Rompay MI, et al. The use of complementary and alternative therapies to treat anxiety and depression in the United States. The American Journal of Psychiatry. 2001;**158**(2):289-294. DOI: 10.1176/appi.ajp.158.2.289

[18] Ajaya S. Healing the Whole Person: Applications of Yoga Psychotherapy. Pennyslvania: Himalayan Institute Press; 2008. p. 3

[19] Bridges L, Sharma M. The efficacy of yoga as a form of treatment for depression. Journal of Evidence-Based Complementary & Alternative Medicine. 2017;**22**(4):1017-1028. DOI: 10.1177/2156587217715927

[20] Muktibodhananda S. Hatha Yoga Pradipika. 3rd ed. Munger: Yoga Publications Trust; 1998. p. 4

[21] Telles S, Singh N, Gupta RKB, A. A selective review of dharana and dhyana in healthy participants. Journal of Ayurveda and Integrative Medicine. 2016;7(4):255-260. DOI: 10.1016/j.jaim.2016.09.004

[22] Mohan AG, Mohan I. Yoga Therapy: A Guide to the Therapeutic Use of Yoga and Ayurveda for Health and Fitness. Boston: Shambhala Publications Inc; 2004. pp. 15-30

[23] Nichols N. How Does Yoga Work? [Internet]. 2021. Available from: medicalnewstoday.com/articles/286745 [Accessed: July 20, 2021]

[24] Alter JS. Yoga in Modern India: The Body between Science and Philosophy. Princeton: Princeton University Press; 2004. p. 73

[25] Williams KA, Petronis J, Smith D, Goodrich D, Wu J, Ravi N, et al. Effect of Iyengar yoga therapy for chronic low back pain. Pain. 2005;**115**(1-2):107-117. DOI: 10.1016/j.pain.2005.02.016

[26] Brisbon NM, Lowery GA. Mindfulness and levels of stress: A comparison of beginner and advanced hatha yoga practitioners. Journal of Religion and Health. 2011;**50**(4):931-941. DOI: 10.1007/s10943-009-9305-3

[27] Conboy LA, Wilson A, Braun T. Moving beyond health to flourishing: The effects of yoga teacher training. Scientific World Journal. 2010;**10**:788-795. DOI: 10.1100/tsw.2010.87

[28] Stiles M. Structural Yoga Therapy: Adapting to the Individual. San Francisco: Red Wheel/Weiser; 2013. pp. 17-20

[29] Butterfield N, Schultz T, Rasmussen P, Proeve M. Yoga and mindfulness for anxiety and depression and the role of mental health professionals: A literature review. The Journal of Mental Health Training, Education and Practice. 2017;**12**(1):44-54. DOI: 10.1108/JMHTEP-01-2016-0002

[30] Polsgrove MJ, Eggleston BM, Lockyer RJ. Impact of 10-weeks of yoga practice on flexibility and balance of college athletes. International Journal of Yoga. 2016;**9**(1):27-34. DOI: 10.4103/0973-6131.171710

[31] Nanthakumar C. The benefits of yoga in children. Journal of Integrative

Medicine. 2018;**16**(1):14-19. DOI: 10.1016/j.joim.2017.12.008

[32] Woodyard C. Exploring the therapeutic effects of yoga and its ability to increase quality of life. International Journal of Yoga. 2011;**4**(2):49-54. DOI: 10.4103/0973-6131.85485

[33] Brown RP, Gerbarg PL. Sudarshan Kriya yogic breathing in the treatment of stress, anxiety, and depression: Part I—Neurophysiologic model. Journal of Alternative and Complementary Medicine. 2005;**11**(1):189-201. DOI: 10.1089/acm.2005.11.189

[34] Collins C. Yoga: Intuition, preventive medicine, and treatment. Journal of Obstetric, Gynecologic, and Neonatal Nursing. 1998;**27**(5):563-568. DOI: 10.1111/j.1552-6909.1998.tb02623.x

[35] Sengupta P. Health impacts of yoga and pranayama: A state-of-the-art review. International Journal of Preventive Medicine. 2012;**3**(7):444-458

[36] Falsafi N. A randomized controlled trial of mindfulness versus yoga: Effects on depression and/or anxiety in college students. Journal of the American Psychiatric Nurses Association. 2016;**22**(6):483-497. DOI: 10.1177/1078390316663307

[37] Falsafi N, Leopard L. Pilot study: Use of mindfulness, self-compassion, and yoga practices with low-income and/or uninsured patients with depression and/or anxiety. Journal of Holistic Nursing. 2015;**33**(4):289-297. DOI: 10.1177/0898010115569351

[38] Simon NM, Hofmann SG, Rosenfield D, Hoeppner SS, Hoge EA, Bui E, et al. Efficacy of yoga vs cognitive behavioral therapy vs stress education for the treatment of generalized anxiety disorder: A randomized clinical trial. JAMA Psychiatry. 2021;**78**(1):13-20. DOI: 10.1001/jamapsychiatry.2020.2496

[39] Doria S, de Vuono A, Sanlorenzo R, Irtelli F, Mencacci C. Anti-anxiety efficacy of sudarshan kriya yoga in general anxiety disorder: A multicomponent, yoga based, breath intervention program for patients suffering from generalized anxiety disorder with or without comorbidities. Journal of Affective Disorders. 2015;**184**:310-317. DOI: 10.1016/j.jad.2015.06.011

[40] Kinser PA, Elswick RK, Kornstein S. Potential long-term effects of a mind-body intervention for women with major depressive disorder: Sustained mental health improvements with a pilot yoga intervention. Archives of Psychiatric Nursing. 2014;**28**(6):377-383. DOI: 10.1016/j.apnu.2014.08.014

[41] de Manincor M, Bensoussan A, Smith CA, Barr K, Schweickle M, Donoghoe LL, et al. Individualized yoga for reducing depression and anxiety, and improving well-being: A randomized controlled trial. Depression and Anxiety. 2016;**33**(9):816-828. DOI: 10.1002/da.22502

[42] Prathikanti S, Rivera R, Cochran A, Tungol JG, Fayazmanesh N, Weinmann E. Treating depression with yoga: A prospective, randomized, controlled pilot trial. PLoS One. 2017;**12**(3):e0173869. DOI: 10.1371/journal.pone.0173869

[43] Shohani M, Badfar G, Nasirkandy MP, Kaikhavani S, Rahmati S, Modmeli Y, et al. The effect of yoga on stress, anxiety, and depression in women. International Journal of Preventive Medicine. 2018;**9**(1):21-23. DOI: 10.4103/ijpvm.IJPVM_242_16

[44] Uebelacker LA, Tremont G, Gillette LT, Epstein-Lubow G, Strong DR, Abrantes AM, et al. Adjunctive yoga v. health education for persistent major depression: A randomized controlled trial.

Psychological Medicine. 2017;**47**(12): 2130-2142. DOI: 10.1017/S0033291717000575

[45] Desai R, Tailor A, Bhatt T. Effects of yoga on brain waves and structural activation: A review. Complementary Therapies in Clinical Practice. 2015;**21**(2):112-118. DOI: 10.1016/j.ctcp.2015.02.002

[46] Kalyani BG, Venkatasubramanian G, Arasappa R, Rao NP, Kalmady SV, Behere RV, et al. Neurohemodynamic correlates of 'OM' chanting: A pilot functional magnetic resonance imaging study. International Journal of Yoga. 2011;**4**(1):3-6. DOI: 10.4103/0973-6131.78171

[47] Nyer M, O'Hair CM, Hopkins LB, Roberg R, Norton R, Streeter C. Yoga as a treatment for depression: Applications for mental health practitioners. Psychiatric Annals. 2019;**49**(1):11-15. DOI: 10.3928/00485713-20181203-01

[48] Uher R, Mors O, Rietschel M, Rajewska-Rager A, Petrovic A, Zobel A, et al. Early and delayed onset of response to antidepressants in individual trajectories of change during treatment of major depression: A secondary analysis of data from the genome-based therapeutic drugs for depression (GENDEP) study. The Journal of Clinical Psychiatry. 2011;**72**(11):1478-1484. DOI: 10.4088/JCP.10m06419

[49] Kessler RC, Berglund P, Demler O, Jin R, Koretz D, Merikangas KR, et al. National comorbidity survey replication. The epidemiology of major depressive disorder: Results from the national comorbidity survey replication (NCS-R). Journal of the American Medical Association. 2003;**289**(23): 3095-3105. DOI: 10.1001/jama.289.23.3095

Chapter 6

Medicinal Plants Used in the Management of Psychosis

Sunday Oritsetimenyin Otimenyin and Lydia Doosuur Ior

Abstract

Substantial number of studies has been conducted to find alternatives or treatments for psychosis. Psychosis represents a variety of mental disorders characterized by the presence of delusions, hallucinations and grossly disorganized thinking in a clear sensorium. Psychosis is burdensome and difficult to treat given the inability of the typical and atypical antipsychotics to adequately manage it, accompanied by numerous disturbing adverse effects. Therefore, many with chronic mental health problems justifiably feel disappointed by the apparent ineffectiveness of conventional treatment and naturally search for a more holistic approach to treatment and alternative medicines having less or no side-effects. Plants are rich in secondary metabolites which have the ability to interact with the Central nervous system (CNS) to produce effects that can be beneficial for the management of psychosis, these phytochemicals are believed to have minimal adverse effects. A review of some of the medicinal plants used as antipsychotics, indicated that many medicinal plants possess antipsychotic effects that can improve the treatment of psychosis. Apparently, further studies are necessary in order to isolate the active constituents, ascertain their molecular mechanisms and safety, and also to test them in clinical studies for the development of new pharmacotherapies for psychosis.

Keywords: Medicinal plants, Molecular mechanisms, Psychosis, Secondary metabolites, Antipsychotics

1. Introduction

The term "psychosis" denotes a variety of mental disorders: the presence of delusions, various types of hallucinations, usually auditory or visual, but sometimes tactile or olfactory, and grossly disorganized thinking in a clear sensorium. Schizophrenia is an enduring, disabling psychiatric illness affecting about 1% of the population globally. It is characterized by various symptoms classified into positive, negative and cognitive) [1, 2].

Plants provide the essential nutrients and remedy needed by humans, they are healthier compared to animal diets. Over time much benefits have been derived from medicinal plants due to their rich natural phytochemicals that interact favorably with the human body and neurotransmitters to produce effects that are beneficial to man. In this chapter we will look at some medicinal plant used in the pharmacotherapy of psychosis.

IntechOpen

2. Management of psychosis

Psychosis is an immense social and economic problem, but the management of psychosis remains insufficient. Basically typical and atypical antipsychotics are used for the treatment of schizophrenia, the typical antipsychotics such as chlorpromazine and haloperidol are only effective in the treatment of positive symptoms, and are accompanied by disturbing adverse effects such as extrapyramidal side-effects [3], the atypical antipsychotic drugs such as risperidone and olanzapine provide some beneficial effects on negative symptoms and cognitive deficits [4], but they are inadequate and mild. Prolonged use also results in increased oxidative load [5] which could lead to cardiovascular disorders, diabetes, and agranulocytosis seen with clozapine, they also cause moderate to severe weight gain [2, 6–8]. The use of medicinal plants as complementary remedies for the treatment of psychosis have become necessary because of their characteristically high chemical diversity, biochemical specificity, and several other properties that make them favorable lead structures for the treatment of various disorders, including psychosis [9], for example, *Alpinia zerumbet* (Pers.) B. L. Burtt (Zingiberaceae) [10], *Lonchocarpus cyanescens* (Schumach and Thonn.) Benth. (Fabaceae) [11] etc., which have been used in the pharmacotherapy of psychosis. Interestingly many of these plants were studied and found to have lesser side effects e.g. catalepsy [12–15] indicating that these plants may not cause extrapyramidal side effects in humans.

Medicinal plants are either used as an alternative or in addition to orthodox medicine [16], users search for a more holistic approach to treatment, others expect that alternative medicines have less or no side-effects, and many with chronic mental health problems justifiably feel disappointed by the apparent ineffectiveness of conventional treatment [17].

3. Review of relevant pathophysiology

Neuropsychiatric Disorders may occur as a result of a number of factors such as genetic predisposition, lifestyle factors such as substance abuse and recently diet is also believed to be a factor [18] due to certain observations that associated incidence of psychotic episodes in neuropsychiatric diseases with poor dietary patterns, such as a lower intake of omega-3 fatty acids, vegetables, fibers, fruits, vitamins and minerals [19], all these are substances that can be obtained naturally supporting the use of natural products in psychosis especially because of the high antioxidant content of these natural products, since oxidative stress is implicated in psychosis.

4. Secondary metabolites in medicinal plants for psychosis

The discovery of effective plant-based medicinal plants for the treatment of psychosis is constrained by a need to conclusively identify relevant active constituents and understand synergies within them and an inability to sufficiently standardize replicable extracts.

A large number of natural phytochemicals are claimed to have beneficial effects on the adequate functioning of the human brain [20]. Essentially, metabolites produce effects on human brain function probably due to the connection between plant, mammalian biochemistry and molecular functioning. Principally, as a result of the numerous molecular signaling pathways that are conserved between taxa and their role in the synthesis of secondary metabolite [21]. Secondly the effects might be based on the similarities between the prevalent natural herbivores of plants and the nervous systems of humans. Therefore, the phytochemicals whose synthesis has been retained by a process of natural selection and on the basis of their ability to interact with the CNS of herbivorous or symbiotic insects will also interact with the human CNS system via the same mechanisms [22]. Some of the significance of secondary metabolites involve general protective roles (such as antioxidant, ultra violet (UV) light-absorbing, free radical-scavenging and antiproliferative agents) and preservation the plant against microorganisms such as bacteria, fungi, and viruses. More intricate actions involve dictating or modifying the plant's relationship with more complex organisms [23–25]. This is achieved primarily by their role of feeding deterrence, consequently, many phytochemicals are bitter and/or toxic to potential herbivores, with this toxicity often extending to direct interactions with the herbivore's central and peripheral nervous systems [26] identified extracts and constituents from 85 individual medicinal plants that have potential efficacy for treating psychiatric disorder. Accordingly, secondary metabolites often act as agonists or antagonists of neurotransmitter systems [25, 27] or form structural analogs of endogenous hormones [28].

Secondary metabolites can be subdivided into many distinct groups base on their chemical structure and synthetic pathways, furthermore, these groups can be broadly categorized in terms of the nature of their ecological roles and also their eventual effects and comparative toxicity in the consuming animal. The phytochemicals are herewith, discussed base on the chemical nature of their alleged active components. The largest and most widespread of phytochemical groups are the alkaloids, phenolic compounds and terpenes.

4.1 Alkaloids

Alkaloids are a structurally diverse group of over 12,000 cyclic nitrogen-containing compounds that are found in over 20% of plant species [29]. The use of alkaloids for medicinal purposes dates as far back as the Stone Age [20].

The alkaloids are known to be the common poisons, neurotoxins, and traditional psychedelics for example atropine, scopolamine, and hyoscyamine, from *Atropa Belladonna* plant and social drugs such as ephedrine, nicotine, opiates, cocaine, and caffeine widely consumed for recreational purposes [30]. Despite their posoinous nature, this group of chemicals also found application in the treatment of Alzheimer's Disease, because of their cholinesterase inhibiting effects e.g. riverstigmine, huperzine, physostigmine, and huperzine [31].

Gentianine is a major alkaloid extracted from *Swertia chirata* Linn (Gentianaceae), it was reported to possess antipsychotic activity in experimental animals by antagonizing amphetamine induced stereotypy [32]. 11-demethoxyreserpiline, 10- demethoxyreserpiline, α-yohimbine and reserpiline are alkaloids isolated from the leaves of *Rauwolfia tetraphylla* and are found to possess atypical antipsychotic-like actions [33]. alstonine an indole alkaloid isolated from *Picralima nitida* Alstonine was found to possess antipsychotic properties [34, 35].

4.2 Phenolic compounds

Phenolic compounds are universally found across the plant kingdom, with approximately 10,000 structures identified to date. Phenolics are synthesized from precursors produced by the phenylpropanoid pathway with the exception of a few notable compounds. Structurally, they share at least one aromatic hydrocarbon ring with one or more hydroxyl groups attached [22].

Phenolic compounds comprise of simple low-molecular weight compounds, such as the coumarins, simple phenylpropanoids, and benzoic acid derivatives, to more complex structures such as flavanoids, tannins and stilbenes [22]. These compounds play an important role in CNS functioning by interacting directly with neurotransmitter systems. In in vivo models, phenolics enhance cognition through antagonistic gamma-aminobutyric acid (GABA) receptor binding, with resultant cholinergic upregulation and exert antidepressant effects via monoamine oxidase inhibition in the brain, sedative, anxiolytic and antipsychotic effects by binding to GABA receptors, [36–38]. Flavonoids are widely distributed throughout the plant kingdom. They are constituents of medicinal plants used as herbal medicines in traditional medical practice, and are now considered valuable therapeutic agents in modern medicines [39, 40]. Many studies have reported that flavones modulate neurotransmission through enhancement of GABA activity in the central nervous system; which led to the hypothesis that they could exert tranquilizing effects in behavioral hyperactivity such as schizophrenia [41, 42]. Undeniably, a number of evidences have implicated the role of altered GABAergic transmission in the pathophysiology of schizophrenia [43, 44]. Morin a flavonoid isolated from plants was found to exhibit antipsychotic effects [45].

4.2.1 Tannins

Tannins are a group of plant secondary metabolites that have the ability to tan or convert animal skin into leather. These compounds are classified as being water soluble phenolics with the ability to precipitate alkaloids, gelatins, and other proteins. High tannin concentrations are found in nearly every part of many plants, such as in the bark, wood, leaves, fruit, roots, plant galls, and seed. Tannins may exert their biological effects in two different ways: as unabsorbables, these are usually complex structures with binding properties which may produce local effects in the gastrointestinal tract (antioxidant, radical scavenging, antimicrobial, antiviral, antimutagenic, and antinutrient effects), or as absorbable, these are usually low molecular weight structures which are easily absorbed, and produce systemic effects in various organs [46]. Gallic acid, a gallotanin found in many plants was reported to demonstrate anti-schizophrenic activity primarily due to its antioxidant and anti-inflammatory effects [47]. A novel tannin composition effective in treating mental diseases such as acute or chronic schizophrenia, was isolated from Rhubarb (Rhe; Rhi zoma) a kind of crude drug known from the past and has been frequently used as a Japanese-Chinese medicine [48].

4.2.2 Saponins

Saponins are naturally occurring, but functionally and structurally diverse phytochemicals that are broadly distributed in plants. They are a complex and chemically varied group of compounds consisting of triterpenoid or steroidal glycones linked to oligosaccharide moieties. Although there is a scarce documentation on the antipsychotic potential of saponin, polygalasaponins, a saponin isolated from *Polygalae tenuifolia* was reported to possessed antipsychotic effects [49].

4.3 Terpenes

Terpenes are a diverse group of more than 30,000 lipid-soluble compounds. Their structure includes 1 or more 5-carbon isoprene units, Terpenoids are classified base on the number of isoprene units they contain; isoprene, which itself is synthesized and released by plants, comprises 1 unit and is classified as a hemiterpene;

monoterpenes incorporate 2 isoprene units, sesquiterpenes incorporate 3 units, diterpenes comprise 4 units, sesterpenes include 5 units, triterpenes incorporate 6 units, and tetraterpenes 8 units [22]. Some of the recognized antipsychotic terpenoids are myrcene, beta-caryophyllene and limonene. However, these terpenoids do not only have antipsychotic properties but possess anti-depressant effects due to the suppression and activation of the cannabinoid receptor 2 [20].

5. Review of medicinal plants for psychosis

Many medicinal plants are in use both in developed and developing countries for the treatment of psychosis, some of these plants have been studied for their antipsychotic properties whereas most of these plants have no scientific backings for their efficacy. Literature search of the PUBMED and Sciencedirect journals have documented a number of plants studied for their antipsychotic properties in laboratory animals, however, most of the studies carried out are preliminary, and the need for further studies to isolate the active constituents, determine the mechanism of action and conduct clinical trials to verify their efficacy and safety is necessary. **Table 1** gave a list of some of the reviewed antipsychotic plants, their constituents and probable mechanism of action.

6. Efficacy of natural plants in the treatment of psychosis

Many medicinal plants studied for psychosis were found to have efficacy against the positive, negative and cognitive deficit of schizophrenia in laboratory animals, without the disturbing adverse effects seen with conventional antipsychotic drugs. Even those that are thought to act on the dopamine receptors had minimal or no cataleptic tendencies. The tendency for these plants to ameliorate the negative symptoms in schizophrenia, and in some cases also improve psychotic symptoms, may be owing to the ability of most plants to generally exert anti-inflammatory effects [71] and given that inflammation is a risk factor in most neuropsychiatric disorders including schizophrenia [72]. Oxidative stress is also a major factor in psychosis, plants contain diverse constituents which exhibit antioxidant, and neuroprotective effects useful in ameliorating psychotic symptoms [67].

Large number of schizophrenic patients fail to respond adequately to the initial antipsychotic drug treatment necessitating the addition of natural antipsychotic plants to their treatment regimen. As recently reviewed by Hoenders et al. [73] the inclusion of traditional medicine or Ayurvedic herbs to antipsychotics, generally improve the psychopathology of the disease, however, more studies are needed to conclusively support this finding.

7. Molecular mechanisms of antipsychotic action of medicinal plants

Many medicinal plants have been studied for their antipsychotic properties and several mechanisms of action have been proposed for their actions. A number of these plants were believed to act in a similar manner as orthodox medicines but in most cases without the disturbing adverse effects. **Table 1** gave a summary of the probable antipsychotic mechanism of action of the medicinal plants. Various animal models are used to investigate the antipsychotic properties of medicinal plants, some of these models help to determine whether these plants have typical or atypical antipsychotic like effects.

Plant name	Parts used	Constituents and effects	Probable mechanism of action	Author
Albizia zygia (DC.) J.F. Macbr. (Leguminosae)	Roots	The root extract of *Albizia zygia* is used to manage mental disorders in African traditional medicine. Some of the phytochemical constituents are flavonoids, alkaloids, tannins and saponins. The extract exhibited an antipsychotic-like activity in mice with potential to alleviate positive, negative and cognitive symptoms of schizophrenia.	The possible mechanism of action of *Albizia zygia* may be related to enhancement of N-methyl-D-aspartate (NMDA) receptors located on inhibitory GABAergic neurons.	Kumbol, et al. [50]
Alpinia zerumbet	Leaves	The essential oil was extracted from the leaves of *Alpinia zerumbet,* the major constituents are 1,8-cineole and terpinen4-ol which may be responsible for the antipsychotic effects observed from the plant.	The possible mechanism of action might be due to antioxidant effects as well as enhancing NMDA neurotransmission.	de Araújoa et al. [10]
Alstonia scholaris Linn. R.Br. (Apocynaceae)	Leaves	*Alstonia scholaris* is used widely in the treatment of anxiety, depression and other mental illnesses. The plant was found to possess antipsychotic effects.	Mechanism of action may be attributed to dopamine antagonism in the frontal cortical regions of the brain.	Jash & Chowdary. [15]
Bacopa monniera (Linn.) (Scrophularia-ceae)	Whole plant	Triterpenoid, saponins, and bacosides are considered to be the major constituents in the plant. *Bacopa monniera* has been reported to possess antipsychotic, anxiolytic and other medicinal properties.	The antipsychotic properties may be related to its normalization of dopamine and serotonergic neurotransmission and reduction of acetylcholinesterase activity.	Chatterjee et al. [9]
Brassica Oleracea Var. sabellica (Brassicaceae)	Leaf Juice	*Brassica oleracea* possess excellent phytoconstituents such as flavonoids and polyphenols and is widely used as dietary supplements. It has antioxidant and anti-inflammatory properties, and was found to possess antipsychotic properties.	*Brassica oleracea* increase GABA levels resulting in the control of dopaminergic neurotransmission which may be its possible mechanism of action.	Yadav et al. [51]
Cannabis sativa Linn. (Cannabaceae)	Leaves	Cannabidiol one of the major constituent of *Cannabis sativa* leaves possesses atypical antipsychotic-like properties in humans and laboratory animals.	The possible mechanism of *C. sativa* may be due to enhancement of NMDA receptors located on inhibitory GABAergic neurons in the limbic and subcortical brain regions.	Zuardi et al. [52]

Plant name	Parts used	Constituents and effects	Probable mechanism of action	Author
Crassocephalum bauchiense (Hutch.) Milne-Redh (Asteraceae)	Leaves	*Crassocephalum bauchiense* is a medicinal herb effective in the cases of cerebral deficit, anxiety, epilepsy, cerebral malaria, neuropathic pain, and behavioral disturbances in mentally retarded children. The plant contains alkaloid that was found to possess promising antipsychotic properties.	The antipsychotic properties are possibly mediated via the GABAergic neurotransmission as well as blockade of dopamine D-2 receptors	Taıwe et al. [53]
Crinum Giganteum (Amarylli-daceae)	Bulb	alkaloids, saponins and tannins were found to be some of the major constituents of *Crinum giganteum*, the plant is used traditionally for various medicinal purposes including psychiatric illnesses. The extract of *C. giganteum* was found to possess antipsychotic effects in laboratory animals	The possible mechanism of action of Crinum giganteum may be limited to dopamine D_1 antagonism.	Amos et al. [54]
Desmodium adscendens (Sw.) DC (Fabaceae)	Whole plant	The major constituent in *Desmodium adscendens* is alkaloid, it is a medicinal herb with several uses including psychosis. The extract was found to possess antipsychotic effects against apomorphine induced climbing and stereotypic behavior.	The possible mechanism of action may be due to dopamine receptor antagonism	Amoateng et al. [13]
Embelia ribes Burm.f (Myrsinaceae)	Ber-ries	Embelin was isolated from Embelia ribes and found to be responsible for the antipsychotic effect of the plant. Embelin reversed apomorphine induced stereotypic behavior, confirming its antipsychotic potential.	Embelin action may be due dopamine antagonism and decreased level of neurotransmitters such as dopamine, serotonin and noradrenaline as well as antioxidant effects.	Durg et al. [55]
Guiera senegalensis J. F. Gmel (Combretacea)	*Stem bark*	*Guiera senegalensis* is rich in tannin and known to possess varying medicinal effects. The extracts attenuated amphetamine-induced stereotyped behavior in mice suggesting that the plant possess antipsychotic properties that can be useful as a safe alternative.	The effect of the extract amphetamine-induced stereotyped behavior in mice suggest anti-dopaminergic actions on the limbic system	Amos et al. [56]

Plant name	Parts used	Constituents and effects	Probable mechanism of action	Author
Lonchocarpus cyanescens (Schumach and Thonn.) Benth. (Fabaceae)	Leaves	*Lonchocarpus cyanescens* is reputed for its used in traditional medicine for the treatment of Psychosis. Studies have shown that *Lonchocarpus cyanescens* contains various active principles such as quercetin, kaempferol, loncocarpin, and rhamnetin which may be responsible for its antipsychotic activity. *Lonchocarpus cyanescens* was found to possess antipsychotic properties.	The probable mechanism of action of *Lonchocarpus cyanescens* might be due to antidopaminergic effects.	Arowona et al. [57]
Maytenus obtufisolia Mart. (Celastraceae)	Roots	Triterpenes has been identified in *Maytenus obtufisolia,* it is known that terpenes have pharmacological actions on animal behavior. Findings revealed the antipsychotic effects of *M. obtufisolia*	The probable mechanism of action of *Maytenus obtufisolia* might be via a central dopaminergic action	de Sousa & de Almeida. [58]
Morinda citrifolia Linn (Rubiaceae)	Fruits	scopoletin, rutin and quercetin are the major constituents of *Morinda citrifolia*. The plant has so many Uses for CNS disorders. The fruit juice was found to possess antipsychotic properties.	The probable mechanism of antipsychotic effect of *M. citrifolia* extract is attributed to antidopaminergic activity.	Pandy et al. [59]
Nauclea laltifolia Smith (Rubiaceae)	Root bark	Saponins are present in abundance in the extract and might contribute in part for the observed CNS effects. The extract demonstrated antipsychotic effects by attenuating apomorphine induced stereotypic behavior	The effect of the extract against apomorphine is suggestive of possible interference with central dopaminergic neurotransmission.	Amos et al. [60]
Newbouldia laevis Seem. (Bignoniaceae)	Stem bark	*Newbouldia laevis* is a medicinal plant used in the treatment of various ailments. The plant contains alkaloids and saponins which might be responsible for its neuroleptic effects. The extract of *N. laevis* was found to possess antipsychotic effects.	The probable mechanism of action might be due to dopamine D_1 and D_2 antagonism.	Amos, et al. [61]

Plant name	Parts used	Constituents and effects	Probable mechanism of action	Author
Ocimum sanctum (Lamiaceae)	Leaves	*Ocimum sanctum* have been reported for their pharmacological actions including anti-oxidant, anti-stress, and anticonvulsant. The plant contains flavonoids, essential oil, Caffeic acid and vitamins. *Ocimum sanctum* leaves possesses anti-psychotic like property.	The Probable mechanism of action include antioxidant action and enhancement of NMDA neurotransmission as well as neuroprotection.	Sharma et al. [62]
Panax quinquefolium Linn (Araliaceae)	Leaves	The plant's major compound is ginseng which is known to possess numerous pharmacological effects. *Panax quinquefolium* extract was effective against negative and cognitive dysfunctions induced by ketamine	The antipsychotic properties may be related to its normalization of dopamine and serotonergic neurotransmission and reduction of acetylcholinesterase activity.	Chatterjee et al [14]
Picralima nitida Stampf Th. et H.Dur. (Apocynaceae)	Fruits	alstonine an indole alkaloid isolated from *Picralima nitida* a plant commonly used by traditional psychiatrist as part of the treatment of psychosis. Alstonine was found to possess antipsychotic properties experimental profile comparable with that of clozapine and is compatible with the alleged effects in mental patients.	Alstonine indirectly modulates DA receptors, specifically by modulating DA uptake, it also decreases glutamate uptake in acute hippocampal slices. Alstonine also increases serotonergic transmission and increases intraneuronal dopamine catabolism.	Linck et al. [34, 35]
Piper guineense Schum & Thonn (Piperaceae)	Fruits	*Piper guineense* is a medicinal plant used in the Southern States of Nigeria to treat fever, mental disorders and febrile convulsions. β-sesquiphellandren is an essential oil isolated from the plant and was found to possess antipsychotic effects.	The antipsychotic activity may be mediated through augmentation of GABA at the GABAA–benzodiazepine receptor complex pathway, or inhibition of dopamine neurotransmission at dopamine D1/D2 receptors	Oyemitan et al. [63]
Polygala tenuifolia Willdenow (Polygalaceae)	Roots	*Polygala tenuifolia Willdenow* has been prescribed for hundreds of years to treat psychotic illnesses in Korean traditional medicine. Studies have found polygasaponin to be the major constituent responsible for its antipsychotic effect.	polygalasaponin molecular mechanism of action is dopamine (D_2) and serotonin ($5HT_2$) receptor antagonism	Chung et al. [49]

Plant name	Parts used	Constituents and effects	Probable mechanism of action	Author
Rauwolfia tetraphylla L. (Syn. *R. canescens/R. heterophylla/ R. hirsuta*; (Apocynaceae)	Leaves	11-demethoxyreserpiline, 10- demethoxyreserpiline, α-yohimbine and reserpiline are alkaloids isolated from the leaves of *Rauwolfia tetraphylla* and are found to possess atypical antipsychotic-like actions	The mechanism of action of the plant is due to the blockade of dopamine (D_2) and serotonin ($5HT_2$) receptor.	Gupta et al. [33]
Rhodiola rosea Linn. (Crassulaceae)		The extracts of *R. rosea* are used in traditional medicine for various conditions related to nervous system function. Studies has shown that the extract has beneficial antipsychotic properties.	The probable antipsychotic mechanism of *R. rosea* is due to reversal of prepulse inhibition deficits in laboratory rodents.	Coors et al. [64]
Saururus cernuus Linn. (Sauru-ruraceae)		*Saururus cernuus* has been used in folk medicine as a sedative and to treat other illnesses. Manassantin A. a neolignoid isolated from *Saururus cernuus* was found to demonstrate neuroleptic activity	The antipsychotic effect of *Saururus cernuus* may be due to weak antagonism of dopamine receptors.	Rao et al. [65]
Securinega virosa (Roxb ex. Willd) Baill.	Root Bark	Securinega virosa has been described as "cure all" in Africa traditional medicine because of its use widely in the treatment of many illnesses. The plant contains saponins, flavonoids, alkaloids and tannins, and was found to possess antipsycotic activity	The probable mechanism of action may be due to dopamine D_1 and D_2 antagonism.	Magaji et al. [66]
Spinacia oleracea Linn Chenopo-diaceae	Seeds	*Spinacia oleracea* is reported to have beneficial effect against several neurodegenerative disorders. Phytoconstituents such as ascorbic acid, apigenin, astragalin, caffeic, lutein, β-carotene, ferulic acid, kampeferol, rutin, querecetin were isolated from the plant. The seed extract of *Spinacia oleracea* showed antipsychotic activity.	*Spinacia oleracea's* protective effect in schizophrenia may be associated with its regulating effect on dopamine, GABA, acetylcholinesterase, glutathione, malondialdehyde levels	Yadav [67]
Spondias mombin Linn. (Anacar-diaceae)	Leaves	*Spondias mombin* is a medicinal plant widely use in the treatment of various ailments including mental illness. The extract contains tannins, flavonoids and saponins as its major constituents. *S. mombin* possess typical antipsychotic-like effects.	The antipsychotic mechanism of *S. mombin* may be due to dopaminergic receptor antagonism.	Ayoka et al. [68]

Plant name	Parts used	Constituents and effects	Probable mechanism of action	Author
Swertia chirata Linn Gentianaceae)	Leaves	Gentianine is a major alkaloid isolated from *Swertia chirata* and was found to possess antipsychotic properties by antagonizing amphetamine induced stereotypy.	It probable mechanism of action might be due to dopamine antagonism.	Bhattacharya et al. [32]
Synedrella nodiflora (Linn.) Gaertn (family Asteraceae)		The extract of the whole plant has demonstrated anticonvulsant, sedative, in vitro antioxidant and free radical scavenging properties as well as antinociceptive properties in acute and neuropathic pain. *Synedrella nodiflora* also possess antipsychotic properties.	The probably mechanism of the antipsychotic properties of *Synedrella nodiflora* might be due to central dopamine receptor antagonism.	Amoateng et al. [69]
Terminalia macroptera Guill. & Perr. (Combreta-ceae)	Leaves and roots	The plant contains Flavonoids, saponins and tannins in abundance which may be responsible in part for the observed activities. *T. macroptera* has been used traditionally for the treatment of hallucinations, and has also being found to possess antipsychotic properties in the ketamine-induced psychosis model.	*T. macroptera* possible mechanism of action may be due to enhancement of NMDA receptors located on inhibitory GABAergic neurons in the limbic and subcortical brain regions and also its antioxidant properties.	Ior et al. [12]
Viscum album Linn. (Lorantha-ceae)		*Viscum album* is claimed in traditional medical practice, to be useful in the treatment of psychosis and insomnia. Some of the major constituents of the extract are flavonoids and tannins. *V. album* was found to possess antipsychotic properties.	The mechanism of action of *Viscum album* maybe due to dopamine antagonism.	Guptaa et al. [70]

Table 1.
Some medicinal plants, their constituents, effects and probable mechanisms of action.

Dopaminergic deregulation, hypofunction of NMDA receptors and GABAergic activity, diminished cholinergic firing, neuroinflammation and increased oxidative stress has been demonstrated to play a pathophysiological role in schizophrenia [67].

The dopamine and amphetamine animal models are basically used to study the typical antipsychotic effects of drugs, their action are similar to the conventional antipsychotics such as haloperidol, chlorpromazine, fluphenazine and thioridazine. The stereotypic behavior observed in animals following the administration of apomorphine a dopaminergic agonist, are attributed to stimulation of D_1 and D_2 receptors [74, 75]. Mesolimbic and nigrostriatal dopaminergic pathways play key roles in the mediation of locomotor activity and stereotyped behavior. Animal models used for assessing antipsychotic drugs are established on the neurochemical hypothesis of schizophrenia, which involve largely the neurotransmitters dopamine and glutamate [76]. The antagonism of dopamine D_2 receptors in the mesolimbic-mesocortical system is thought to be the basis of the therapeutic actions of the antipsychotic drugs, especially those active against hallucinations and delusions [77]. The dopamine-based models usually employ apomorphine, a direct agonist, or amphetamine, a drug that increases the release of this neurotransmitter and blocks its re-uptake.

The term atypical refers to the reduced propensity of the of an agent to cause undesirable motor side effects, but it is also used to describe agents with a different pharmacological profile from the typical antipsychotics; several of these newer antipsychotics improve the negative as well as the positive symptoms [78]. The atypical antipsychotics are categorized base on their pharmacological properties. These include serotonin–dopamine antagonists, multi-acting receptor- Targeted antipsychotics, and dopamine partial agonists. [79]. Examples include clozapine, quetiapine, risperidone, amisulpride, sertindole, zotepine and aripiprazole. The dopamine dysregulation with hyperfunction of the mesolimbic dopamine system was the original tenet theory underlying the basis of schizophrenia [80] and the earliest animal models were established on the basis of pharmacological manipulation in an endeavor to simulate this feature [81], which respond to agents that affect primarily the dopaminergic system, but does not demonstrate the negative or cognitive symptoms seen in schizophrenia [82]. In contrast, a widely used animal model of schizophrenia involves the acute or repeated administration of subanesthetic doses of ketamine [83]. In rodents, N-methyl-Daspartic acid receptor (NMDAR) blockade induces hyperactivity, stereotypy, deficits in prepulse inhibition [84], social interaction and memory (Becker and Grecksch [85]), which models the positive, negative and cognitive symptoms of schizophrenia, respectively [9]. Furthermore, studies have revealed that reactive oxygen species have a significant role in the pathogenesis of many illnesses, particularly neurological and psychiatric illnesses. [86] Oxidative stress may be a common pathogenic mechanism underlying many major psychiatric disorders as the brain is relatively susceptible to oxidative damage [87]. Previous study confirmed that oxidative stress damage occurs in patients with schizophrenia and one possible therapeutic solution is to use antioxidants [88]. Reports from some of the medicinal plants studied that delineate some of the animal models used and their molecular mechanism of action are highlighted.

7.1 *Morinda citrifolia* Linn (Rubiaceae)

Morinda citrifolia (noni) is an evergreen tree that grows in open coastline areas at sea level and in forest regions. Four doses (1, 3, 5, 10 g/kg) of the fruit extract of noni were administered prior to apomorphine/ amphetamine administration and observed for climbing behavior and stereotypy. The extract significantly decreased the apomorphine-induced cage climbing behavior and climbing time in mice in a dose dependent manner. Demonstrating the antidopaminergic effect of the plant. The plant was found to be rich in rutin and scopoletin which might have played a role in the antipsychotic mechanism [60].

7.2 *Securinega virosa* (Roxb ex. Willd) Baill

Securinega virosa is a medicinal plant commonly used in Africa in the management of epilepsy and other mental illnesses. The antipsychotic prospect of the residual aqueous fraction of the plant was assessed by means of the apomorphine induced stereotypic climbing behavior model and the swim induced grooming model, all in mice. The effect of the fraction on haloperidol-induced catalepsy was also assessed. The fraction inhibited the grooming behavior and attenuated the climbing behavior of the mice. These action of *S. virosa* extract was associated to its involvement with the dopamine D1 receptor. Therefore, the study confirmed the antipsychotic potential of *S. virosa* in traditional medicine [66]. The observed effects were ascribed to the presence of alkaloid, saponin, flavonoid and tannin in the leaves.

7.3 *Picralima nitida* Stampf Th. et H. Dur.

Picralima nitida is the only species of the genus Picralima and it is related to Hunteria and Pleiocarpa. it belongs to the apocynaceae family. *P. nitida* has widely varied applications in West Africa folk medicine. The indole alkaloid alstonine was identified as the major component of the fruit rind of *P. nitida*, a plant-based treatment administered to psychotic patients in Nigeria [34]. Alstonine was given prior to apomorphine/ amphetamine administration and observed for climbing behavior and stereotypy, the effect of the alkaloid on haloperidol-induced catalepsy was also assessed [89]. Further studies of alstonine showed a clear antipsychotic profile in rodents, closer to atypical than to typical antipsychotics. Apparently, apomorphine induced stereotypy and amphetamine-induced lethality were significantly reduced by alstonine, suggesting a decrease in mesolimbic dopamine, alstonine reversed haloperidol-induced catalepsy, indicating that nigrostriatal dopamine transmission is not lessened [89]. Alstonine was found to reduce negative symptoms, through a mechanism involving $5HT2_{A,C}$ receptors, and reverses interaction deficits induced by MK801 [90]. Further studies by Linck et al. [35] indicated that alstonine indirectly modified DA receptors, precisely by modifying DA uptake. This unique mechanism for DA transmission modulation backs the antipsychotic-like effects of alstonine and is attuned with its behavioral profile in mice and apparent effects in patients. These findings may signify an innovation in the antipsychotic development field [35].

7.4 *Panax quinquefolium* Linn

Panax quinquefolium is a native plant of North America, but is now cultivated widely and used in many countries. The plant contains dammarane type ginsenosides as the major biologically active constituents particularly Rb1, Rd. and Re ginsenoside saponins [91] which are responsible for most of its bioactive properties. A graded dose study with *P. quinquefolium* revealed differential effects against the ketamine induced hyperactivity in the Digiscan animal activity monitor, and blocked ketamine induced memory impairment in the passive avoidance paradigm. In the chronic studies, *P. quinquefolium* attenuated the ketamine-enhanced immobility in the forced swim test and did not produce extra-pyramidal side effects in bar test and wood block test of catalepsy. These behavioral effects were compared with standard drugs haloperidol and clozapine. *P. quinquefolium* was also found to reduced DA and 5-HT content after prolonged treatment. Furthermore, *P. quinquefolium* extract reduced acetylcholinesterase activity and nitrate levels, conversely it increased glutamate levels in hippocampus. Ultimately, the study revealed that *P. quinquefolium* possess antipsychotic like properties, which may be beneficial in predominant negative and cognitive symptoms of schizophrenia [9].

7.5 *Spinacia oleracea* Linn

Spinacia oleracea commonly known as spinach is endowed with a number of medicinal properties [92]. Ethnopharmacological studies proposed that *Spinacia oleracea* seeds have promising antioxidant, neuroprotective, anti-epileptic, anti-alzheimer and anti-inflammatory effects [93–95]. The study evaluated the protective effects of *Spinacia oleracea* seed extract in an experimental model of ketamine-induced schizophrenia in mice. Ketamine was used to induce stereotyped psychotic symptoms in mice. Behavioral studies (locomotor activity, stereotypy, immobility duration and memory retention) were carried out followed by biochemical, neurochemical and cellular alterations in the brain. Chronic treatment with *Spinacia oleracea* seed extract significantly attenuated stereotyped behavioral symptoms in mice. Biochemical estimations revealed that the extract reduced lipid peroxidation and restored total brain proteins. Likewise, *Spinacia oleracea* remarkably reduced dopamine levels, acetylcholinesterase activity & inflammatory surge serum tumor necrosis factor (TNF-α) and increased the levels of GABA and reduced glutathione in mice. The results of the study indicated that the extract could ameliorate ketamine-induced psychotic symptoms in mice, signifying a protective effect in the treatment of schizophrenia. Moreover, its protective effect in schizophrenia may be associated with its regulating effect on dopamine, GABA, acetylcholinesterase enzymes, glutathione and malondialdehyde levels [67].

7.6 *Terminalia macroptera* Linn

Terminalia macroptera Guill. & Perr. (Combretaceae) is a medicinal plant used commonly in Africa. Ethnomedicinal report from Mali mentions the decoction of leaves of *T. macroptera* in treatment of epilepsy [96], and anxiolytic effects of *T. macroptera* has also been reported by [97]. The study was carried out to investigate the antipsychotic effects of *T. macroptera* in an experimental model of ketamine-induced psychosis in mice. Ketamine and apomorphine were used to induce stereotyped psychotic behavioral symptoms in mice. Behavioral studies (stereotype behavior, locomotor activity, immobility duration and memory retention) were carried out to investigate the protective effect of the ethyl acetate fraction of *T. macroptera* on ketamine-induced psychotic symptoms, repeated treatment with the ethyl acetate fraction for 7 consecutive days significantly attenuated stereotyped behavioral symptoms, immobility duration and memory deficit in mice. The study revealed that *T. macroptera* could ameliorate psychotic symptoms indicating protective effects in psychosis. Agent that ameliorate ketamine induced psychotic symptoms are generally thought to act in a similar manner as atypical antipsychotics [12].

7.7 *Crassocephalum bauchiense* (Hutch.) Milne-Redh

Crassocephalum bauchiense is a medicinal plant with diverse medicinal uses. The leaves decoction of *C. bauchiense* is effective in the treatment of epilepsy, cerebral malaria, cerebral deficit, anxiety and behavioral disturbances in mentally retarded children. Likewise, an aqueous extract of the whole plant is useful in the treatment of insomnia, psychosis and other central nervous system disorders, [98, 99]. The antipsychotic effects of *C. bauchiense* extracts were evaluated using the apomorphine animal model of psychosis. The ability of the leaves extracts of *C. bauchiense* to modify the duration of akinesia was observed in the catalepsy test. Furthermore, gamma-aminobutyric acid concentrations in the brain of treated mice were also estimated. The aqueous extract and the alkaloid fraction of *C. bauchiense* attenuated the apomorphine-induced stereotypy and fighting, and had significant fall of the body temperature. In biochemical experiments, the concentration of the inhibitory amino acid, gamma-aminobutyric acid, was significantly increased in the brain of animals treated with the aqueous extract of *C. bauchiense*. The results revealed that the antipsychotic and sedative properties of *C. bauchiense* are possibly mediated via the blockade of dopamine D-2 receptors and GABAergic activation [54].

7.8 *Alpinia zerumbet* (Pers.) Burtt. et Smith

Alpinia zerumbet has important physiological and pharmacological functions, such as antioxidative [100], anticancer [101], anti-inflammatory [102], and anti-anxiety [103]. In phytotherapy, *A. zerumbet* is used to treat neuropsychiatric symptoms such as depression, stress and anxiety, but it is only recently that the central nervous system (CNS) effects of the essential oil from the plant leaves have been studied [10]. The essential oil of *A. zerumbet* (50, 100 and 200 mg/kg i.p.) was administered once to mice to evaluate antipsychotic activity assessed by ketamine-induced hyperlocomotion, hypnotic activity induced by sodium pentobarbital, antioxidant effects (determination of lipid peroxidation and GSH levels), as well as variations in nitric oxide levels (determination of nitrite content). The result revealed that the extract at doses of 100 and 200 mg/kg prevented ketamine hyperlocomotion, and at a dose of 200 mg/kg decreased sleep latency, while all doses increased sleeping time. The in-vitro antioxidant capacity of the oil caused a reduction in lipid peroxidation and increase in glutathione levels. The extract also prevented the decrease in nitrite content caused by oxidative stress. The findings indicate antipsychotic and antioxidant effects of the essential oil of *A. zerumbet* that may have promising efficacy for the treatment of schizophrenia [10].

7.9 *Albizia zygia* (DC.) J.F. Macbr. (Leguminosae)

Albizia zygia is one such plant with numerous medicinal uses. A decoction of the roots is used for the treatment of insanity [104]. Several compounds including two novel oleanane-type saponins, zygiaosides A and B, were lately isolated from the roots of *A. zygia* [105].

A. zygia effects were assessed against apomorphine-induced cage climbing, ketamine induced hyperlocomotion, −enhanced immobility, −impaired social interaction as well as novel object recognition. The propensity of the extract to induce catalepsy and to attenuate haloperidol-induced catalepsy were also investigated. Findings revealed that *A. zygia* extract significantly attenuated apomorphine-induced climbing behavior as well as ketamine-induced hyperlocomotion, immobility and object recognition deficits. Furthermore, the extract had no cataleptic effect. The root extract of *A. zygia* therefore exhibited antipsychotic-like activity in mice with potential to alleviate positive, negative and cognitive symptoms of schizophrenia [51].

8. Conclusions

Plants have been the mainstay for the treatment of diseases all over the world before the development of conventional medicines. The interest in the therapeutic uses of plants have been revived due to obvious reasons such as their safety, availability, and affordability as well as their efficacy. Research on medicinal plant have provided evidences for their use, and further studies in order to isolate the active constituents and also to test them in clinical studies is important for the development of new pharmacotherapies for psychosis.

Acknowledgements

The authors acknowledge all sources, and are grateful to the authors/editors of all the articles, journals, and books from where the literature for this article has been reviewed.

Conflict of interest

The authors declare no conflict of interest.

Author details

Sunday Oritsetimenyin Otimenyin and Lydia Doosuur Ior*
University of Jos, Jos, Nigeria

*Address all correspondence to: lidyshal@gmail.com

References

[1] Bhugra D (2005) The global prevalence of schizophrenia. PLoS Med 2:e151 quiz e175

[2] Reus VI. Mental disorders. In: Fauci AS, Braunwald E, Kasper DL, Hauser SL, Longo DL, Jameson JL, Loscalzo J, editors. Harrison's principles of internal medicine. McGraw-Hill, New York. 2008.

[3] Lieberman JA. Effectiveness of antipsychotic drugs in patients with chronic Schizophrenia. N Engl J Med 2005;353 Suppl 12: S1209-S1217.

[4] Harvey PD, Green MF, Keefe RS, Velligan DI. Cognitive functioning in schizophrenia: a consensus statement on its role in the definition and evaluation of effective treatments for the illness. J Clin Psychiatry. 2004; 65:361–372

[5] Kumari R, Chatterjee M, Singh S. Oxidative stress: A novel treatment target in psychiatric disorder. Int J Pharm Sci Rev Res. 2011; 9:165–172

[6] Meltzer H. Antipsychotic agents and lithium. In: Katzung BG, Masters SB, Trevor AJ, editors. Basic and clinical pharmacology. McGraw-Hill Companies, New York. 2010.

[7] Meyer JM. Pharmacotherapy of psychosis and mania. In: Brunton L, Chabner B, Knollman B (eds) Goodman and Gilman's The pharmacological basis of therapeutics. McGraw-Hill, New York. 2011.

[8] Newcomer JW. (2005). Second-generation (atypical) antipsychotics and metabolic effects: A comprehensive literature review. CNS Drugs 19: 1–93.

[9] Chatterjee M, Singh S, Kumari R, Verma KA, Palit G. Evaluation of the Antipsychotic Potential of Panax quinquefolium in Ketamine Induced Experimental Psychosis Model in Mice. Neurochemical Research. 2012;37: 759-770.

[10] de Araújoa F, de Oliveira G, Gomes P, Soares M, Silva M, Carvalho A, Macêdo D. Inhibition of ketamine-induced hyperlocomotion in mice by the essential oil of Alpinia zerumbet: possible involvement of an antioxidant effect. Journal of Pharmacy and Pharmacology. 2011;63:1103-1110.

[11] Arowona IT, Sonibare MA, Umukoro S. Antipsychotic property of solvent-partitioned fractions of Lonchocarpus cyanescens leaf extract in mice. J Basic Clin Physiol Pharmacol. 2014;25(2):235–240.

[12] Ior LD, Otimenyin SO, Okwuasaba FK. Antipsychotic-like effect of ethyl acetate fraction of Terminalia macroptera leaf in mice. IBRO Neurosci. Reports. 2021; 10, 10: 83-89.

[13] Amoateng P, Adjei S, Osei-Safo D, Kukuia KK, Karikari TK, Nyarko AK. An ethanolic extract of Desmodium adscendens exhibits antipsychotic-like activity in mice Amoateng P, Adjei S, Osei-Safo D, Kukuia KK, Karikari TK, Nyarko AK. An ethanolic extract of Desmodium adscendens exhibits antipsychotic-like activity in mice. J Basic Clin Physiol Pharmacol. 2017;1-12.

[14] Chatterjee M, Verma R, Kumari R, Singh S, Verma A, Palit G. Antipsychotic activity of standardized Bacopa extract against ketamine-induced experimental psychosis in mice: Evidence for the involvement of dopaminergic, serotonergic, and cholinergic systems. Pharmaceutical Biology. 2015;1-11.

[15] Jash R, Chowdary kA. Ethanolic extracts of Alstonia Scholaris and Bacopa Monniera possess neuroleptic activity due to anti-dopaminergic effect. Phcog. Res. 2014;6(1):46-51.

[16] Zimmerman RA. Thomspon IM Jr. Prevalence of complementary medicine in urologic practice. A review of recent studies with emphasis on use among prostate cancer patients. Urology Clinics of North America. 29, 1-9.

[17] Werneke U, Turner T, Priebe S. Complementary medicines in psychiatry, Review of effectiveness and safety. British Journal of Psychiatry. 2006;188:109-121.

[18] Skalicka-Woz'niaka K, Gertsch J. Antipsychotic natural products. Annual reports in medicinal chemistry. 2020;1-35.

[19] Aucoin M, LaChance L, Cooley K, Kidd S. Functional food for the management of of Autism Spectrum Disorders and SchizophreniaNeuropsychobiology. 2018; 25:1–23.

[20] Ajao AA, Alimii AA, Olatunji OA, Balogun FO, Saheed SA: A synopsis of anti- psychotic medicinal plants in Nigeria. Trans Royal Soc. S.A. 2017;1-9.

[21] Schultz JC. Shared signals and the potential for phylogenetic espionage between plants and animals. Integr Comp Biol. 2002; 42:454–462.

[22] Kennedy D, Whiteman E. Herbal Extracts and Phytochemicals: Plant Secondary Metabolites and the Enhancement of Human Brain Function. American Society for Nutrition. Adv. Nutr. 2011;2:32–50.

[23] Gershenzon J. The cost of plant chemical defense against herbivory: a biochemical perspective. In: Bernays EA, editor. Insect-plant interactions. Boca Raton (FL): CRC Press; 1994. p. 105–173.

[24] Tahara S. A journey of twenty-five years through the ecological biochemistry of flavonoids. Biosci Biotechnol Biochem. 2007; 71: 1387–1404.

[25] Wink M. Evolution of secondary metabolites from an ecological and molecular phylogenetic perspective. Phytochemistry. 2003; 64:3–19.12. Rattan RS. Mechanism of action of insecticidal secondary metabolites of plant origin. Crop Prot. 2010; 29:913–920

[26] Zhang ZJ. Therapeutic effects of herbal extracts and constituents in animal models of psychiatric disorders. Life Sci. 2004; 75:1659–1699.

[27] Wink M. Interference of alkaloids with neuroreceptors and ion channels. Stud Nat Prod Chem. 2000; 21:3–122

[28] Miller AE, Heyland A. Endocrine interactions between plants and animals: Implications of exogenous hormone sources for the evolution of hormone signaling. Gen Comp Endocrinol. 2010; 166:455–461

[29] Zulak K, Liscombe D, Ashihara H, Facchini P. Alkaloids. Plant secondary metabolism in diet and human health. Oxford: Blackwell Publishing; 2006. p. 102–136.

[30] Zenk MH, Juenger M. Evolution and current status of the phytochemistry of nitrogenous compounds. Phytochemistry. 2007; 68:2757–2772.

[31] Mukherjee PK, Kumar V, Mal M, Houghton PJ. Acetylcholinesterase inhibitors from plants. Phytomedicine. 2007; 14:289–300

[32] Bhattacharya SK, Ghosal S, Chaudhuri RK, Singh AK, Sharma P: (1974). Chemical Constituents of Gentianaceae XI: Antipsychotic Activity of Gentianine. J. Pharm. Sci. 1974;63(8): 1341-1342.

[33] Gupta S, Khanna V, Maurya A, Bawankule D, Shukla R, Pal A, Srivastava SK. Bioactivity guided isolation of antipsychotic constituents from the leaves of Rauwolfia tetraphylla L. Fitoterapia. 2012;83:1092–1099.

[34] Linck VM, Herrmann AP, Piato AL, Detanico BC, Figueiró M, Flório J, Iwu MM, Okunji CO, Leal MB, Elisabetsky E. Alstonine as an antipsychotic: Effects on brain amines and metabolic changes. Evid. Based Complement. Alternat. Med. 2011;1–7.

[35] Linck VM, Ganzella M, Herrmanna AP, Okunji OC, Souza DO, Elisabetskya E. Original mechanisms of antipsychotic action by the indole alkaloid alstonine (Picralima nitida). Phytomedicine. 2015;22:52–55.

[36] Dhawan K, Dhawan S, Sharma A. Passiflora: a review update. J of Ethnopharmacol. 2004; 94:1–23.

[37] Kim DH, Jeon SJ, Son KH, Jung JW, Lee S, Yoon BH, Lee JJ, Cho YW, Cheong, JH. The ameliorating effect of oroxylin A on scopolamine-induced memory impairment in mice. Neurobiology of Learning and Memory. 2007; 87:536–546.

[38] Xu Y, Wang Z, You W, Zhang X, Li S, Barish P, Vernon M, Du X, Li G. Antidepressant-like effect of trans-resveratrol: involvement of se- rotonin and noradrenaline system. European Journal of Neuropsychopharmacology. 2010; 20:405–413.

[39] Havsteen BH. The biochemistry and medical significance of the flavonoids. Pharmacol Ther 2002; 96: 67–202

[40] Fang SH, Hou YC, Chang WC. "Morin sulfates/glucuronides exert anti-inflammatory activity on activated macrophages and decreased the incidence of septic shock". Life Sci 2003; 74: 743–756

[41] Marder M, Paladini AC. GABA-A receptor ligands of flavonoid structure. Curr Top Med Chem 2002; 2: 853–867

[42] Wang F, Shing M, Huen Y. Neuroactive flavonoids interacting with GABAA receptor complex. Curr. Drug Targets CNS Neurol. Disord 2005; 4: 575–585

[43] Benes FM, Vincent SL, Alsterberg G. Increased GABAA receptor binding in superficial layers of cingulate cortex in schizophrenics. J Neurosci 1992;12: 924–929

[44] Lewis DA, Pierri JN, Volk DW et al. Altered GABA neurotransmission and prefrontal cortical dysfunction in schizophrenia. Biol Psychiatry 1999; 46: 616–626

[45] Ben-Azu BA, Omogbiya IA, Ajayi AM, Iwalewa EO: Morin Pretreatment Attenuates Schizophrenia-Like Behaviors in. Drug Res 2017; 6: 1-9.

[46] Sieniawska E, Baj T. Tannins. In Plant Metabolites: Their Chemistry. Elsevier. 2017;199-232.

[47] Yadav M, Jindal DK, Dhingra M, Kumar A, Parle M, Dhingra S. Protective effect of gallic acid in experimental model of ketamine-induced psychosis: possible behaviour, biochemical, neurochemical and cellular alterations. Inflammopharmacol.2018; 26:413-424.

[48] Nishioka I, Nonaka G, Fujiwara M, Ueki S: Novel tannin composition - Google Patents. 1985. Available fromhttps://patents.google.com/patent/WO1986005180A1/en [accessed:2021/July/2021].

[49] Chunga I, Moore NA, Ohc W, O'Neillb MF, Ahn J, Park J, Kime YS. Behavioural pharmacology of polygalasaponins indicates potential antipsychotic efficacy. Pharmacology, Biochem Behav. 2002;71:191-195.

[50] Kumbol VW, Abotsi WK, Ekuadzi E, Wood E. Albizia zygia root extract exhibits antipsychotic-like properties in murine models of schizophrenia. Biomedicine & Pharmacotherapy. 2018;106:831–841.

[51] Yadav M, Parle M, Dhingra MS. Protective effect of Brassica oleracea juice against Ketamine-induced stereotypic behaviours in mice. Journal of Medicinal Plants Studies. 2017;5(1): 200-204.

[52] Zuardi A, Crippa J, Hallak J, Moreira F, Guimarães F. Cannabidiol, a Cannabis sativa constituent, as an antipsychotic drug. Cannabidiol as an antipsychotic drug Brazilian Journal of Medical and Biological Research. 2006; 39:421-429.

[53] Taıwe GS, Bum EN, Talla E, Dawe A, Moto FC, Ngoupaye G, De Waard M. Antipsychotic and sedative effects of the leaf extract of Crassocephalum bauchiense (Hutch.) Milne-Redh (Asteraceae) in rodents. Journal of Ethnopharmacology. 2012; 143:213–220.

[54] Amos S, Binda L, Akah P, Wambebe C, Gamaniel K. Central inhibitory activity of the aqueous extract of Crinum giganteum. Fitoterapia. 2003;74:23-28.

[55] Durg S, Kumar N, Vandal R, Dhadde SB, Thippeswamy BS, Badami S. Antipsychotic activity of embelin isolated from Embelia ribes: A preliminary study. Biomedicine & Pharmacotherapy. 2017;90:328–331.

[56] Amos S, Binda L, Vongtau HC, Abbah J, Sambo N, Odim E, Gamaniel, K. Sedative effefcts of the methanolic extract of Newbouldia laevis in mice and rats. Bollettino Chimico Farmaceutico. 2002; 471-475.

[57] Arowona IT, Sonibare MA, Umukoro S. Antipsychotic property of solvent-partitioned fractions of Lonchocarpus cyanescens leaf extract in mice. J Basic Clin Physiol Pharmacol. 2014;25(2):235–240.

[58] de Sousa D, de Almeida RN. Neuroleptic-Like Properties of the Chloroform Extract of Maytenus obtusifolia MART. Roots. Biol. Pharm. Bull. 2005;224-225.

[59] Pandy V, Narasingam M, Mohamed Z. Antipsychotic-like activity of Noni (Morinda citrifolia Linn.) in mice. BMC Complementary and Alternative Medicine. 2012;12:186-194.

[60] Amos S, Abbah J, Chindo B, Edmonda I, Binda L, Adzu B, Buhari S, Odutola AA, Wambebea C Gamaniel K; Neuropharmacological effects of the aqueous extract of Nauclea latifolia root bark in rats and mice. JEP. 2005: 53–57.

[61] AMOS S, Binda L, Vongtau HC, Abbah J, Sambo N, Odim E, Gamaniel K. Sedative effefcts of the methanolic extract of Newbouldia laevis in mice and rats. Bollettino Chimico Farmaceutico. 2002;471-475.

[62] Sharma K, Parle M, Yadav M. Evaluation of antipsychotic effect of methanolic extract of Ocimum sanctum leaves on laboratory animals. Journal of Applied Pharmaceutical Science. 2016;6: 171-177.

[63] Oyemitan IA, Olayera OA, Alabi A, Abass L, Elusiyan CA, Oyedeji AO, Akanmu MA. Psychoneuropharmacological activities and chemical composition of essential oil of fresh fruits of Piper guineense (Piperaceae) in mice. Journal of Ethnopharmacology, 2015;0378-8741.

[64] Coors A, Brosch M, Kahl E, Khalil R, Michel B, Laub A, Fend M. Rhodiola rosea root extract has antipsychotic-like effects in rodent models of sensorimotor gating. Journal of Ethnopharmacology. 2019;235:320–328.

[65] Rao KV, Puri VN, EI-Sawaf HA. Further studies on the neuroleptic profile of manassantin A. European Journal of Pharrnacology. 1990;179: 367-376.

[66] Magaji MG, Mohammed M, Magaji RA, Musa AM-A, Hussaini IM. Evaluation of the antipsychotic potential of aqueous fraction of Securinega virosa root bark extract in mice. *Metabolic Brain Disease*. 2014.

[67] Yadav M, Parle M, Sharma N, Jindal DK, Bhidhasra A, Dhingra MS, Dhingra S. Protective effects of Spinacia oleracea seeds extract in an experimental model of schizophrenia: Possible behavior, biochemical, neurochemical and cellular alterations. Biomedicine & Pharmacotherapy. 2018; 105:1015–1025.

[68] Ayoka A, aAkomolafe RO, Iwalewa E, Akanmu M, Ukponmwan O. Sedative, antiepileptic and antipsychotic effects of Spondias mombin L. (Anacardiaceae) in mice and rats. Journal of Ethnopharmacology. 2006;103:166-175.

[69] Amoateng PA, Osei-safo D, Kukuia KK, Bekoe EO, Karikari TK, Kombian SB. Extract of Synedrella nodiflora (L) Gaertn exhibits antipsychotic properties in murine models of psychosis. BMC Complementary and Alternative Medicine. 2017;17:389- 40.

[70] Guptaa G, Kazmi I, Afzal M, Rahman M, Saleem S, Ashraf S, Anwar F. Sedative, antiepileptic and antipsychotic effects of Viscum album L. (Loranthaceae) in mice and rats. Journal of Ethnopharmacology. 2012;141:810-816.

[71] Gertsch J. Viveros-Paredes JM. Taylor P; Plant immunostimulants-scientific paradigm or myths. JEP. 2011; 136:385–391

[72] Aricioglu, F.; Ozkartal, C. S.; Unal, G.; Dursun, S.; Cetin, M.; Muller, N. Bull. Clin. Psychopharmacol. 2016, 26, 329–444.

[73] Hoenders, H. J. R.; Bartels-Velthuis, A. A.; Vollbehr, N. K.; Bruggeman, R.; Knegtering, H.; de Jong, J. T. V. M. J. Nerv. Ment. Dis. 2018, 206, 81–101.

[74] Seeman P: Brain dopamine receptor. Pharmacol Rev 1980, 32:229–313.

[75] Stoff JC, Kebabian JW: Two dopamine receptor: biochemistry physiology and pharmacology. Life Sci 1984, 35:2281–2296.

[76] Lipska BK, Weinberger DR: To model a psychiatric disorder in animals: schizophrenia as a reality test. Neuropsychopharmacol 2000, 23:223–239.

[77] Gardner DM, Baldessarini RJ, Waraich P: Modern antipsychotic drugs: a critical overview. Can Med Assoc J 2005, 172:1703–1711.

[78] Remington G. Understanding antipsychotic "atypicality": a clinical and pharmacological moving target. J Psychiatry also necessary in terms of distinguishing between Neurosci 2003; 28: 275-284

[79] Horacek, J., Bubenikova-Valesova, V., Kopecek, M., Palenicek, T., Dockery, C., Mohr, P., & Hoschl, C. (2006). Mechanism of Action of Atypical Antipsychotic Drugs and the Neurobiology of Schizophrenia. In CNS Drugs (pp. 389-409). Czech Republic: Adis Data Information BV.

[80] Murray RM, Lappin J, Di Forti M. Schizophrenia: From developmental deviance to dopamine dysregulation. Eur Neuropsychopharmacol. 2008;18: 129- 134.

[81] Jones PB, Barnes TR, Davies L, Dun G, Lloyd H, Hayhurst KP, Murray RM, Markwick A, Lewis SW. Randomized controlled trial of the effect on quality of life of second- vs first-generation antipsychotic drugs in schizophrenia: Cost Utility of the Latest Antipsychotic Drugs in Schizophrenia Study (CUtLASS 1). Arch Gen Psychiatry. 2006; 63:1079-1087.

[82] Featherstone RE, Rizos Z, Kapur S, letcher PJ. A sensitizing regimen of

amphetamine that disrupts attentional setshifting does not disrupt working or longterm memory. Behav Brain Res. 2008; 189:170

[83] Bubenikova-Valesova V, Horacek J, Vrajova M, Hoschl C. Models of schizophrenia in humans and animals based on inhibition of NMDA receptors. Neurosci Biobehav Rev. 2008; 32: 1014-1023.

[84] Jentsch JD, Roth RH. The neuropsychopharmacology of phencyclidine: From NMDA receptor hypofunction to the dopamine hypothesis of schizophrenia. Neuropsychopharmacology. 1999; 20: 201-225.

[85] Becker A, Grecksch G. Ketamine-induced changes in rat behavior: A possible animal model of schizophrenia. Test of predictive validity. Prog Neuropsychopharmacol Biol Psychiatry. 2004; 28:1267- 1277.

[86] Ng FB, Dean O, Bush A; Oxidative stress in psychiatric disorders: evidence base and therapeutic implications. Int J Neuropsychopharmacol 2008; 11: 851–876.

[87] Yao JK, Reddy RD, van Kammen DP. Oxidative damage and schizophrenia: an overview of the evidence and its therapeutic implications. CNS Drugs 2001; 15: 287–310.

[88] Padurariu M, Ciobica A, Dobrin I, Stefanescu C. Evaluation of antioxidant enzymes activities and lipid peroxidation in schizophrenic patients treated with typical and atypical antipsychotics. Neurosci Lett. 2010. 2; 479(3):317-20.

[89] Costa-Campos L, Elisabetsky E, Lara DR, Carlson TJ, King SR, Ubillas R, Nunes DS, Iwu MM, Nkemjika CO, Ozioko A, Agwu CO. Antipsychotic profile of alstonine: ethnopharmacology of a traditional Nigerian botanical remedy. " Anais da Academia Brasileira de Ci^encias. 1990;71(2):189-201.

[90] de Moura Linck V, Herrmann AP, Goerck GC et al. "The putative antipsychotic alstonine reverses social interaction withdrawal in mice," Progress in Neuropsychopharmacology and Biological Psychiatry. 2008;32(6): 1449–1452.

[91] Zhu S, Zou K, Fushimi H, Cai S, Komatsu K. Comparative study on triterpene saponins of Ginseng drugs. Planta Med. 2004; 70:666–677.

[92] Yadav, M. Parle, M. Kadian, K. Sharma, A review on psychosis and anti-psychotic plants, Asian. J. Pharm. Clin. Res. 8 (2015) 24–28.

[93] Kumar GR, Hypolipidemic activity of *Spinacia oleracea* L. in atherogenic diet induced hyperlipidemic rats, J. Bio. Pharm. Res. 1 (2012) 39–43.

[94] Verma R, Sisodia R, Bhatia AL. Role of Spinacia oleracea as antioxidant: a biochemical study on mice brain after exposure of gamma radiation, Asian. J. Exp. Biol. Sci. 17 (2003) 51–57.

[95] Sultana R, Perluigi M. Butterfield, Protein oxidation and lipid peroxidation in brain of subjects with Alzheimer's disease: insights into mechanism of neurodegeneration from redox proteomics, Antioxid. Redox Signal. 8 (2006) 2021–2037.

[96] Pham, AT, Malterud, K. E., Paulsen, B. S., Diallo, D., & Wangensteen, H. (2011). DPPH Radical Scavenging and Xanthine Oxidase Inhibitory Activity of Terminalia macroptera Leaves. Natural Product Communications, 6(8), 1125 - 1128.

[97] Bum EN, Neteydji S, Djafsia G, Njifutie N, Taiwe GS, Rakotonirina SV, Rakotonirina A; The aqueous extract of *Terminalia macroptera* possess

anxiolytic and antipyretic activities in mice. Asian J. Pharm. Health Sci. 2012; 2,4: 555–561.

[98] Adjanohoun JE, Aboukakar N, Dramane K, Ebot ME, Ekpere JA, Enow-Orock EG, Focho D, Gbile ZO, Kamanyi A, Kamsu KJ, Keita A, Mbenkum T, Mbi CN, Mbiele AL, Mbome IL, Mubiru NK, Nancy WL, Nkongmeneck B, Satabu B, Sofowora A, Tamze V, Wirmum CK. Traditional medicine and pharmacopoeia. Contribution to Ethnobotanical and Floristic Studies in Cameroon. Centre de Production de Manuels Scolaires, Porto-Novo (Rep. Du Benin). 1996; 133

[99] Biholong M, Contribution a l'e ´tude de la flore du Cameroun: les Aste'race'es. These de doctorat. Universite ´ de Bordeaux III, Bordeaux. France. 1986;10–50

[100] Xuan TD, Khanh TD, Khang D, Quan NT, Elzaawely AA. Changes in chemical composition, total phenolics and antioxidant activity of Alpinia (Alpinia zerumbet) leaves exposed to UV. Int Lett Nat Sci. 2016; 55:25–34.

[101] Junior WA, Gomes DB, Zanchet B, Schönell AP, Diel KA, Banzato TP, et al. Antiproliferative effects of pinostrobin and 5,6-dehydrokavain isolated from leaves of Alpinia zerumbet. Rev Bras Farmacogn. 2017;27(5):592–598.

[102] Anuthakoengkun A, Itharat A. Inhibitory effect on nitric oxide production and free radical scavenging activity of Thai medicinal plants in osteoarthritic knee treatment. J Med Assoc Thai. 2014 Aug;97 Suppl 8:S116–S124.

[103] de Sousa DP, de Almeida Soares Hocayen P, Andrade LN, Andreatini R. A systematic review of the anxiolytic-like effects of essential oils in animal models. Molecules. 2015;20(10):18620–18660.

[104] Bouquet A, Debray M. Plantes médicinales de la Côte d'Ivoire. Travaux et Documents de l'orstom No. 32, orstom, Paris, 1974.

[105] Noté OP. Simo L, Mbing JN. Guillaume D, Aouazou SA, Muller CD, Pegnyemb DE, Lobstein A.Two new triterpenoid saponins from the roots of *Albizia zygia* (DC.) JF Macbr, Phytochem. Lett. 18 (2016) 128–135, https://doi. org/10.1016/j. phytol.2016.09.010.

Section 3

Complementary Therapies and Clinical Rehabilitation

Chapter 7

Non-pharmacological Therapies in Integrative Rehabilitation and Physiotherapy

Andrés J. Ursa Herguedas

Abstract

Although pharmacological therapy is a resource to be taken into account in rehabilitation medicine and physiotherapy (RMP), a series of therapies, techniques, and empirical practices have been available since time immemorial, some with scientific publications, which play an important role in healthcare current health worldwide. Some millennials like Traditional Chinese Medicine (TCM) and medicinal plants (MP), and other centenarians like Homeopathic Medicine (HM) and Osteopathic Medicine (OM). In the twentieth century, numerous medical techniques were developed, framed under the term of Biological Medicine in Europe such as Antihomotoxic Medicine (AM), Neural Therapy (NT), Catalytic Oligotherapy (CO). Throughout the twentieth and twenty-first centuries, the wealth of experiences and knowledge on the application of Growth Factors in therapeutics, Oxygen-Ozone Therapy, and other related techniques that have enriched medical practice has increased. The objective of this chapter is to highlight the convenience of incorporating unconventional therapies (UT) techniques with scientific evidence into RMP that enjoy efficacy, efficiency, and economic and environmental sustainability. It would be desirable to allocate more financial resources to continue researching these therapies, implement them in Health Sciences studies and continue working to comply with the maxim of medicine that is "primum non nocere" (first do no harm).

Keywords: rehabilitation medicine, integrative physiotherapy, unconventional therapies, integrative medicine

1. Introduction

RMP, developed from the Hippocratic doctors of the fourth century to C, and technically and scientifically perfected to this day, with its holistic, non-organicist, and multidisciplinary nature, is a continuation of the process of recovery from multiple human conditions, from traumatic to degenerative, at all ages of life. Its mechanism of action, which is becoming better known, is based on the tendency to spontaneous healing that the organism has (Vis medicatrix naturae of the Hippocrats), today explained by the multiple homeostatic mechanisms available to the human economy, some of them collected in **Table 1**.

Rehabilitation medicine, physiotherapy, and the like (speech therapy, occupational therapy, orthopedics, psychology) have been enriched in recent decades by

System/phenomenon	Mechanism	Function
Neuroendocrine regulation	Hypothalamic-pituitary-adrenal/gonadal axis	Growth menstrual cycle birth. lactation, metabolism stress, etc.
Immune system	Natural and adaptive	Defends against hostile external and internal agents
Blood coagulation system	Coagulation cascade (12 factors)	Prevents spontaneous bleeding Wound healing process
Bone regeneration after fracture	Remodeling	Restitutio ad integrum
HLA system	T cells: examine peptides and distinguish whether they are self or foreign	Recognizes peptides and presents them on the surface of antigen-presenting cells (macrophages)
Renin-angiotensin-aldosterone system	Kidney-lung/heart-adrenal	Regulates blood pressure
Thermoregulation	Hypothalamus	Adaptation to the environment
Bicarbonate-carbonic acid system	Breathing	Maintains pH
Kidney function	Nephron	Electrolyte and acid-base balance
Endocrine pancreas	Insulin-glucagon	Glycemic regulation
Food digestion	Digestive secretion	Nutrient absorption
Gut microbiota	Absorption of nutrients, synthesis of vitamins, production of short-chain fatty acids, etc.	Immune, neurotransmitters, etc.
Neuroplasticity	Establishment of neural connections due to the effect of various stimuli	Recovery after brain injuries, cerebrovascular accidents, etc.

Table 1.
Some of the homeostatic systems of the organism (taken from Guyton and Hall's medical physiology, 2016 and completed by A. Ursa) [1].

a series of techniques and methods, with implantation determined according to different countries and public or private practice, such as acupuncture, osteopathy (joint manipulations), neural therapy, different manual techniques (Cyriax, etc.), dry needling, etc., as well as concepts such as Bobath's or methods such as Perfetti's or Therasuit's, the aims being an assistance comprehensive customer service and functional recovery.

Although it is true that physiotherapy has been gaining in attributions in recent years, such as the capacity for diagnosis and treatment, the scheme "the rehabilitating doctor diagnoses and prescribes and the physiotherapist executes" is still valid.

A legal obstacle for physiotherapists is the limitation in their therapeutic actions. Although it varies from country to country, these health professionals are generally denied access to the internal environment to introduce substances with pharmacological activity. As in other professional groups (Odonto-stomatology, podiatry, etc.), they have a limitation in the pharmacological prescription, covering a reduced group of drugs.

A good number of physiotherapists, especially those who work on their own in the private sphere, knowing about drug iatrogenesis, have adopted unconventional therapies (UT), such as phytotherapy, acupuncture, osteopathy, etc., or conventional ones such as diet therapy, in order to facilitate the healing processes.

This chapter deals with UTs that can contribute to a better response in the field of RMP, either by shortening the recovery time, reducing pain, or achieving good functionality, enriching their scope of action. Some of these techniques can be used in physiotherapy.

2. Complementary techniques in rehabilitation medicine and physiotherapy

2.1 Acupuncture

It is one of the techniques used in Traditional Chinese Medicine (TCM). Introduced and disseminated in Europe by Soulié de Morant, French ambassador to China in the nineteenth century [2]. The Canon of this discipline is the Nei King, written in the time of Emperor Huang Ti around the year 2610 BC. This treatise includes the conception of life according to Chinese philosophy, the theory of Yin and Yang (the TAO), etc., which is also applied in therapeutics. In the doctrinal exposition of the Nei King, collected in the treatise called Sou Wen, he talks about the Tch'i (Chi) energy that, circulating through some channels (meridians), would fill all the organs of the body with vital energy. The energy from the breath, the cosmic, and others would be added to this energy. All these approaches lead to the Theory of the Five Elements. At first, they coincided with the four elements of the Hippocratic Tradition (water, fire, earth, and air). Later, during the reign of Emperor Wou (1122–255 BC), a fifth element was added. These five elements would be governed by specific laws forming the Ko cycle [3].

The disease in TCM is an alteration of the energy balance, with physical and/or mental impairment. By means of certain techniques, the therapist must be able to restore the energy balance that results in the restoration of health [3].

Table 2 shows the techniques most used in TCM to restore health, in addition to acupuncture.

Technique	Procedure	Rationale
Moxibustion	Combustion of mugwort (plant) on specific points	Provides heat to stimulate or inhibit
Diet Therapy	Food Yin and Yang	Energy balance
Chinese Materia Medica	Medicinal plants in capsules, tablets, infusion, etc.: minerals, etc.	Specific effects
Digitopuncture	Massage in certain points	Symptomatic relief in acute conditions
Auriculomedicine, manopuncture, etc.	Puncture of the pinna, hand, etc.	Represents the entire organism
Tui Na massage	Stimulation of meridians	Circulation of Chi
Suction cups	A vacuum is created (negative pressure)	Decongests in depth
Chi-kung	Specific movements with a certain speed	Preventive and curative purposes through the mobilization of energy

Table 2.
Techniques most used in TCM (taken from the complete book of Chinese medicine) [4].

Acupuncture is a physical therapy based on the millenary observation that needle puncture in certain areas of the skin lining can lead to the re-establishment of certain conditions. Several mechanisms of action have been proposed, one of the most investigated being the analgesic effect produced by the release of endogenous opioids, already described in the 70s of the twentieth century [5].

In 1979 the World Health Organization (WHO) made public that acupuncture was effective in 49 conditions. With the standardization of the STRICTA criteria for clinical trials with acupuncture, the indications for chronic painful conditions such as headaches, osteoarthritis, low back pain, etc., were reduced [6].

Acupuncture, as a therapy, has its contraindications and side effects. Because of this, it is recommended that a health professional apply it.

2.2 Homeopathy (homeopathic medicine)

Although Homeopathic Medicine (HM) is in low hours, it has been used from the nineteenth century to the present day.

The law of similarity on which homeopathy is based appears already in the Hippocratic writings. In the Renaissance, Paracelsus made his observations on the minimum doses, but it was necessary to arrive at its implementation with the German physician Samuel Hahnemann (1755–1843). Disappointed by the medicine of the time based on bloodletting and other ineffective and highly iatrogenic procedures, he abandoned the medical practice. To continue caring for his large family, he had 11 children, since he was fluent in several languages, he dedicated himself to translating medical books into other languages. In translating a book by Cullen, he called her attention to a procedure that he tried on himself and on his family with good results. Encouraged by the successes, he developed and perfected the homeopathic method. He compiled his observations in a treatise the organon of the art of healing that saw its first edition in 1810. He made numerous disciples and spread homeopathy to the rest of Europe, America, and other countries [7].

The procedure for obtaining the homeopathic remedy follows a series of steps until the desired dilution is obtained. Its mechanism of action is still unknown. Due to this, in recent years a smear campaign has been orchestrated qualifying homeopathy as pseudoscience.

The truth is that homeopathy is still used throughout the world, its results are acceptable – although the demands have been made in clinical trials – it does not produce iatrogenesis, its cost is affordable, and its environmental impact is acceptable.

Homeopathy should continue to be investigated with its own method since as it does not consist of weight doses such as pharmacology, and is individualized treatment, the scientific method for its validation is not always valid.

Possibly the day will come when science and technology have advanced and the mechanism of action of this therapy can be unraveled. When requiring a clinical diagnosis, the prescription of the homeopathic remedy should be exclusive to the doctor. This is not the case in the vast majority of cases, and this could be the reason for the smear campaign.

2.3 Osteopathy (osteopathic medicine)

The term Osteopathic medicine (OM) of osteo (bone) and ducks (disease) is not a graceful name to name this preventive and therapeutic method, with its own diagnostic techniques. Its main field of application is the joints. OM was developed in the United States (USA), its pioneer being the physician Andrew Taylor Still (1828–1917), who stated its principles [8].

Still claimed that human diseases originate from problems of the musculoskeletal system, and that manual manipulation could solve these problems by taking advantage of the body's self-healing potential [8]. Like many other empiricists, he developed this method after his wife and daughters died of meningitis. The remedies of the time were not enough to save their lives.

OM can be considered as an integral medicine that cares for the person in all its dimensions, unlike allopathy that fragments the organism into patches. It enhances or favors the body's self-healing processes (the vis medicatrix naturae of the Hippocrats) in order to restore homeostasis [8].

OM is based on the knowledge of the anatomy and physiology of tissues and organs, biomechanics, as well as the functional/dysfunctional interrelation between the different tissues. In the diagnosis and treatment, it uses conventional processes and others specific to the method [8]. The WHO and the European Union, the latter with the European standard on Osteopathy (UNE-EN 16689) defined the academic, professional, scientific, and ethical parameters years ago [8].

The OM is widely disseminated throughout the world. There are countries with official studies (USA, England, France, Belgium, Portugal, etc.). Regarding the professional figure, there are countries that are taught exclusively to doctors, such as Russia. In Italy, they train doctors and physiotherapists respectively in OM. In Spain and Latin America, there are OM schools where physiotherapists are taught above all [8]. In Australia, the United Kingdom, and New Zealand, non-medical osteopaths are regulated by law. In Canada and Germany, both doctors and non-doctors can practice OM, with the corresponding authorizations. In Spain, the order of the Ministry of Science and Innovation CIN/2135/2008, of July 3, established the requirements for the verification of official university degrees that would qualify for the exercise of the profession of physiotherapist and established osteopathy as a subject of the Degree in Physiotherapy. Several Spanish universities offer postgraduate courses in Osteopathy.

The most prominent OM types are listed in **Table 3.**

The indications for OM, therefore, are broad and focus on the treatment of spinal pain and diseases, visceral dysfunctions (hiatal hernia, gastroesophageal reflux, intestinal transit disorders, etc.), and cranial dysfunctions (neuralgia, migraines, dizziness, etc.) [8].

Despite the criticism of OM for its scientific evidence, more and more quality publications are being made.

OM meets the appropriate conditions to integrate it into the health systems in the near future since it is decisive in musculoskeletal and joint diseases, often without pharmacological intervention, and may contribute to the reduction of health costs. It does not require large facilities and is environmentally sustainable.

Good training, whether medical or non-medical, would be desirable, as it has indications, contraindications, and the possibility of side effects.

	Place of actions	Aims/objectives
Structural	l Focuses on the spine	Restore the musculoskeletal, articular, and postural systems
Cranial	Nervous system (through the mobility of the cranial sutures)	Action on cerebrospinal fluid and circulation
Visceral	Organs and viscera	Through improved blood flow, obtain a benefit in the organ/viscera

Table 3.
Types of O/MO (taken from the book osteopathy based on evidence).

2.4 Phytotherapy

The word comes from the Greek – phytós (plant or vegetable) and therapeia (therapy). It is the part of the therapy that uses products of plant origin (medicinal plants) for the prevention, cure, or relief of certain human conditions.

The WHO defines phytotherapy as the science in charge of studying plant products for their subsequent use in the therapy of pathological states [9]. It refers, above all, to the empirical use of medicinal plants (MP), with a long tradition in all cultures. Phytomedicine, however, involves a transformation of MP into drugs or phytopharmaceuticals, after clinical trials in order to guarantee the quality, safety, and efficacy [10].

The medicinal use of plants dates back to the mists of time. Used in all great civilizations to restore health, the contributions of Ancient Egypt, Greece, and Classical Rome stand out. There were no great advances in the Middle Ages until the Renaissance, where Paracelsus discovered that the properties of MP lie in the active principles [11].

WHO recommends to health authorities that each country include medicinal plants in health systems and especially in primary health care [9].

In some countries of the European Union, phytotherapy is applied mainly by doctors, although its use is very extensive, and the legislation does not hinder anyone who wants to use it. In the United States, only licensed physicians are allowed. In general, training on phytotherapy is provided in all countries, although their degree of officiality varies: some have specialties for doctors or postgraduate programs at the university, as in Germany, Italy, or Spain. In other countries, training is carried out by non-university entities such as Sweden or Canada [11].

WHO recognizes the importance of medicinal plants in the treatment and prevention of multiple diseases [9].

In general, health professionals qualified as primary and specialized care physicians have little knowledge on this subject and, at times, it is a reason for discord with patients, since many MPs cause interactions with commonly prescribed drugs. Phytotherapy is a resource to consider for multiple reasons: MP is found in nature, it is easy to prepare, etc. If we want to obtain better results, we have to go to Phytomedicine which, with standardized preparations, backed by clinical studies, guarantees quality, safety, and efficacy.

2.5 Neural therapy

The brothers Ferdinand and Walter Huneke, German doctors, in 1928 made known to the world of medicine the existence of "unknown distant effects of local anesthetics." Surprising results had been achieved since 1923 by applying procaine to certain areas (scars, etc.). Ferdinand Huneke observed in 1940 the so-called phenomenon in seconds. By applying a procaine injection in the area of periostitis in the context of chronic osteomyelitis in a lower limb, he managed to cure in a few seconds a persistent and painful disease in the shoulders that had been treated without success with the so-called segment therapy. With this fact, he deduced that the states of nervous irritation, called interference fields (IF), located outside the metamere can cause and maintain different diseases. By applying procaine, these IFs and pathologies that are reluctant to conventional therapies can be eliminated [12].

The purpose of Neural Therapy (NT) is to facilitate the self-healing mechanisms of the diseased organism through stimuli in specific points/areas that act on the autonomic or vegetative nervous system (VNS) [12].

The scientific bases of NT have their beginnings in the investigations of Pavlov and Speransky. Later the contributions of Ricker, Pischinger, and Virchow [12] were decisive.

To understand the neural therapeutic effect, it is necessary to take into account the concept of the basic system (BS), described by Pischinger, which is the carrier of non-specific defense functions. Its regulatory system is located in the extracellular space and behaves as a functional unit. The whole organism is connected through this BS and this also connects with the cells of the parenchyma. In chronic diseases, there is a dysfunction of the BS.

BS consists of undifferentiated soft connective tissue cells (reticulocytes or fibroblasts), extracellular tissue fluid, capillaries, and nerve terminal vegetative fiber plexuses [12].

The levels of integration of VNS, with feedback systems, explain many of the effects of NT. **Table 4** lists these levels of integration.

Although in NT chemical substances such as procaine or lidocaine are used, in very low concentrations, I wanted to introduce this therapy in this chapter since there are many advantages it offers to restore health as long as it is applied by an experienced therapist.

The "irritations" in the nervous system can be produced by infections, surgical interventions, scars, fractures, dental problems, mental trauma, eating disorders, etc. These events can generate the conditions for the appearance of certain conditions that can manifest locally or remotely, depending on the predispositions of each person. The goal of NT is to neutralize these irritations that affect VNS and cause health problems. To neutralize these irritations, a local anesthetic is used, one of the most common being procaine hydrochloride at a concentration of 0.5 to 1%. This substance is used since it has a high electrical potential. Procaine repolarizes and stabilizes the cell membrane potential (previously altered) thus allowing the recovery and stabilization of VNS. Furthermore, VNS can be acted upon through the cuti-visceral sympathetic reflex. Although there are other neural therapies, procaine offers more advantages due to its vasodilator effect, short half-life, and low toxicity [12].

The improvement achieved with NT can be immediate (phenomenon in seconds), although the most common is the repetition of several sessions until recovery is achieved. Although NT can be used in any condition, the fields in which it is most used are in the musculoskeletal system and in chronic pain. NT has its indications, contraindications, and side effects, so it is advisable to practice it by a health professional (medicine, nursing, odonto-stomatology) with experience in the technique. It can be used in all ages and for any disease. Physiotherapists cannot use NT but it is important for them to know the technique for good coordination within a multidisciplinary

Level	Location	Action/effects
Autonomous periphery	Basic system (Pischinger)	Nonspecific defense
Peripheral-spinal	Reflex segment	Physical (muscle) and psychic (emotions, etc.) levels
Rhombus-mesencephalic	Medulla, protuberance, reticular formation, tectum, etc.	Cardiocirculatory, alertness, muscle tone, etc.
Diencephalic	Thalamus and hypothalamus	Neuro-endocrine coordination
Cortical	Limbic system	Psychic phenomena in somatic pathology

Table 4.
Integration levels of VNS (taken from the book by L. Fischer, neural therapy according to Huneke, 2012).

team. NT is therapy with good results, safe and economically and environmentally sustainable. It would be desirable to include it in the national health system of the different countries in order to obtain rapid results, reduce iatrogenesis and health costs.

2.6 Homotoxicology (antihomotoxic medicine)

According to the International Academy of Homotoxicology (IAH) Antihomotoxic Medicine (AM) is a regulatory therapy devised by the German physician Hans-Heinrich Reckeweg (1905–1985). In 1952, he published the theory of Homotoxicology based on homeopathic medicine. The foundation of this therapy is the fight against homotoxins since they would be the cause of diseases. Reckeweg's goal was to establish a comprehensive perspective of medical science at the time and to establish a bridge between conventional and unconventional medicine [13].

According to Reckeweg, all the processes, syndromes, and manifestations that we know as diseases are the expression of the body's fight against toxins and its intention to neutralize and excrete them. To achieve this end he uses homeopathic products, medicinal plants, organic, and pharmacological products, etc., in various homeopathic dilutions to apply them in the phase in which the disease is found according to the table of six phases [13].

The "biological cut" is the separation between the cell and the extracellular environment [13].

Homotoxicosis would be a pathophysiological state that would originate after the action of a homotoxin on cells and tissues. It would manifest itself in a humoral or cellular way (see table of the six phases) and can be accompanied by morphological changes in the tissues. This state induces defense measures of the organism in order to eliminate homotoxins and restore health. To do this, it acts on the extracellular matrix (basic system) described by Pischinger (as in Neural Therapy according to Huneke). The body, depending on various factors, can achieve this balance by itself. If this is not possible, there are several possibilities for action. If we use the principle of opposites (anti-inflammatory, etc.) there is the possibility of a progressive vicariation (it would evolve to a disease of greater caliber), on the other hand, if we use AM, the advancement of the disease would not occur but the regression (vicariation regressive) [13].

The different components of the antihomotoxic preparations stimulate the body's defense system, through the immune assistance reaction (IAR), this being its main mechanism of action. IAR is based on low-dose antigen reactions (D1 to D14). When administering antihomotoxic products orally, parenterally, sublingually, etc., the nonspecific defense (monocytes/macrophages) acts in interaction with the specific one. In areas of dysregulation, especially where there is inflammation, Th3 cells that secrete cytokines such as the transforming tissue growth factor-beta with broad anti-inflammatory effect are attracted [14].

Antihomotoxic preparations must be prescribed in the phase in which the patient is, so an appropriate anamnesis and examination will be necessary. Sometimes techniques such as autohemotherapy, isotherapeutic (nosodes), etc., are used to achieve the objectives. The combined technique of TA with neural therapy achieves better results and in less time [13].

AM, well applied, has shown its effectiveness in most pathological processes, especially in the area of inflammation. In specialties such as sports medicine, it accelerates the healing of injuries and does not produce doping.

2.7 Catalytic oligotherapy

The concept "trace element (trace element)" was first used in 1885 by Gabriel Bertrand, who later deduced that trace elements were vital to all cells in minute

Number	Diathesis	Behavior	Clinical	Therapeutic
I	Arthritic/allergic	Morning asthenia. Memory impairment. Optimistic	Migraines. Allergy. Heart disease	Mn I/S
II	Hypostenic	Fatigue. Pessimistic	Respiratory, digestive, and skin fragility	Mn-Cu
III	Dystonic	Morning asthenia Difficult to focus. Anxiety	Neuro-vegetative dystonia. Circulatory disorders	Mn-Co
IV	Anergic	Asthenia. Memory disorders Depression	Acute infections Rheumatism	Cu-Au-Ag
	Maladjustment syndrome	Periodic asthenia. Depression	Endocrine dysfunction	Zn-Cu/ Zn-Ni-Co

Table 5.
Diathesis according to Ménétrier (taken from Colonques [17]).

quantities. The use of trace elements for therapeutic purposes (oligo therapy) began in France with the research of Bertrand (nineteenth century) and Jacques Ménétrier in the middle of the twentieth century [15].

Jacques Ménétrier (1908–1986) is considered the founder of functional medicine, of Catalytic Oligotherapy (CO), and one of the main representatives of field medicine, pioneered by the French scientist Claude Bernard [16]. CO activates a trace element present in the body in order to regulate a specific metabolic pathway [17].

Ménétrier classified groups of diseases according to the inherited terrain, their receptivity or resistance to certain diseases according to their physical and mental behaviors, and defined a series of "terrains" that he called "diathesis." With his practice, he demonstrated the relationship of a specific diathesis with one or more trace elements that, in case of disease, its administration achieved improvement/recovery, acting on the metabolic pathways of said terrain. **Table 5** shows the Ménétrier diathesis, behavior, symptoms, and regulatory trace elements [17].

According to Ménétrier, functional diseases present very different and vague clinical pictures, with imprecise signs, compared to classic diseases. They do not present lesions in radiology, nor alterations in clinical analysis. He affirmed that "most diseases do not belong to the sector of true and proper pathology, but they do belong to functional diseases, which are simple dysfunctions of the organism and that, if they are not corrected at this stage, lead to specific diseases [18].

CO, as it can be used for preventive or curative purposes. The highly diluted and ionized preparations are administered. Among the different routes of administration, the sublingual is one of the most widely used. The dosage is the same for all ages. It can be associated with drugs with very few incompatibilities and with most complementary therapies (acupuncture, Phytotherapy, etc.). The European Medicines Agency, in a review a few years ago, left some diathesics treatments for CO out of hand by removing some trace elements for being supposedly "toxic".

3. Prevention in integrative rehabilitation and physiotherapy (IRP)

A task little known by users of health systems but insisted ad nauseam by IRP professionals is the preventive aspect. Users, in general, go to IRP services in case of injury and most are unaware of the preventive aspect of IRP in both athletes and non-athletes. On the other hand, the WHO has issued a document in 2017 (Rehabilitation 2030) in which it warns of the need for IRP in the world and that due to the lack of these professionals, the inhabitants of less developed countries will be left unprotected. This will lead, posteriori, to higher healthcare costs since illnesses and/or injuries have not been detected, assessed, and treated which, if they had done so, would have contributed to reducing morbidity and mortality. In developed countries, the services offered by IRP are not sufficiently valued for various reasons. It is not uncommon for a stroke to be included in an IRP program late, due to service saturation or other reasons, obtaining worse functional recovery.

According to the WHO, greater access to rehabilitation services is required to "ensure healthy lives and promote well-being for all at all ages". This coincides with point 3 of the Sustainable Development Goals (SDG) and specifically SDG 3.8: "Achieve universal health coverage, including protection from financial risks, access to quality basic medical services and access to safe, effective, quality and affordable basic medicines and vaccines..." [19].

The role of rehabilitation is essential for the effective implementation of the Global Strategy and Plan of Action on Aging and Health (2016–2020) [20], the Plan of Action on Mental Health (2013–2020) [21], and the Framework on people-centered integrated health services, and as a contribution to the WHO [22].

4. Conclusions

There are approximately one billion people with disabilities on the planet, most of whom lack access to medical care and RMP services. Because of this, these people have more problems achieving and maintaining an adequate level of autonomy and health. The deficit of RMP services hinders inclusion and participation in all aspects of life, leading to misery and poverty.

The processes and procedures employed in RMP are intended to allow people with disabilities to achieve and maintain an optimal level of physical, sensory, intellectual, psychological, social, and spiritual performance. RMP encompasses a wide range of therapeutic possibilities, some with scientific evidence and others with less scientific evidence, but widely used by the world population and with wide acceptance. The WHO has been recommending for decades that all available therapeutic resources should be used and that research is continued for their validation [23].

Persons with disabilities should have access to general medical care and adequate RMP services.

The Convention on the Rights of Persons with Disabilities states that countries must ensure that persons with disabilities have access to appropriate health services, including general health care and RF services, and do not suffer discrimination in the provision of health services. WHO actively supports the application of the Convention, having ratified it in successive meetings with representatives of member countries.

Conflict of interest

There is no conflict of interest.

Abbreviations

RMP	Rehabilitation medicine and physiotherapy
UT	Unconventional Therapies
TCM	Traditional Chinese Medicine

USA	United States of America
WHO	World Health Organization
MP	Medicinal plants
OM	Osteopathic Medicine
AM	Antihomotoxic medicine
IAH	International Academy for Homotoxicology
IAR	Immune assist reaction
NT	Neural Therapy
IF	Interference field
BS	Basic system (Pischinger)
VNS	Vegetative nervous system
CO	Catalytic Oligotherapy
IRP	Integrative Rehabilitation and Physiotherapy
SDG	Sustainable Development Goals

Author details

Andrés J. Ursa Herguedas[1,2,3]

1 Teaching officer (health area) Junta de Castilla y León, Spain

2 Illustrius Academy of Health Sciences Dr. Ramón y Cajal, Madrid, Spain

3 Institute of Integrative Medicine, Valladolid, Spain

*Address all correspondence to: ajursa@educa.jcyl.es

References

[1] Guyton y Hall. Treaty of Medical Physiology. 13th ed. Amsterdam, Netherlands: Elsevier; 2016

[2] Soulié de Morant G. Compendium of true Chinese acupuncture. Madrid: Alhambra S.A.; 1984

[3] Álvarez-Simó E. Acupuncture Treaty. Volumes I and II. 2nd ed. Madrid: PAR; 1983

[4] Wong Kiew Kit. The Complete Book of Chinese Medicine. Barcelona: Urano; 2003

[5] Han JS. Acupuncture: Neuropeptide release produced by electrical stimulation of different frequencies. Trends in Neurosciences. 2003;**26**(1):17-22. DOI: 10.1016/s0166-2236(02) 00006-1

[6] Muñoz-Ortego J et al. Medical indications for acupuncture: Systematic review. Clinical Medicine. 2016;**147**(6): 250-256. DOI: 10.1016/j.medcli.2016. 02.029

[7] Mure C, Giordan A, Raichvarg D. The Origins of Homeopathy. Madrid: Boiron; 2010

[8] Ricard F, y Oliva Pascual, A. Evidence-Based Osteopathy. 1nd ed. Madrid: Medos Edition S.L; 2017

[9] World Health Organization. Strategy on Traditional Medicine. Geneva: World Health Organization; 2014-2023

[10] Vanaclocha B, Cañigueral S. Phytotherapy, Prescription Formulary. 5th ed. Barcelona: Elsevier; 2019

[11] Marcia Abello L, Isabel Cisternas F. Phytotherapy, its origins, characteristics and situation in Chile. Revista Medica de Chile. 2010;**138**:1288-1293. DOI: 10.4067/ S0034-98872010001100014

[12] Fischer L. Neural Therapy According to Huneke. México; 2012. ISBN: 03 2001 03011 2555 200 01

[13] Academy for Homotoxicology. Introdution to Homotoxicology. International Academy for Homotoxicology. London (UK), 2017. www.bioregmed.com /bhomf.org

[14] Heine H. Neurogenic Inflammation as the Basis of Chronic Pain. Relationships with Antihomotoxin Therapy. Lecture 31. Baden-Baden (Germany): Med Woche; 1997

[15] Ramirez J et al. Proposal for a new classification of trace elements for their application in nutrition, oligotherapy and other therapeutic strategies. Hospital Nutrition. 2015;**31**(3):1020-1033. DOI: 10.3305/nh.2015.31.3.8325

[16] Torti A. Principles of Oligotherapy Trace elements as catalysts and functional medicine. Natura Medicatrix. Medical Journal for the Study and Dissemination of Alternative Medicines. 2000;**58**:18-25

[17] Douart JP. Oligotherapy in functional pathology. París: Maloine Editions; 1994. ISBN: 2 229 02324-3

[18] Picard H. Therapeutic Use of Trace Elements. Málaga (Spain): Sirio Publishing House; 2000. ISBN: 978 8486221126

[19] United Nations. A/RES/70/1. Transforming Our World: The 2030 Agenda for Sustainable Development. New York: United Nations; 2015

[20] WHO. Global Strategy and Plan of Action on aging and health 2016-2020: Towards a World in Which All People Can Live a Long and Healthy Life. A69/A/CONF./8. Agenda item 13.4; 2016

[21] WHO. Plan of Action on Mental Health 2013-2020. Geneva: WHO; 2013

[22] WHO. Disability and rehabilitation. WHO Global Action. Plan 2014-2021. Geneva, 2015

[23] WHO. Strategy on Traditional Medicine 2014-2023. Geneva: WHO; 2013

Chapter 8

An Introduction to Chiropractic BioPhysics® (CBP®) Technique: A Full Spine Rehabilitation Approach to Reducing Spine Deformities

Deed E. Harrison and Paul A. Oakley

Abstract

Chiropractic Biophysics® (CBP®) technique is a full-spine and posture correcting method that incorporates mathematical principles into a unique approach to treat spinal disorders. It considers that the identification of postural rotations and translations of human postures are first evaluated and compared to the radiographic assessment of the spine alignment. Mirror image® postural positions and movements are utilized including spinal extension positions to improve the spine and posture towards a normal/ideal alignment. Specifically, corrective exercises, corrective traction and chiropractic adjustments are performed encompassing a multimodal rehabilitation program with the goal of improving the posture and spine alignment. CBP Rehabilitation programs are typically performed in-office with supportive at-home measures. Repeat assessment including radiographs are used to quantify and monitor structural improvements. CBP technique is an evidence-based approach to treat spine deformities and is supported by all forms of clinical evidence including systematic literature reviews, randomized controlled trials, non-randomized controlled trials, case reports/series as well as is supported by biomechanical posture-spine coupling validity, radiographic and posture analysis reliability/repeatability and use of a validated biomechanical spinal model as the outcome goal of care. CBP technique is a proven method to improve pain, disability and quality of life in those with structural deformities.

Keywords: spine deformity, structural rehabilitation, traction, exercise, chiropractic

1. Introduction

Chiropractic Biophysics® (CBP®) technique is a full-spine and posture correcting method that incorporates engineering and mathematical principles into a unique approach in the treatment of spine disorders [1–5]. CBP technique is best described as a 'structural' rehabilitation approach as opposed to 'functional' rehabilitation that typically encompasses physiotherapeutic modalities, stretching and exercises to regain function. The goal in structural rehabilitation is to restore the spine alignment and posture to as near normal as possible.

CBP operates on three main premises: 1. There is a normal/ideal static spinal configuration; 2. Abnormal alterations of the spine/posture result in abnormal function disrupting homeostatic balance; 3. Altered static spine/postural alignment results in abnormal dynamics [1]. The contemporary spine literature supports all three of these premises (See Section 4). CBP technique has published research on many facets of the technique including defining what normal/ideal spine alignment is, how to measure spine alignment parameters with reliable and repeatable methods, how to correct/re-align spinal displacements, and evidence proving correcting spine and postural displacements correlates with improvements in pain, disability and quality of life (QOL) measures (These studies are detailed later).

Herein, an overview is given of the scientific approach to treating spine disorders (i.e. subluxation) by the unique approach of CBP technique. A review will be given of the historical beginnings of CBP, rotations and translations of posture, the Harrison normal spinal model, radiographic analysis, posture and spinal coupling, the CBP protocol, clinical evidence of efficacy as well as the safety of the use of X-rays (The term 'X-rays' imply the use of plain radiographs throughout this chapter).

2. Historical beginnings

Donald D. Harrison, who had a Master's degree in Mechanical Engineering and a Doctorate degree in Applied Mathematics developed a devote urgency to bring contemporary science to chiropractic. In the late 1970s, Harrison was the main instructor for the chiropractic technique named 'Pettibon.' Dissatisfied with the failure to produce spinal correction, he often incorporated his own methods in certain cases to better attain spine and posture improvements. It was in the treatment of one particular case (circa 1980) where he discovered that the body must be treated using the principles of mathematics; the term 'mirror image®' adjusting he later coined to describe these new approaches [1].

A 1974 paper by Panjabi et al. describes a Cartesian coordinate system for use in the description and study of joint biomechanics (**Figure 1**) [6]. Harrison was the first to apply this system of analysis to upright human posture (**Figures 2** and **3**). Harrison began discovering the rotations and translations of human posture in 1980. During the early 1980s, the analysis system evolved to incorporate a full spine analysis of the

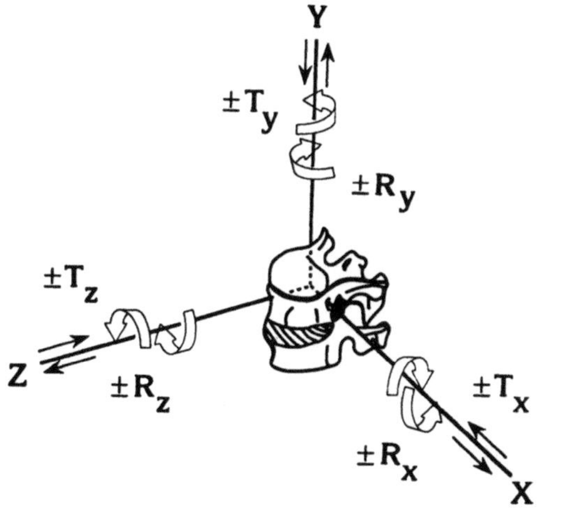

Figure 1.
A vertebra described in terms of rotations about and translations along the x, y, and z-axes on a cartesian coordinate system as proposed by Panjabi (courtesy CBP seminars).

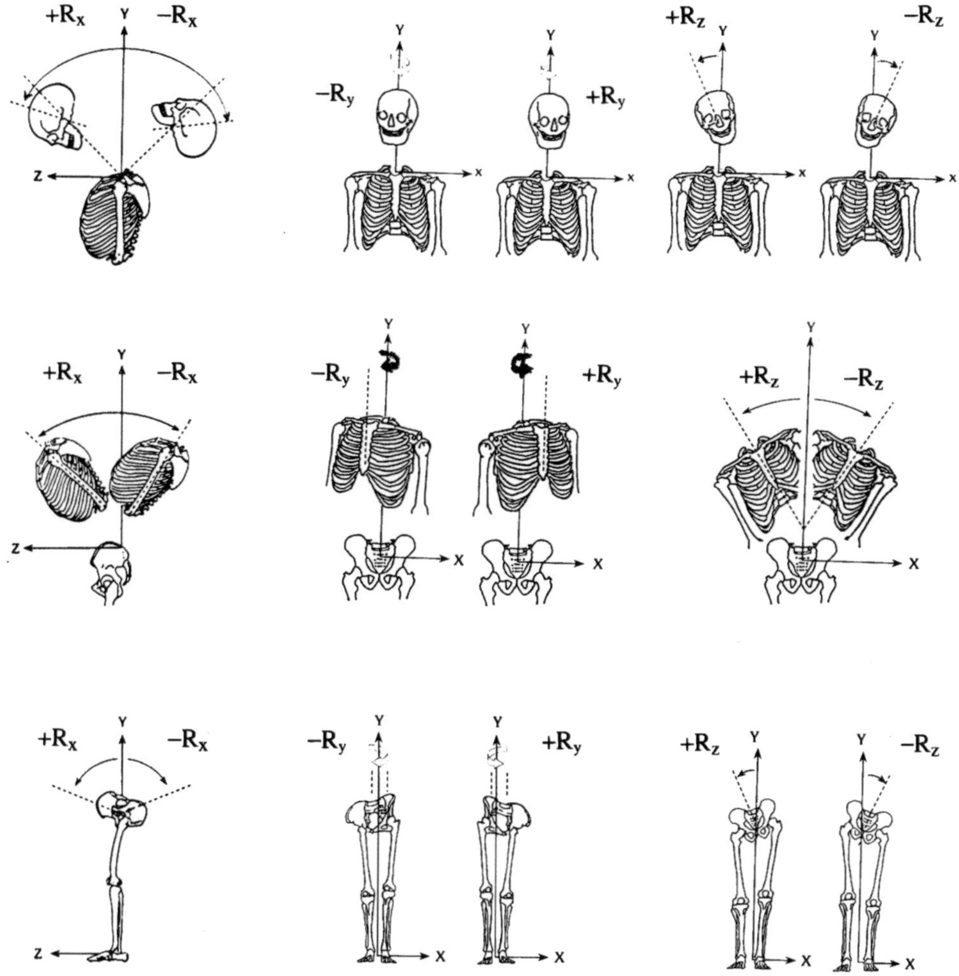

Figure 2.
If the head, thoracic cage, and pelvis are considered rigid bodies, then the possible rotations in three-dimensions are illustrated. Flexion and extension are rotations on the x-axis, axial rotation is about the y-axis, and lateral flexion is rotation about the z-axis (courtesy CBP seminars).

head, rib cage and pelvis in three-dimensions. The technique methods continued to evolve with intellectual contributions from early practitioners of CBP including among others, Drs. DeGeorge, Gambale, Pope and Deed Harrison (founder's son).

One of the unique methods within CBP is the use of 'extension traction' to restore the normal cervical or lumbar lordosis (**Figures 4** and 5). The first cervical extension traction was with use of an inclined bench that utilized a camlock and pulley system to hyperextend the neck by pulling on the forehead [7]. This is the traction used in the first CBP non-randomized controlled clinical trial (nRCT) that showed that no traction either by no treatment or only cervical manipulation but no traction resulted in no improved alignment, while the traction group (also receiving cervical spinal manipulation) achieved improved lordosis [7].

Further development in cervical traction involved the addition of a posterior-to-anterior (PA) pull through the mid cervical spine with simultaneous extension and distraction of the head while sitting in a chair, so-called 'Pope's 2-way' traction (**Figure 4**) [8]. A slight modification of this traction involves the use of a chin-forehead strap to add weight directly to the patients head as an extension-compression 2-way traction (**Figure 4**) [9]. More recently, a cervical extension

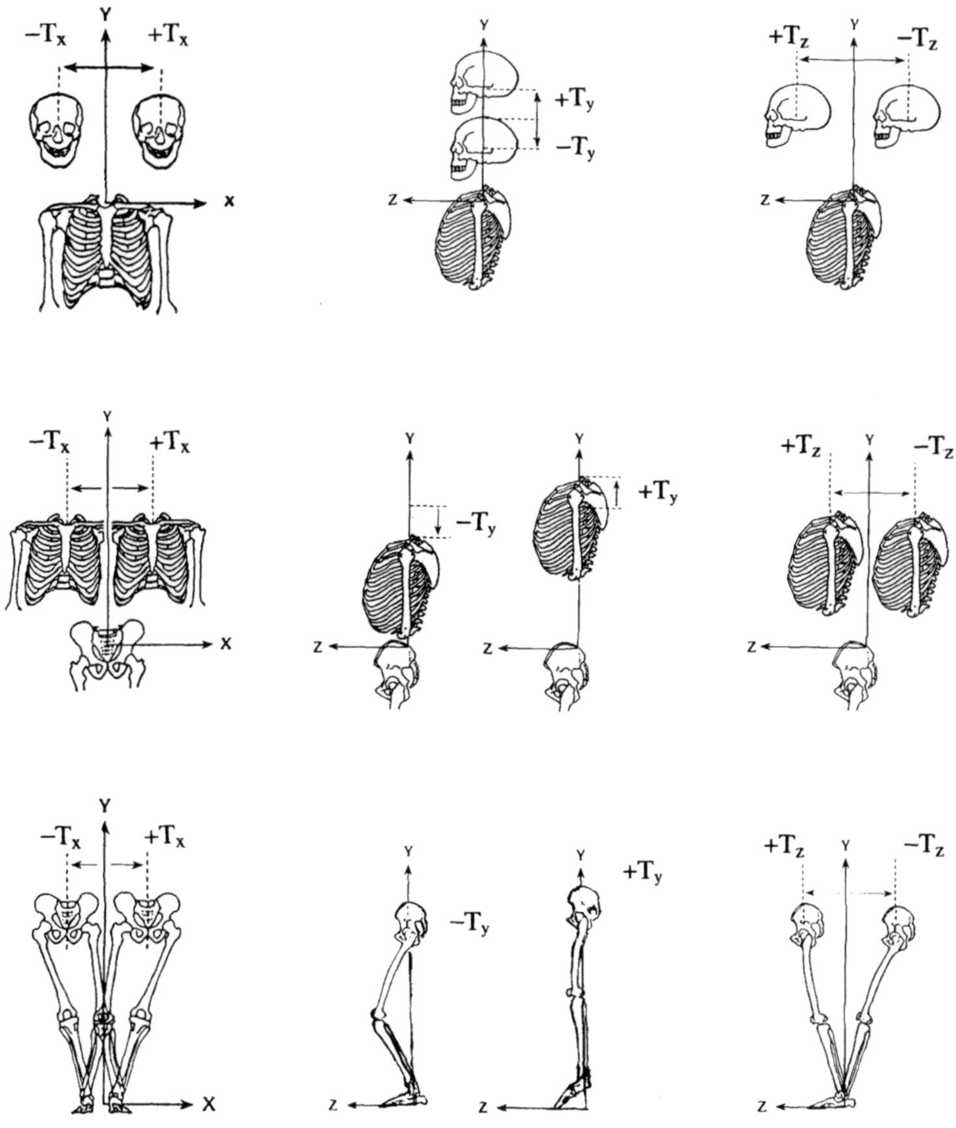

Figure 3.
If the head, thoracic cage, and pelvis are considered rigid bodies, then the possible translations in three-dimensions are illustrated. Lateral translations occur along the x-axis, vertical translations occur along the y-axis, and anterior–posterior translations (protraction-retraction) occurs along the z-axis (courtesy CBP seminars).

orthotic (Denneroll) has been shown to be effective at increasing cervical lordosis (**Figure 4**).

In the mid 1990s, Deed Harrison helped to develop precision vectors for lumbar extension traction (**Figure 5**), where the first nRCT showing lumbar curve restoration was published in the *Archives of Physical Medicine and Rehabilitation* in 2002 and concluded: "This new method of lumbar extension traction is the first nonsurgical rehabilitative procedure to show increases in lumbar lordosis in chronic LBP *(low back pain)* subjects with hypolordosis" [10]. A lumbar extension orthotic device by Denneroll is also used for lumbar extension traction (**Figure 5**).

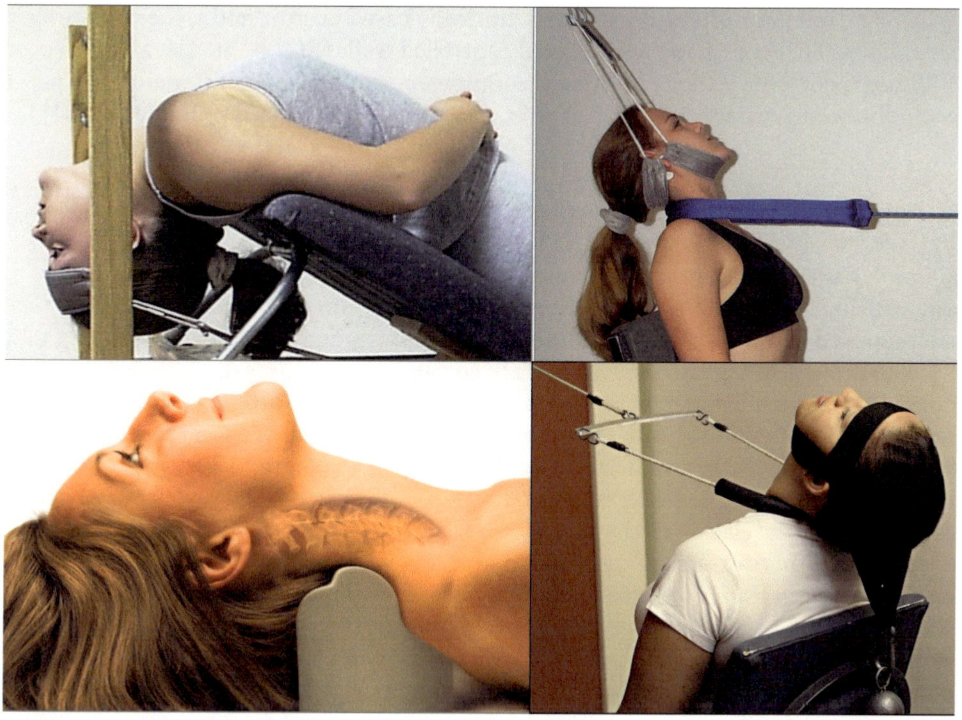

Figure 4.
Cervical extension traction (courtesy CBP seminars).

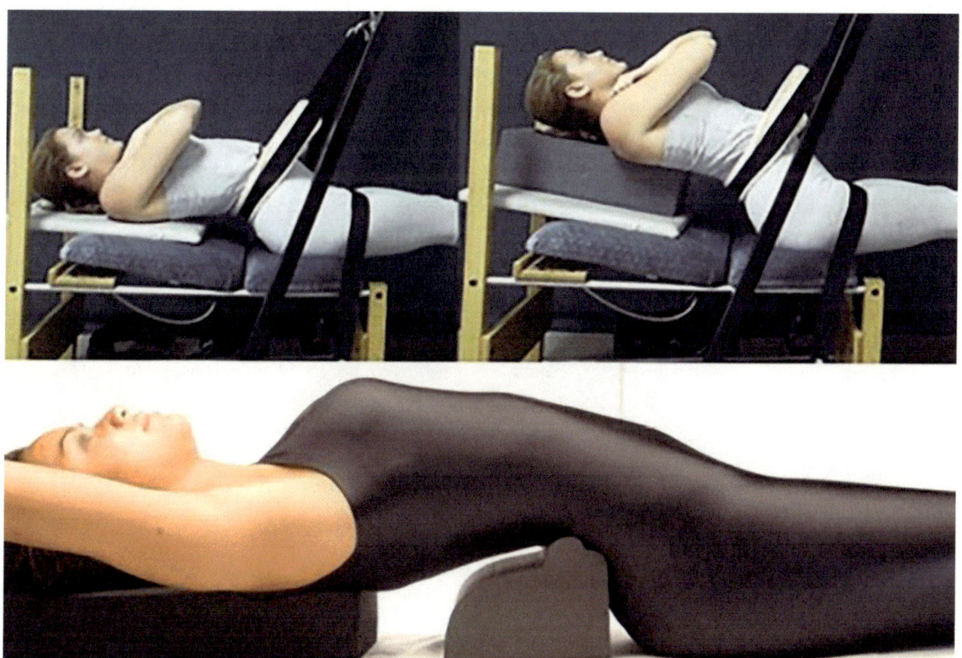

Figure 5.
Lumbar extension traction (courtesy CBP seminars).

CBP technique is one of the most scientifically based posture and spine correcting techniques. There are many randomized controlled trials (RCTs), nRCTs, and well over 100 case reports/series documenting the improvement of diverse spine deformity patterns with concomitant reduction of pain, disability and increased QOL measures [11].

3. Rotations and translations of posture

The main strength of CBP technique is its fundamental underpinnings in engineering and mathematics [1]. It is a general theorem that any object can be decomposed as a rotation, a translation and a deformation [12]. Acknowledging that deformation of living tissues occurs, as in compressing of discs, ligaments, muscles etc., we divert attention to rotations and translations of posture. The main masses of the body, namely the head, thorax and pelvis can be described in relation to the body mass below within a Cartesian coordinate system (**Figures 2** and **3**). That is, the head is described in relation to the thorax, the thorax in relation to the pelvis, and the pelvis in relation to the feet [1, 13].

Any rotations or translations of the body masses as seen in neutral posture via external observation or internally by X-ray is acknowledged as abnormal. Therefore, no offset of the masses equates to the normal postural alignment (i.e. un-subluxated position). It is important to note that in the assessment of a patient, it is the presence of a rotation or translation in the neutral standing position that is abnormal. When Harrison first applied this method of analysis, the treatment became apparent with the postural diagnosis. That is, for any rotation or translation apparent in neutral standing posture, the opposite position would need to be the treatment as applied during exercises, spinal traction or spinal adjustments, as this is the mathematical solution, "the exact reversing of the patient's abnormal posture" [1]. In fact, because the soft tissues require a significant magnitude of stress and strains to attempt to correct the spinal position via mirror image methods, Harrison suggested that postural reflections (i.e. 'mirror image' adjustments) need to be applied in "twice the negative of the translation distances and rotation angles" [1].

It should be noted when Harrison finally developed the full spine analysis of rotations and translations of posture in the mid 1980s, he discovered that virtually

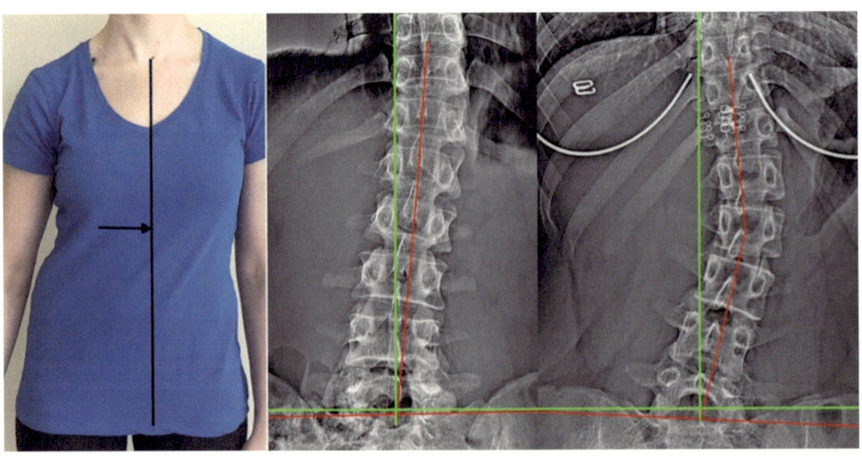

Figure 6.
Posture image and antero-posterior lumbar radiographs depicting a left lateral thoracic translation (side shift). Both patients in the radiographs have a 20 mm left lateral shift of T10 off midline. Left patient has a pure left lateral thoracic translation posture, aka 'pseudo-scoliosis.' Right patient has a true left lumbar scoliosis (vertebral rotation). Green line is vertical; red line highlights patient alignment (courtesy CBP seminars).

50% of all human movements had never been studied (except forward head posture). Thus, the Harrison research group performed several studies to evaluate the normal range of motion for several translation postures including lateral head and thoracic postures as well as anterior and posterior thoracic translation postures (Discussed in Section 6) [2, 3]. Clinically, the spinal coupling patterns as discovered to be associated with these common postural positions are of utmost importance in the treatment of these spinal disorders.

Importance of the study of these never previously studied translation postures can be highlighted in the distinction between true scoliosis and 'pseudo-scoliosis' (**Figure 6**) [14] Pseudo-scoliosis is a lateral thoracic translation posture that characteristically features little to no vertebral rotation (simple to correct) [15, 16], whereas, true scoliosis characteristically features significant vertebral rotation (and is typically much more difficult to treat). X-ray screening of the spine is the only way to differentiate true scoliosis from pseudo-scoliosis.

As mentioned, the absence of rotations and translations of the body masses in standing posture is normal. However, the shape of the spine position, particularly in the sagittal plane has traditionally been debated.

4. The Harrison normal spine model

In the mid 1990s to the mid 2000s, the Harrison research team performed a series of spine modeling studies of the sagittal spinal curves (**Figure 7**) [17–24]. To

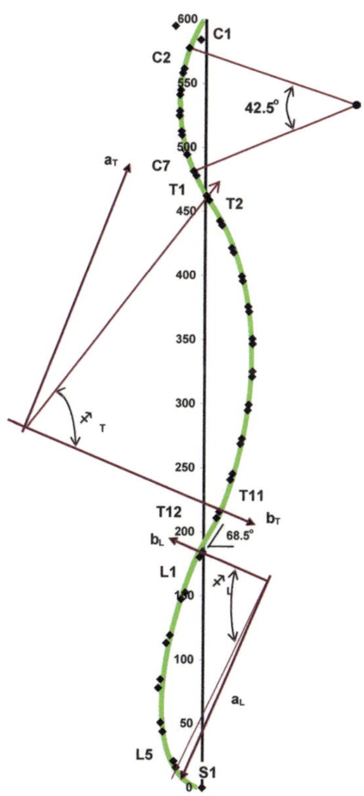

Figure 7.
The Harrison normal sagittal spine model as the path of the posterior longitudinal ligament. The cervical, thoracic and lumbar curves are all portions of an elliptical curve having a unique minor-to-major axis ratio. The cervical curve is circular meaning the minor and major axes are equal (courtesy CBP seminars).

this day, this seminal work serves as the treatment outcome goal (i.e. gold standard) for providing structural rehabilitation by CBP methods (**Figure 8**). In a series of systematic studies, elliptical shape modeling of the path of the posterior longitudinal ligament was performed as it could be easily compared to the posterior vertebral body margins on X-rays, the same anatomical region used for measuring the sagittal spinal curves (i.e. Harrison posterior tangents (**Figure 9**) [25–28]).

Computer iterations of spine shape modeling were applied to determine the best-fit geometric spinal shapes by fitting ellipses of varying minor-to-major axis ratios to the digitized data points from the posterior vertebral body corners from X-ray samples for each of the three regions of the spine (cervical [17–19], thoracic [20, 21], and lumbar spine [22–24]). As shown in **Figure 7**, the Harrison normal spinal model features a circular cervical lordosis, an elliptical thoracic curve featuring greater curvature cephalad with a straightened thoraco-lumbar junction and an

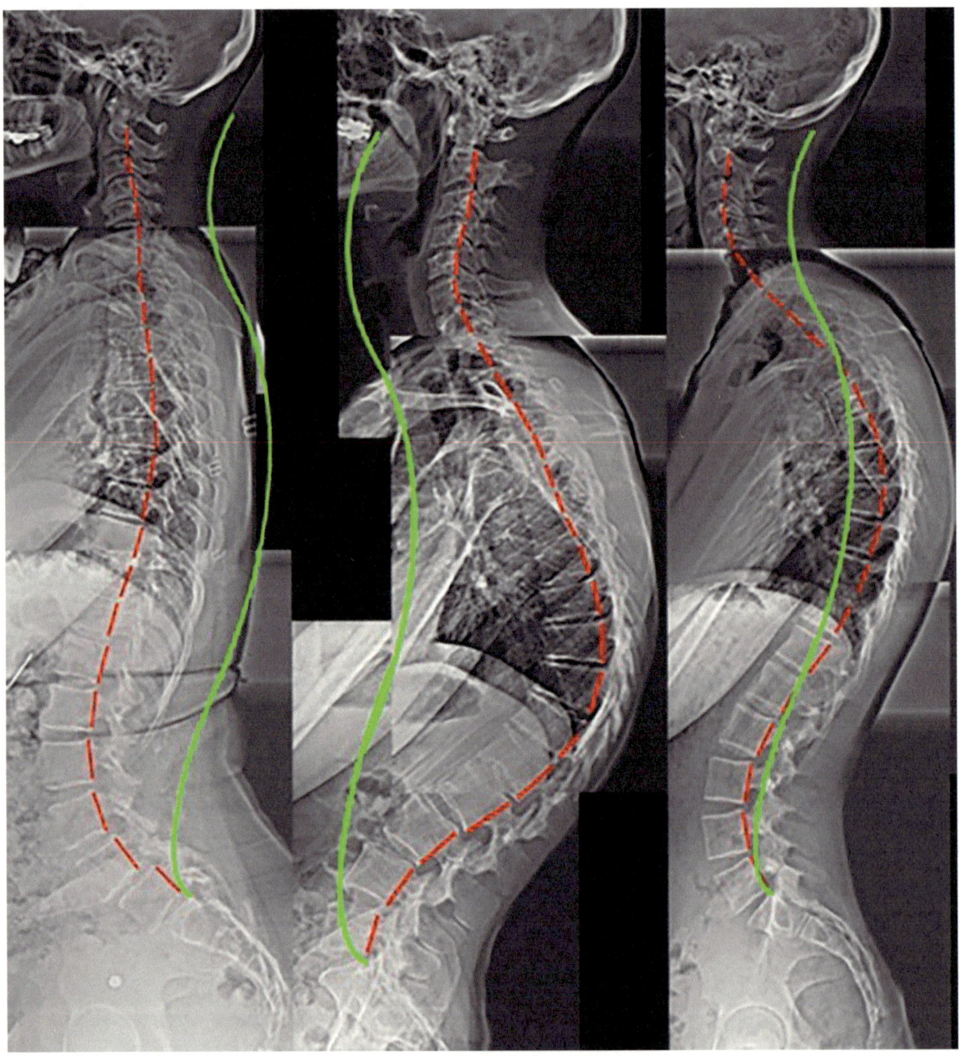

Figure 8.
Three patients demonstrating dramatically different spine alignment patterns. Left: excessive lumbar hyperlordosis, L4 anterolisthesis, and excessive anterior sagittal balance in a mid-aged female with disabling low back pain; middle: excessive thoracolumbar kyphosis and early degenerative changes in a mid-aged male; right: excessive thoracic hyperkyphosis in a young male with Scheuermann's disease. Red line is contiguous with posterior vertebral body margins; green line represents Harrison normal spinal model (courtesy PAO).

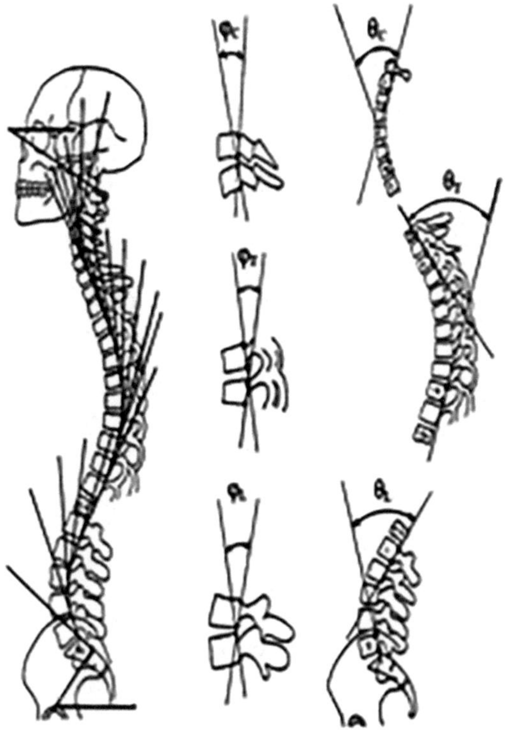

Figure 9.
Harrison posterior tangent method involves lines drawn contiguous with the posterior vertebral body margins. Intersegmental as well as regional sagittal curves are easily quantified having a standard error of measurement within about 2° (courtesy CBP seminars).

elliptical lumbar lordosis showing a greater distal lumbar curvature. The spine is assumed to be vertical in the front view.

Although some have attempted to criticize the Harrison normal spinal model, it is important to acknowledge that it has been validated in several ways. Simple analysis of alignment data on samples of normal, asymptomatic populations have been done [17–24]. Comparison studies between normal samples to symptomatic samples have been performed [17, 29]. Comparisons between normal samples to theoretical ideal models have been done [17, 18, 20, 23]. Statistical differentiation of asymptomatic subjects from symptomatic pain group patients based on alignment data has been performed [19, 24].

In subsequent biomechanical modeling studies, the Harrison group used a validated postural loading model to verify that sagittal spinal balance and the sagittal curves of the spine are critical biomechanical parameters for maintaining postural load balance in healthy subjects [30]. Keller et al. [30] stated "because the pattern of [intervertebral disc] IVD postural stresses mirrored the sagittal curvatures and sagittal displacement of the spine, a failure of the IVD's hydrostatic mechanism under these sustained loads could occur". In a similar biomechanical modeling study, Harrison et al. determined that anterior sagittal thoracic posture (anterior thorax translation relative to the pelvis) resulted in significant increases in disc loads and stresses for all vertebral levels below T9 and that the extensor muscle loads required to maintain static equilibrium in upright anterior posture increased almost five times that of normal [31]. In another study Keller et al. [32] determined that "postural forces are responsible for initiation of osteoporotic spinal deformity in elderly subjects".

The Harrison group also used an elliptical shell model to evaluate the loads and bending moments on the cervical vertebrae in varying cervical spine deformity alignments [33, 34]. They found that in normal lordosis the anterior and posterior vertebral body stresses are nearly uniform and minimal, whereas, in cervical deformity configurations having kyphosis (S-shape kyphosis high or low, total kyphosis), the vertebral body stresses are 'very large' and opposite in direction compared to normal lordosis [33]. They concluded "This analysis provides the basis for the formation of osteophytes (Wolff's Law) on the anterior margins of vertebrae in kyphotic regions of the sagittal cervical curve. This indicates that any kyphosis is an undesirable configuration in the cervical spine" [33]. Anterior head translation and a 'military' neck also displayed significantly increased vertebral body stresses that are reverse in direction from C5-T1 and are also proven to be "undesirable configurations in the cervical spine" [34].

5. Radiographic analysis

All radiographs should be taken in the 'neutral' standing position with the feet positioned with the heels at hips width apart. This is to avoid any induced postural deviations due to foot position. Also, to ensure a reproducible neutral (i.e. natural) body position, the subject should close their eyes and nod the head back and forth a couple times to where the subject should stop in their preferred position and then open their eyes while maintaining this adopted stance. Any postural misalignments seen in the subject should not be corrected. The lower body mass on the particular view being taken should be centered to the bucky. All X-rays should be taken without footwear.

It should be mentioned that the measurement of different sagittal spinal contours including regional curves or absolute rotation angles (ARAs) (i.e. cervical/lumbar lordosis; thoracic kyphosis) and intersegmental relative rotation angles (RRAs) between adjacent vertebrae can be easily quantified by use of the Harrison posterior tangent (HPT) lines (**Figure 9**) [25–28]. The HPT method is preferred for three main reasons, 1. The posterior margins of the vertebral bodies are less affected by osteoarthritic changes as compared to the anterior margins which makes anatomical measurements more reliable and valid; 2. The posterior tangents are contiguous with the slope of the spinal curves and represent the first derivative in an engineering analysis and therefore, their intersection accurately depicts the sagittal configuration; 3. The HPT method has a small standard error of measurement (SEM) of approximately 2° versus higher SEMs with the Cobb (4.5–10°) [25–27]. This is why the HPT method is superior to other methods of sagittal spine mensuration including the popular Cobb method.

Generally, the global curves are measured as C2-C7, T1-T12, and L1-L5, however since the inflection of the cervical lordosis to thoracic kyphosis occurs at T1, some clinicians prefer to measure the cervical curve from C1-T1, and the thoracic curve from T2-T11 or T3-T10. Anterior sagittal translation distances are simply measured by the horizontal displacement offset between comparison vertebrae such as C2-S1, C2-C7 or T1, T1-T12, etc.

The anterior-to-posterior (AP) or PA X-rays are taken using the same postural positioning. The modified Risser-Ferguson method is employed to measure coronal plane alignment (**Figure 10**) [28]. On the AP/PA cervicothoracic view an upper angle is created as the angle between the best fit line of the upper cervical segments and intersection with the bite line, and a lower angle is formed between the best fit lines of the upper to lower spine segments [28]. The Rz angle is the angle formed by a vertical axis line (VAL) drawn from T4 and the lower cervicothoracic best fit line. Normal upper angle, lower angle and Rz cervicothoracic angles are 90°, 0° and 0°, respectively. The AP/PA thoracic view may show an angle. The lumbo-pelvic view has an upper angle, the angle between the best fit line of the upper versus lower lumbar segments, and a lower angle, the angle between the best

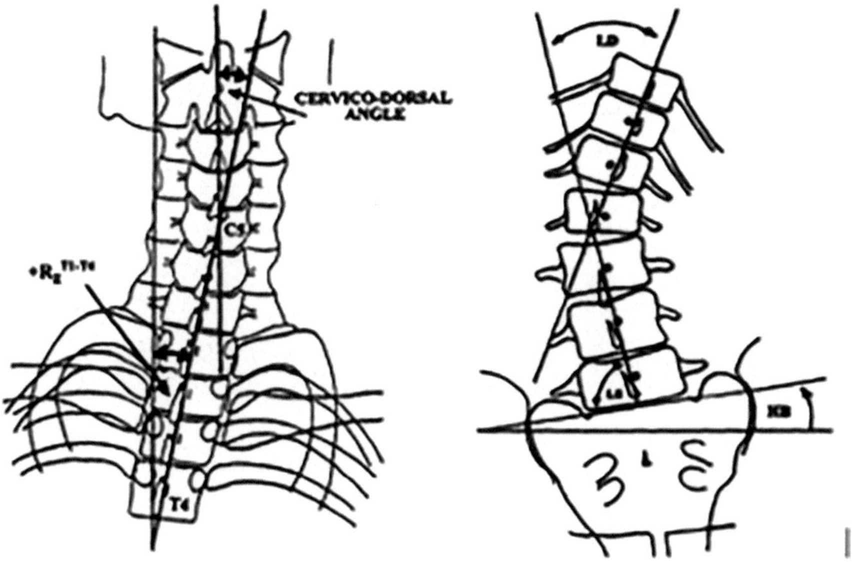

Figure 10.
AP radiographic line drawing by modified Risser-Ferguson method.

fit line between the lower segments and the horizontal pelvic line [28]. The upper angle and lower angle should be 0° and 90°, respectively. Any regional or full-spine coronal balance offset (i.e. imbalance) can be easily quantified as the horizontal distance between the uppermost segment to the lowermost segment (e.g. C2-T2, T1-T12, T12-S1, C2-S1).

6. Posture and spinal coupling

Postural rotations and translations as described by Harrison (**Figures 2** and **3**) are understood as 'main motions' and the corresponding spinal displacements to accommodate the postural positions are termed 'coupled motions' [2, 3, 35–38]. In CBP, a considerable clinical significance is placed on the correlation between the patient's three-dimensional postural presentation (posture displacement in terms of rotations and translations) and the two-dimensional X-ray coupled motion (spinal rotations and translations) [2, 3, 38].

Of prime importance is the appreciation that unless there is buckling, anomalies or ligament damage, standing neutral postural rotation and translation displacements of the head or thorax *cause* the vertebral spinal coupling patterns as seen on X-ray. If a patient's rotations and/or translations of posture 'match' the associated spinal coupling pattern as expected (i.e. normal coupling), then it is considered an 'easy' or typical case and the intuitive mirror image application of CBP methods would apply. When the patient's rotations and/or translations of posture do not match the expected spine coupling pattern (i.e. spinal coupling does not match postural displacement), then it is considered an atypical case where the clinician needs to consider alternative (i.e. more complicated) strategies for spine rehabilitation.

A classic demonstration of the 'matching' versus 'mismatching' of rotations and translations of posture and spine coupling patterns can be illustrated with forward head posture, aka, anterior head translation (AHT) (**Figure 11**). The natural and expected spine coupling with a forward translated head posture involves lower cervical spine flexion and upper cervical spine extension. As seen in **Figure 11**, many

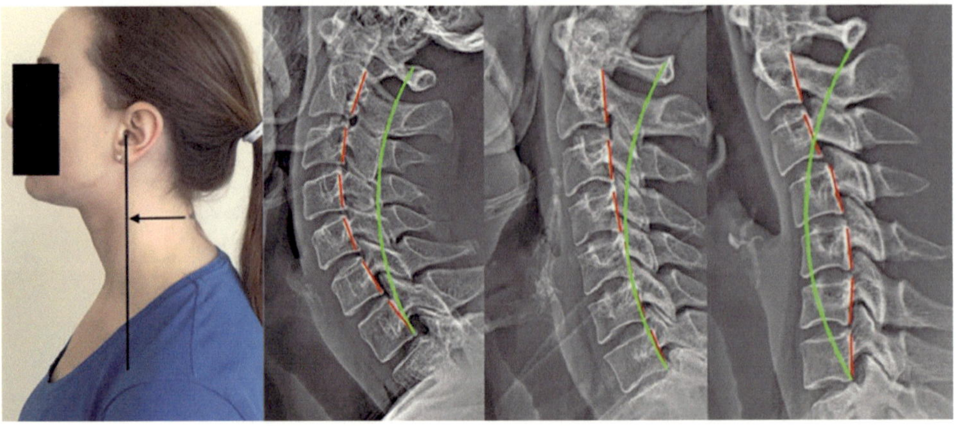

Figure 11.
Forward head translation as shown in posture and in three unique lateral cervical radiographs. All three X-ray images have about 25 mm of forward head translation. Left: hyperlordosis; middle: hypolordosis; right: kyphosis. Green line is normal alignment; red line highlights patient alignment.

spine different vertebral coupling patterns are possible including hyperlordosis, hypolordosis, or kyphosis and accordingly, each cervical configuration requires its own unique application of CBP methods for its ideal correction.

These cervical spine patterns have been termed harmonics and their presence can only be determined by radiography [2, 39]. Importantly, in CBP treatment approaches, each cervical spine coupling pattern (harmonic) requires its own unique treatment protocol. This is why many manual therapy approaches (e.g. Mackenzie head retractions) are inadequate at correcting posture and spine alignment as these are prescribed universally (i.e. 'blackbox treatment') resulting in many patients receiving treatment protocols that are contraindicated. A patient with a hyperlordotic cervical spine should never be prescribed neck extension exercises as this would dynamically hyperextend the cervical joints. A patient with a complete cervical kyphosis should never be prescribed head retraction exercises as this often 'buckles' the spine into further kyphosis.

Also, as mentioned and illustrated in **Figure 6**, 'pseudo-scoliosis' or pure lateral translations of the thorax (or head) must be distinguished from true scoliosis by examination of the spinal coupling patterns [14]. If there is minimal or no vertebral rotation then this represents a typical case requiring CBP mirror image postural correction [3]. If there is vertebral rotation then it is considered true scoliosis and a completely different application of CBP methods (i.e. non-commutative properties of finite rotation angles [40, 41]). Case examples of the special application of CBP methods in the treatment of scoliosis is described later.

7. CBP protocol

The CBP patient management protocol [2–4] involves all typical initial patient examination procedures including the consultation, examination as well as pain, disability and quality of life questionnaires (**Figure 12**). In addition, CBP treatment consideration requires, without exception, a full-spine posture assessment as well as full-spine AP and lateral standing radiographs. Posture needs to be either qualitatively, but ideally quantitatively assessed as rotations and translations of the head, thorax and pelvis in three-dimensions (**Figures 2** and **3**). The X-rays need to be digitized and quantified, ideally with the Harrison posterior tangent method for the sagittal images and with the modified Risser-Ferguson on the AP images.

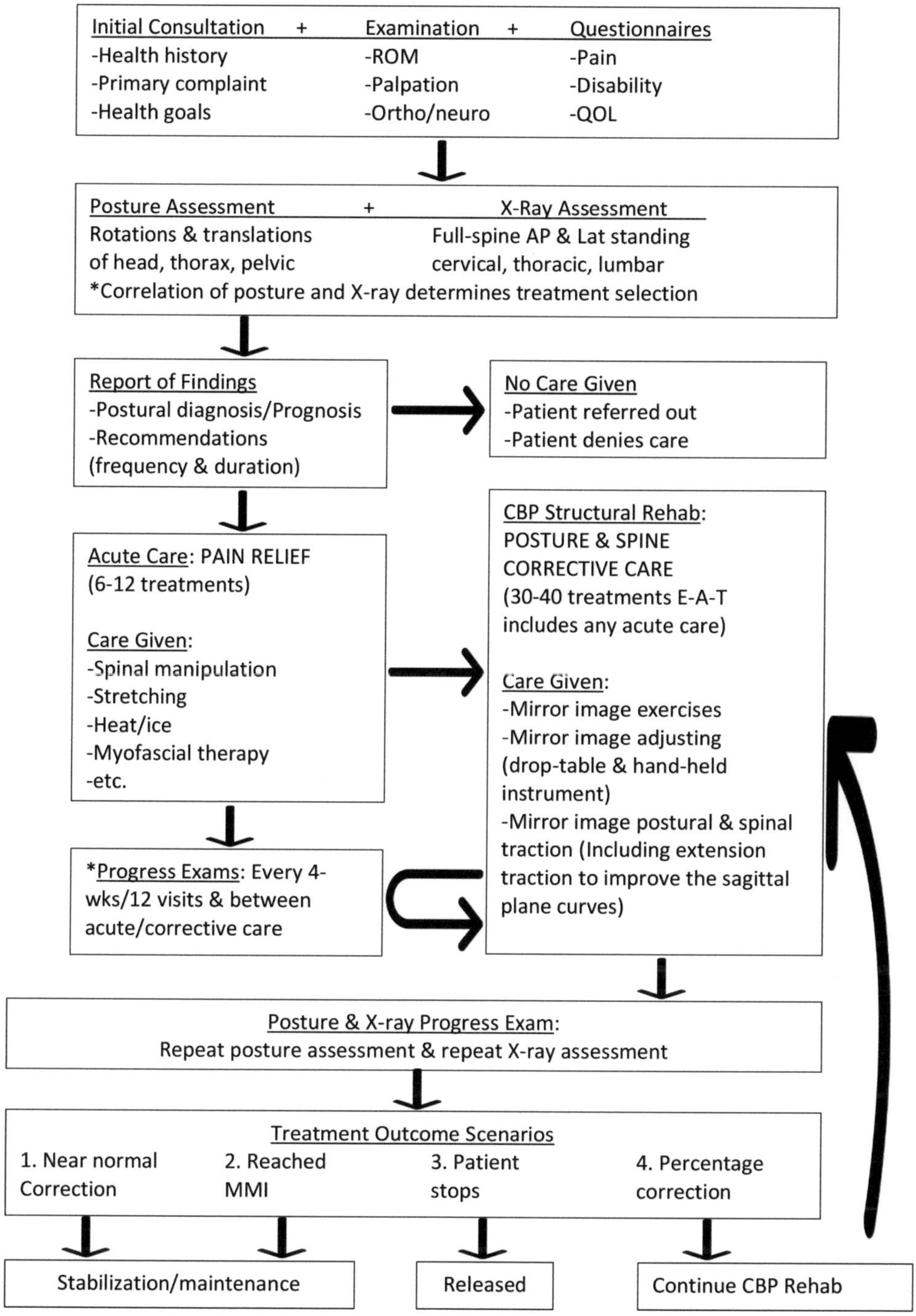

Figure 12.
CBP protocol treatment algorithm.

As seen in **Figure 12**, if appropriate, a new patient should be treated for their acute pain that is distinct and separate from CBP methods. It is recommended that the acute 'pain care' treatment include spinal manipulation, stretching (e.g. proprioceptive neuromuscular facilitation (PNF), Yoga, etc.), heat/ice, soft tissue myofascial therapy (e.g. transverse friction, Nimmo-receptor tonus technique, etc.). Once the patient

Study	Journal	Traction method	Traction time	Number of treatments	Change (°)	Change/txt (°)	Theoretical treatment extrapolation		
							Hypolordotic -20°	No curve 0°	Kyphotic +20°
RCTs									
Moustafa	Sci Reports	Denneroll	20m	30	13.9	0.46	32	76	119
Moustafa	Heliyon	Denneroll	15–20m	30	13.4	0.45	34	78	123
Moustafa	J Athl Train	Denneroll	20m	30	14.7	0.49	31	71	112
Moustafa	APMR	Denneroll	20m	30	13.1	0.44	34	80	126
Moustafa	EJPRM	Denneroll	20m	30	13.7	0.46	33	77	120
Moustafa	BFPTCU	Denneroll	20m	36	12.8	0.36	42	98	155
nRCTs									
Harrison	JMPT	Pope 2-way	20m	38	17.9	0.47	32	74	117
Harrison	APMR	2way	20m	35	14.2	0.41	37	86	136
Harrison	JMPT	Ext-comp	10m	60	13.2	022	68	159	250

**Note: Correction is estimated to achieve -35 of cervical lordosis.*

Table 1.
Summary of cervical lordosis improvement by number of treatments, magnitude correction/treatment and the extrapolation to typical sagittal cervical curve subluxation types and the theoretical treatment number required for their correction to -35° C2-7 ARA.

DOI: http://dx.doi.org/10.5772/intechopen.102686

Study	Journal	Traction method	Traction time	Number of treatments	Change (°)	Change/ txt (°)	Theoretical treatment extrapolation		
							Hypolordotic -30°	Hypolordotic -15°	No curve 0°
RCTs									
Moustafa	JBMR/JMPT	LET	20m	30	6.2	0.21	48	121	194
Moustafa	Clin Rehab	LET	20m	30	8.7	0.29	34	86	138
nRCTs									
Harrison	APMR	LET	20m	36	11.3	0.31	32	80	127

**Note: Correction is estimated to achieve -40 of lumbar lordosis.*

Table 2.
Summary of lumbar lordosis improvement by number of treatments, magnitude correction/treatment and the extrapolation to typical sagittal lumbar curve subluxation types and the theoretical treatment number required for their correction to -40° L1-5 ARA.

Study	Journal	Traction method	Traction time	Number of treatments	Change (mm)	Change/txt (mm)	Theoretical treatment extrapolation		
							Mild offset ±10mm	Moderate offset ±20mm	Severe offset ±30mm
nRCTs									
Head trans Harrison	JRRD	Lat trans	20 m	37	6.9	0.19	54	107	161
Thorax trans Harrison	Eur Sp J	Lat trans	20 m	36	7.7	0.21	47	94	140

Note: Correction is estimated to achieve 0mm of offset.

Table 3.
Summary of AP head and thorax lateral translation reduction by number of treatments, magnitude correction/treatment and the extrapolation to larger coronal plane offset subluxations and the theoretical treatment number required for their correction.

experiences some initial pain relief (e.g. 6–12 treatments) they can be re-assessed and graduated to CBP structural rehabilitation. The decision to first treat a new patient with 'acute' pain care is a clinical decision that is mainly for patients that have either never seen a chiropractor previously or they have not been previously treated for their acute condition. For patients who have received recent previous treatment without relief, CBP rehabilitation care is recommended from the start of treatment [2–4].

CBP structural rehabilitation is suggested as either three times per week for 12-weeks (36 treatments) or four times per week for 9-weeks (36 treatments), however, the controlled trial data support treatment blocks of 30–40 treatment sessions [7–10, 15, 42–55]. An initial patient who has acute or chronic pains and who has not been treated recently or at all for their current spine issue should be treated for an initial 6–12 sessions to provide pain relief. After signs of relief have occurred, a progress exam should be performed and the patient should be transitioned or 'graduated' to CBP corrective care.

CBP treatment occurs in 'blocks of care.' Numerous CBP controlled clinical trials (RCTs [43–55] and nRCTs [7–10, 15, 42]) provide evidence for spine altering changes to occur in the range of 30–40 treatment sessions; thus, it is the practitioners' choice to set their protocol within this range (i.e. treatment blocks). The end of each 'block' of CBP care requires a progress exam which includes all of the typical assessment procedures as well as a posture and X-ray assessment. Exam results may either dictate the need for further CBP treatment or the recommendation for 'supportive' or maintenance care. An initial block of CBP structural rehabilitation will include any acute care provided in the first 2–4 weeks. It is always recommended that ongoing 'progress exams' be performed regularly, at either 4-week or 12 treatment intervals, or as frequently as recommended by each practitioner's regional regulatory board requirements.

CBP does not specifically support 'long-term' care plans. However, based on the data, an adult typically needs 6-months of corrective care (e.g. 72 treatments over 6-months at 3x/week) which is an evidence-based recommendation. Although, any given patient may require a shorted (i.e. 3-month) or longer treatment program based on their initial presenting postural parameters—approximate treatment extrapolations can be made by studying **Tables 1–3**. There is also support for supportive/maintenance care at a frequency of approximately 2×/month [8–10].

8. Clinical evidence of efficacy

As mentioned, CBP technique has an abundance of clinical evidence supporting its effectiveness in correcting spine deformity and posture [7–10, 15, 42–55]. Recently, systematic reviews have summarized the clinical evidence as reported in the published controlled trials on these methods [56, 57]. We summarize the evidence here in four parts: cervical lordosis, lumbar lordosis, lateral translation (pseudo-scoliosis) postures of the head and thorax, and finally, evolving evidence from case reports/series on other important spine deformities including lumbar spondylolisthesis, cervical spondylolisthesis, thoracic hyperkyphosis, thoraco-lumbar junctional kyphosis, thoracic hypokyphosis (straight back syndrome), anterior sagittal balance, lumbar kyphosis (flat back syndrome), lumbar hyperlordosis, post-surgical cervical spine fusion and scoliosis.

8.1 Cervical lordosis

A recent systematic review found that of the RCTs and nRCTs on CBP extension traction methods, a 12–18° improvement in cervical lordosis can be achieved in

10–15 weeks after 30–36 treatment sessions [57]. Most RCTs have used the cervical Denneroll [43–47, 49, 50], and the three nRCTs all used different CET methods (**Table 1**) [7–9].

Table 1 shows the improvement in degrees per treatment as well as theoretical numbers of treatments for various presenting cervical spine subluxations. On average, there appears to be just less than a half degree improvement per treatment session; obviously, there are patients that will have both more correction and less correction than this. Using this estimation as an initial guideline, evidence-based treatment numbers can be predicted. For example, a patient presenting with a cervical kyphosis of 20° would require over 100 treatments to restore the neck to a curve of 35°.

Figures 13 and **14** show the long-term outcomes in patients receiving cervical extension traction versus comparative groups not receiving the traction. The patients restoring lordosis via CBP traction methods show improved cervical alignment which is maintained at a years' follow-up (**Figure 13**) whereas, comparative groups receiving various physiotherapeutic treatments less the extension traction do not experience cervical improvement (**Figure 13**) and also show that any initial pain relief regresses back towards baseline levels after the cessation of treatment (**Figure 14**). Patient's with improved lordosis retain their initial pain relief a year later (**Figure 14**). This is alarming as it shows patients receiving various physiotherapeutic treatments who do not improve their cervical lordosis (in hypolordotic patients) will have a future regression of symptoms post-treatment and may be misled by 'apparent treatment efficacy' [5, 57].

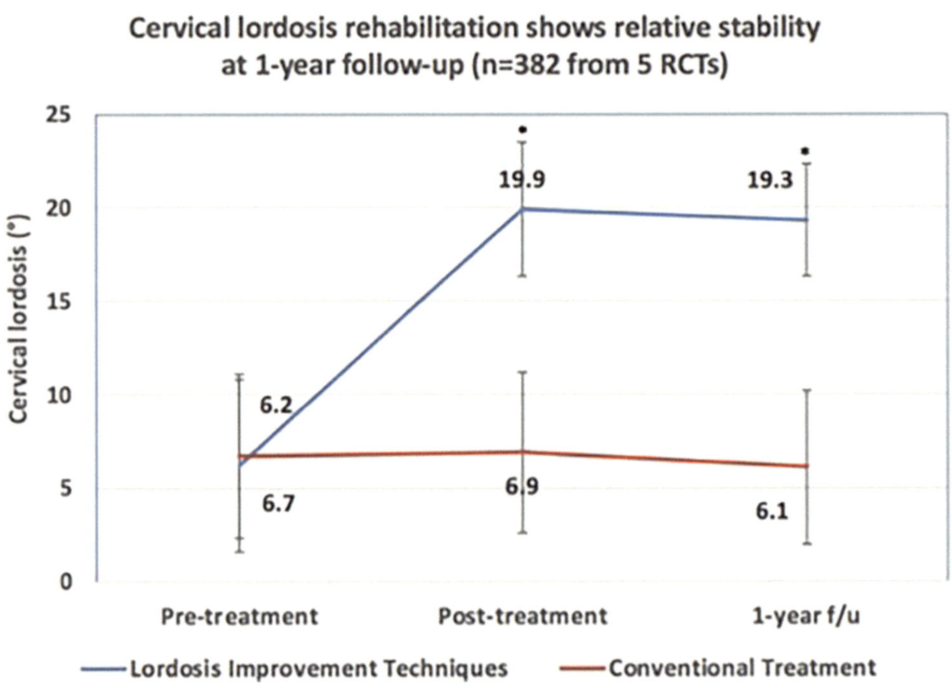

Figure 13.
*Data from five RCTs demonstrates patients achieving cervical lordosis improvement (via extension traction) as well as conventional treatments have lordosis improvements that are sustained for 1 year after stopping treatment versus the cervical curve of comparative groups (controls not achieving lordosis improvement) remain unaffected by conventional treatments (weighted averages from five RCTs [44, 45, 47, 49, 50]). * indicates a significant group difference as specified in each of the five trials; brackets represent weighted standard deviation.*

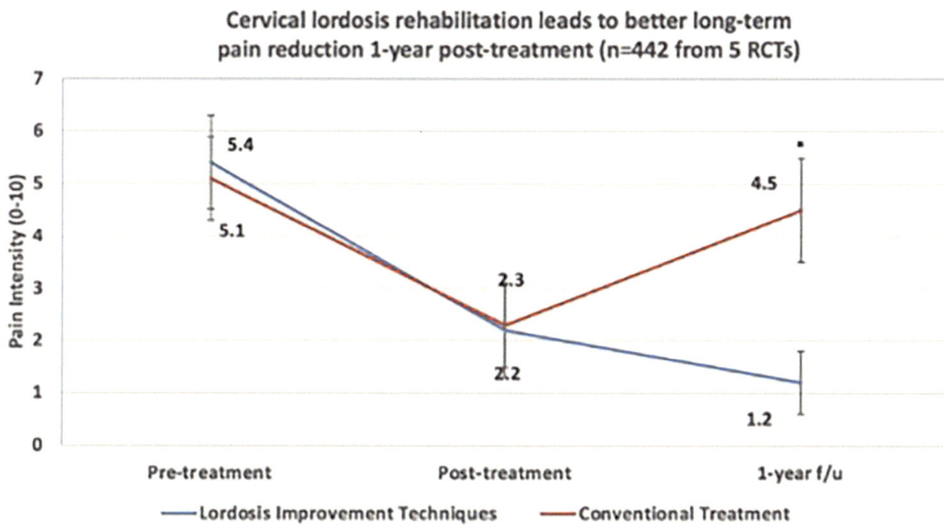

Figure 14.
*Data from five RCTs demonstrates patients achieving cervical lordosis improvement (via extension traction) as well as conventional treatments have pain reductions that are sustained for 1 year after stopping treatment versus comparative groups (controls not achieving lordosis improvement) who show a regression (increase) of pain intensity towards baseline after stopping treatment (weighted averages from five RCTs [45–47, 49, 50]). * indicates a significant group difference as specified in each of the five trials; brackets represent weighted standard deviation.*

8.2 Lumbar lordosis

A recent systematic review found "Limited but good quality evidence substantiates that the use of extension traction methods in rehabilitation programs definitively increases lumbar hypolordosis" [56]. The authors further stated: "Preliminarily, these studies indicate these methods provide longer-term relief to patients with low back disorders versus conventional rehabilitation approaches tested" [56]. On average, a 7–11° increase in lordosis can be achieved over 10–12 weeks after 30–36 treatment sessions (**Table 2**).

It must be mentioned that lumbar extension traction is necessary to increase the lumbar lordosis. Importantly, using the data from published trials [10, 53–55], one can extrapolate approximate treatment duration (**Table 2**). As seen, a mild hypolordotic lumbar spine of 30° (L1-L5 ARA) may only require 32–48 treatments, whereas, a flat lumbar curve would require 127–194 treatments to achieve a normal 40° lordosis.

The same trend as observed in patients receiving cervical lordosis correction versus comparative groups not receiving lordosis improvement is seen in the trials on the lumbar spine [5, 56]. Lordosis increase in patients receiving lumbar extension traction is achieved and maintained at 6-months follow-up (**Figure 15**); these patients also retain their initial pain relief whereas, comparative patient groups not receiving lordosis improvement (**Figure 15**) lose their initial pain relief by 6-months after cessation of treatment (**Figure 16**). Again, this is alarming and shows how active low back treatment, although offering transient pain relief, will likely regress after treatment if not receiving concurrent lordosis correction in those suffering from hypolordotic-related LBP [5, 56].

8.3 AP head and thorax postures

Coronal plane lateral translations of the head and thorax also referred to as 'pseudo-scoliosis' each has an nRCT published [15, 42] and many case reports

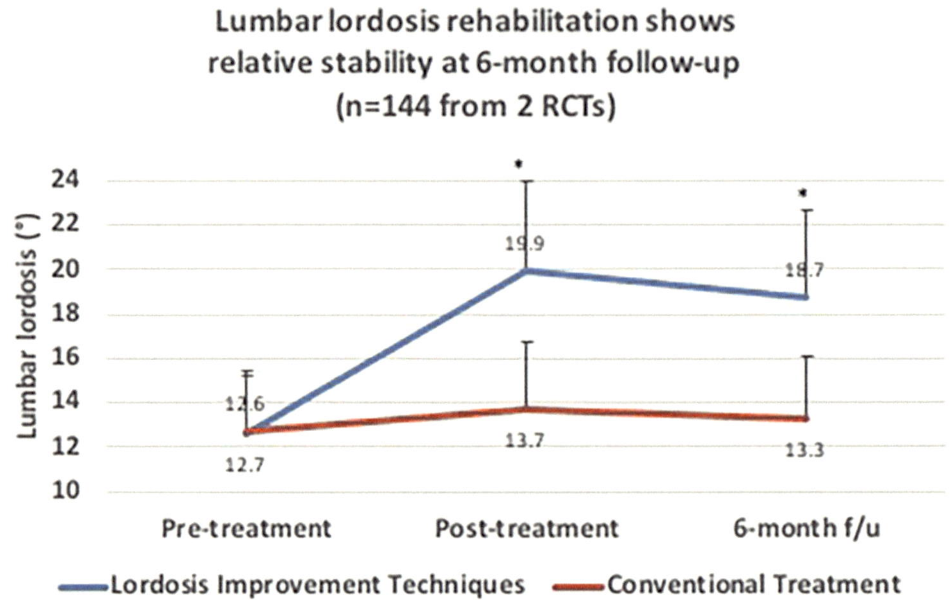

Figure 15.
*Data from two RCTs demonstrates patients achieving lumbar lordosis improvement (via extension traction) as well as conventional treatments have lordosis improvements that are sustained for 6-months after stopping treatment versus the lumbar curve of comparative groups (controls not achieving lordosis improvement) remain unaffected by conventional treatments (weighted averages from two RCTs [53, 54]). * indicates a significant group difference as specified in each of the two trials; brackets represent weighted standard deviation.*

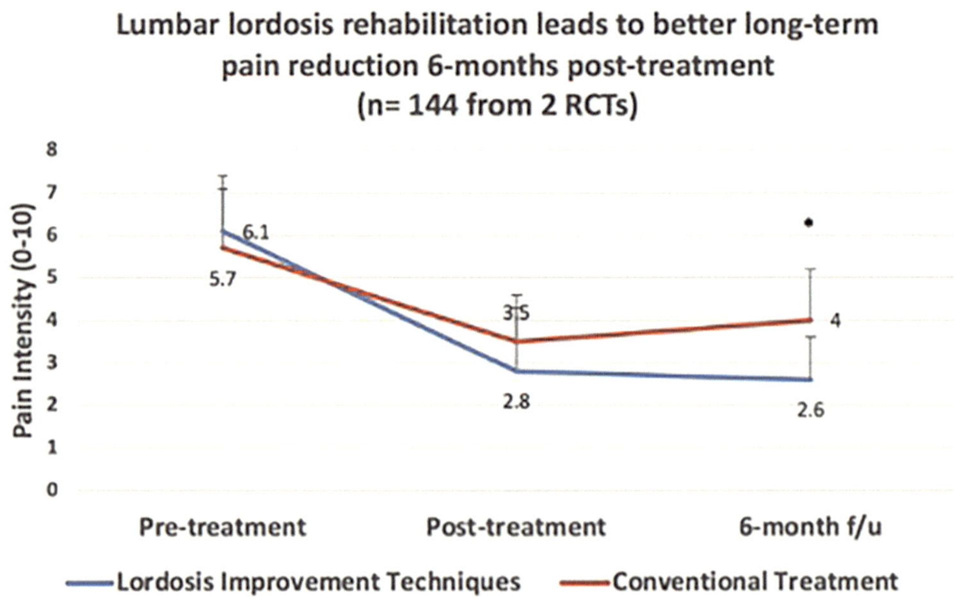

Figure 16.
*Data from two RCTs demonstrates patients achieving lumbar lordosis improvement (via extension traction) as well as conventional treatments have pain reductions that are sustained for 6-months after stopping treatment versus comparative groups (controls not achieving lordosis improvement) who show a regression (increase) of pain intensity towards baseline after stopping treatment (weighted averages from two RCTs [53, 54]). * indicates a significant group difference as specified in each of the two trials; brackets represent weighted standard deviation.*

demonstrating its reduction [16, 58–63]. As discussed earlier, the differentiation from true scoliosis is that the involved vertebrae have minimal to no rotation, whereas, true scoliosis has substantial vertebral rotation (**Figure 6**). Also, the spinal coupling pattern of a laterally translated body mass (head or thorax) will demonstrate the lower involved spinal region to laterally flex towards the side of the translation and the upper involved spinal region to laterally flex back towards the vertical [35, 36].

Based on the data, a laterally translated body mass can be reduced about 7–8 mm after about 35 treatments. On average, correction of a laterally translated head or thorax can be corrected at about 0.2 mm per treatment, or about 1 mm per five treatments. Extrapolations of treatment numbers to patient subluxation presentation are shown in **Table 3**. From the data in each of the nRCTs, an approximate 50% reduction of the initial laterally translated head and thorax postures occurred; therefore, an average patient having an approximate 15 mm translation posture (head or rib cage) requires 6-months of corrective care (approximately 72 treatments). It must also be mentioned that many case reports have demonstrated larger lateral translation postural corrections/reductions with CBP methods in similar time frames [16, 58–63], thus, these serve as approximate treatment extrapolations.

8.4 Other spine deformities

It is known that the science for manual therapies is lacking [64]. Therefore, lesser forms of evidence must be considered when evaluating various treatment approaches used to treat various spinal conditions by manual therapists [65, 66]; this includes treatment utilizing CBP methods. We now highlight more recent case studies and series showing structural spinal correction for a variety of relatively common disorders.

8.4.1 Lumbar spondylolisthesis

Fedorchuk et al. [67] reported on an 11 mm reduction (13.3–2.4 mm) of an L4 anterolisthesis in a 69-year old suffering from LBP and leg cramping. Pain relief was achieved after 60 treatments over 45 weeks. This was the first documented report of a reduction of a Grade 2 lumbar spondylolisthesis by CBP methods, as well as any other non-surgical method.

Oakley and Harrison reported on the reduction of multiple retrolistheses from L1-L4 ranging from 4.5 to 5.9 mm in a 32-year old male with LBP [68]. These were all reduced to within normal (<4.5 mm) after approximately 36 treatments over 14-weeks. A 13-month follow-up indicated the patient remained well and reported no back pain and the corrections had remained stable.

Fedorchuk et al. [69] reported on the reduction of L1 (−6.6 to −1.7 mm) and L2 (−6.1 to −2.0 mm) retrolistheses and an L5 anterolisthesis (+6.8 to −2.5 mm) in a 63-year old female bodybuilder with severe LBP and osteoarthritis. Thirty treatments were given over 10-weeks which resulted in normalizing all spondylolistheses as well as a dramatic reduction in pain and an ability to leg press 60 more pounds in the gym.

Fedorchuk et al. reported the complete reduction of an L3 retrolisthesis and L4 anterolisthesis after 50 treatments over a 7-month period [70]. The patient was 57-years old with severe LBP and sciatica. The L3 retrolisthesis reduced from −5.3 to −1.7 and the L4 anterolisthesis reduced from +5.4 to +1.0 mm. After treatment the patient was able to return to playing hockey and experienced full resolution of the back pain which had forced him to retire from sport. A 1-year follow-up showed the patient had remained well and maintained the corrections.

8.4.2 Cervical spondylolisthesis

Recently, Fedorchuk et al. present a case series of eight female patients with concomitant cervical hypolordosis, forward head translation and spondylolistheses [71]. All were in motor vehicle collisions, each having at least one, and at most four simultaneous cervical vertebral spondylolistheses ranging in magnitude from >2 mm up to 4.5 mm. All cases experienced a reduction in translational offset of the spondylolistheses, and increase in cervical lordosis and a decrease in forward head translation as well as an increase in spinal canal diameter at the location of the spondylolisthesis after 30 treatment sessions that included cervical extension traction over a duration of 12-weeks. On average, the spondylolistheses reduced by 2.6 mm and there was an average drop in neck disability by 30%.

In another case, Fedorchuk et al. presented a single case of a 52-year old with chronic neck pain [72]. The patient had a C4 anterolisthesis of 2.4 mm which was reduced to 0.7 mm as well as an increase in cervical lordosis and reduction in forward head translation after 30 treatments over 12-weeks. The patient reported a resolution of their neck pain and stiffness.

8.4.3 Thoracic hyperkyphosis

Thoracic hyperkyphosis is a relatively common subluxation pattern in the aging. Although there is one RCT on CBP methods showing reduction of the deformity, it is yet to be formally published [52]. A systematic review of CBP methods used to reduce thoracic hyperkyphosis was published [73] and summarized the outcomes of several case reports and series [74–79]. In **Table 2** of the Oakley and Harrison review an average 12° reduction in thoracic kyphosis occurred after 32 treatments over 14.5 weeks from a total of 17 patients [52]. The improved posture correlated with reduced pain, disability and improved QOL [52]. **Figures 17** and **18** show various CBP mirror image spinal exercises and traction, respectively.

8.4.4 Thoracolumbar junctional kyphosis

Thoracolumbar kyphosis is the forward angled spine at the junction of the thoracic and lumbar spine and is associated with chronic LBP (CLBP). Gubbels et al.

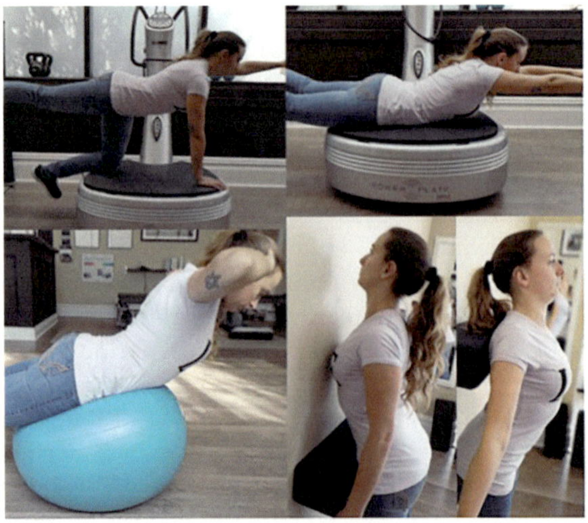

Figure 17.
CBP recommended mirror image exercises for patients with thoracic hyper-kyphosis.

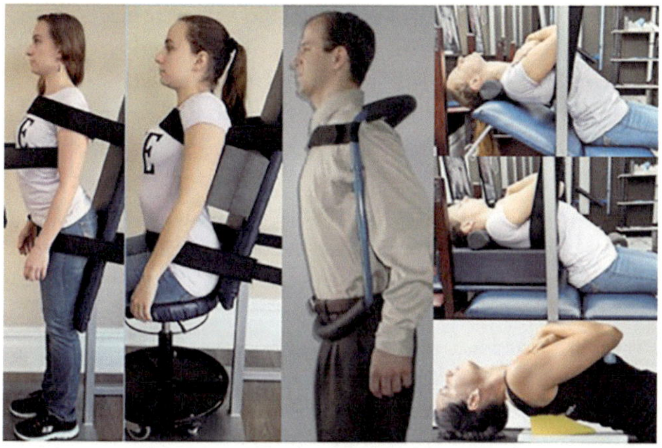

Figure 18.
CBP mirror image traction for patients with thoracic hyper-kyphosis.

presented a case of the minimization of pain in a 16-year old female after a 22° reduction of thoracolumbar kyphosis, a 48 mm reduction of posterior sagittal balance, an 11° increase in lumbar lordosis and a 10° increase in sacral inclination [80]. Twenty-four in office treatments were given over an 8-week period with daily home traction resulting in a minimization of back pains.

8.4.5 Thoracic hypokyphosis (straight back syndrome)

Thoracic spine hypolordosis is termed straight back syndrome (SBS) and is associated with back pains and exertional dyspnea. Fortner et al. [81] reported on an 18-year old male suffering from back pains and exertional dyspnea. Twenty-four treatments over a 9-week period resulted in a 15° increase in thoracic kyphosis, a decrease in pain and improved exertional dyspnea symptoms. A 4-month follow-up showed the patient remained well.

Betz et al. [82] reported the improvement in a 19-year old male who suffered from exertional dyspnea and back pain. Over 12-weeks a 14° increase in thoracic curve was achieved resulting in relief of exertional dyspnea and pain, as well as increases in both the antero-posterior thoracic diameter and the ratio of antero-posterior to transthoracic diameter, both measures critical to the wellbeing of patients with SBS. A 2.75-year follow-up showed the patient remained well.

Fedorchuk et al. [83] reported on a 13° increased thoracic curve in a 26-year old male with back pains and type 1 diabetes. Treatment over 7-weeks included 36 sessions. Back pains reduced and importantly, there was also improvement in blood glucose immediately following the onset of each visit. An improvement in blood glucose averages, percentage of time of blood glucose in a healthy target range, and glycosylated hemoglobin occurred and the patient was able to reduce their basal insulin need by approximately half after the 7-weeks of care.

Mitchel et al. [84] reported a 10° increase in thoracic curve over 16-weeks in a 33-year old male suffering from exertional dyspnea and back pains. The measured lung capacity improved by 2L, the back pain diminished and the exertional dyspnea resolved. A 7-month follow-up indicated the patient remained well.

8.4.6 Anterior sagittal balance

Anterior sagittal balance (ASB) is the forward displacement of the upper body over the pelvis. Haas et al. reported on the dramatic 110 mm reduction in ASB in an 87-year old female with CLBP and sciatica [85]. Treatment consisted of 24 in office sessions over an 8-week period. The patient achieved a dramatic reduction of symptoms, improvements in flexibility and orthopedic testing.

Anderson et al. [86] reported on a 91 mm reduction in ASB in a 59-year old male patient suffering from a variety of symptoms associated with Parkinson's disease. Initial treatment involved 38 treatments over 5 months. The patient experienced significant improvements in multiple postural parameters, gait, balance, hand tremors, low back and knee pains and SF-36 values. A 21-month follow-up showed the patient remained essentially well and most of the initial postural improvements were maintained.

8.4.7 Lumbar kyphosis (flat back syndrome)

Flat back syndrome (FBS) is the anterior translation of the upper body and gross loss (or kyphosis) of the lumbar spine and is associated with high pain and disability. In a case series, Harrison and Oakley describe the significant restoration of lumbar lordosis in two patients suffering from debilitating CLBP from flat back syndrome [87]. One patient had a 50° lordosis improvement in 100 treatments over 20 weeks, the other had a 26° lordosis improvement in 70 treatments over 16.5 weeks. In the discussion section of the report, it was calculated that the treatment costs of the patients receiving CBP treatment versus the projected costs for the surgical procedures recommended to the two patients equated to only 1–8%; the authors stated "at first 70 or 100 treatments may be criticized as 'over-treatment,' however, considering the overall cost-effectiveness and positive patient outcomes, it certainly is not" [87].

8.4.8 Lumbar hyperlordosis

Although lumbar hypolordosis is the most common lumbar misalignment in those presenting with chronic LBP [10], lumbar hyperlordosis is also seen clinically. CBP methods can be directed at decreasing lumbar lordosis and its typically associated anteriorly rotated pelvis. In a recent case, Oakley et al. [88] presented a case demonstrating the relief of CLBP and hip pains after an 8° reduction in lumbar hyperlordosis, a 5° reduction in pelvic tilt and an accompanying 17 mm reduction of forward sagittal balance. This occurred over a period of 13 months and 73 total treatments.

8.4.9 Post-surgical cervical spine fusion

Post-surgical cervical spine intervertebral fusion is not a common finding in clinical practice however, it is occasionally encountered. Many of these patients continue to suffer years after the intervention. Harrison et al. [89] presented a case showing improvement in sagittal postural parameters which corresponded with improved clinical outcome in a 52-year old male. Over a 6-month period, a 6° increase in cervical lordosis was achieved as well as a 13 mm reduction in anterior head translation (AHT). These improvements were maintained at a 2.5-year follow-up.

Fedorchuk et al. [90] also presented a successful outcome in a 43-year old with a C5-6 intersegmental fusion. After 36 treatments over 3-months, there was a 13° increase in cervical lordosis, a 9 mm decrease in AHT and a 5 mm reduction in lateral head translation.

8.4.10 Scoliosis

Although too large of a topic to address in this chapter, CBP technique has a unique approach in the treatment of scoliosis [3]. CBP methods incorporates the 'non-commutative property of finite rotation angles under addition' to ascertain the order of postural movements to be prescribed in the mirror image treatment of this disorder. Harrison and Oakley described reductions in curve magnitude in five lumbar or thoracolumbar scoliosis patients ranging from 5° to 24° after 18–84 treatments [40]. All patients were female and ranged in age from 19 to 45 years.

Haggard et al. reported a 19° reduction in a thoracolumbar curve in a 15-year old female patient after 24 office treatments over 15-weeks. The patient also performed 45 at home spine blocking sessions as prescribed by the attending chiropractor [41]. The patients LBP and headaches were dramatically improved, and the curve was reduced to 8°.

9. Use of X-ray

Use of X-ray for spine analysis is essential for treating spine deformities, including with CBP technique methods. Historically, there has been concerns of carcinogenicity associated with X-ray use. Recently, however, new evidence has come to light showing that anti-X-ray sentiment stemming from the supposed carcinogenicity is based on flawed science [91–93]. The bottom line is the linear no-threshold (LNT) model used to support radiation risk analysis is not scientific as it is not consistent with current radiobiological data [94–98].

X-rays and CT scans deliver low-dose radiation doses (<200 mGy), and because of this they cannot cause cancer. This is because low-dose (versus high-dose) radiation exposures stimulate the adaptive repair systems of the body to repair any damage done [99–101]. Although this topic is important, it is a much larger issue than the scope of this chapter but many recent reviews have found that X-rays (and CT scans) are not harmful. In fact, after a substantial and critical review of higher quality studies on radiation exposure, Schultz et al. concluded: "The evidence suggests that exposure to multiple CT scans and other sources of low-dose radiation with a cumulative dose up to 100 mSv (approximately 10 scans), and possibly as high as 200 mSv (approximately 20 scans), does not increase cancer risk." Thus, there should be no hesitation or misunderstanding surrounding X-ray risks. Doctors and patients need to become updated on X-ray safety and not succumb to the traditional carcinogenicity misinformation.

10. Conclusion

CBP technique is a well-studied approach to the structural improvement of spinal disorders. Many spinal disorders with associated pain and functional syndromes have either well characterized or evolving evidence for their treatment by the mirror image approach that underpins CBP methods. The correlation of the spine alignment and postural rotations and translations of posture are of critical importance and unique in the CBP approach.

Acknowledgements

We acknowledge the pioneering work of Dr. Donald D. Harrison.

Conflict of interest

D.E.H. teaches spine rehabilitation methods and sells products related to the treatment of spine deformities; P.A.O. is a paid consultant to CBP.

Nomenclature

AHT	anterior head translation
ASB	anterior sagittal balance
AP	anterior-to-posterior
ARA	absolute rotation angle
CBP	Chiropractic BioPhysics®
CLBP	chronic low back pain
HPT	Harrison posterior tangent
IVD	intervertebral disc
LBP	low back pain
LNT	linear no-threshold
nRCT	non-randomized controlled trial
QOL	quality of life
PA	posterior-to-anterior
PNF	proprioceptive neuromuscular facilitation
RCT	randomized controlled trial
RRA	relative rotation angle
SEM	standard error of measurement
SBS	straight back syndrome

Author details

Deed E. Harrison[1] and Paul A. Oakley[2]*

1 CBP NonProfit, Inc., Eagle, Idaho, USA

2 Private Practice, Newmarket, Ontario, Canada

*Address all correspondence to: docoakley.icc@gmail.com

References

[1] Harrison DD, Janik TJ, Harrison GR, Troyanovich S, Harrison DE, Harrison SO. Chiropractic biophysics technique: A linear algebra approach to posture in chiropractic. Journal of Manipulative and Physiological Therapeutics. 1996;**19**(8):525-535

[2] Harrison DE, Harrison DD, Haas JW. Structural Rehabilitation of the Cervical Spine. Evanston, WY: Harrison CBP® Seminars, Inc.; 2002

[3] Harrison DE, Betz JW, Harrison DD, et al. CBP Structural Rehabilitation of the Lumbar Spine. Eagle, ID, USA: Harrison Chiropractic Biophysics Seminars; 2007

[4] Oakley PA, Harrison DD, Harrison DE, Haas JW. Evidence-based protocol for structural rehabilitation of the spine and posture: Review of clinical biomechanics of posture (CBP) publications. Journal of the Canadian Chiropractic Association. 2005;**49**(4):270-296

[5] Oakley PA, Moustafa IM, Harrison DE. Restoration of Cervical and Lumbar Lordosis: CBP® Methods Overview. In: Bettany-Saltikov J, Kandasamy G, editors. Spinal Deformities in Adolescents, Adults and Older Adults [Internet]. London: IntechOpen; 2019 [cited 2022 Apr 26]. DOI: 10.5772/intechopen.90713

[6] Panjabi MM, White AA 3rd, Brand RA Jr. A note on defining body parts configurations. Journal of Biomechanics. 1974;7(4):385-387

[7] Harrison DD, Jackson BL, Troyanovich S, Robertson G, de George D, Barker WF. The efficacy of cervical extension-compression traction combined with diversified manipulation and drop table adjustments in the rehabilitation of cervical lordosis: A pilot study. Journal of Manipulative and Physiological Therapeutics. 1994;**17**(7): 454-464

[8] Harrison DE, Cailliet R, Harrison DD, Janik TJ, Holland B. A new 3-point bending traction method for restoring cervical lordosis and cervical manipulation: A nonrandomized clinical controlled trial. Archives of Physical Medicine and Rehabilitation. 2002;**83**(4):447-453

[9] Harrison DE, Harrison DD, Betz JJ, Janik TJ, Holland B, Colloca CJ, et al. Increasing the cervical lordosis with chiropractic biophysics seated combined extension-compression and transverse load cervical traction with cervical manipulation: Nonrandomized clinical control trial. Journal of Manipulative and Physiological Therapeutics. 2003;**26**(3):139-151

[10] Harrison DE, Cailliet R, Harrison DD, Janik TJ, Holland B. Changes in sagittal lumbar configuration with a new method of extension traction: Nonrandomized clinical controlled trial. Archives of Physical Medicine and Rehabilitation. 2002;**83**(11):1585-1591

[11] CBP NonProfit. www.cbpnonprofit.com.

[12] Beer FP, Johnston ER. Vector Mechanics for Engineers: Statics and Dynamics. 4th ed. New York: McGraw-Hill; 1984. p. 95

[13] Harrison DD. Abnormal postural permutations calculated as rotations and translations from an ideal normal upright static spine. In: Sweere J, editor. Chiropractic Family Practice. Gaitherburg, MD: Aspen Publishers; 1992

[14] Harrison DE, Betz JW, Cailliet R, Colloca CJ, Harrison DD, Haas JW, et al. Radiographic pseudoscoliosis in healthy male subjects following voluntary lateral translation (side glide) of the thoracic spine. Archives of Physical Medicine and Rehabilitation. 2006;**87**(1): 117-122

[15] Harrison DE, Cailliet R, Betz JW, Harrison DD, Colloca CJ, Haas JW, et al. A non-randomized clinical control trial of Harrison mirror image methods for correcting trunk list (lateral translations of the thoracic cage) in patients with chronic low back pain. European Spine Journal. 2005;**14**(2):155-162

[16] Henshaw M, Oakley PA, Harrison DE. Correction of pseudoscoliosis (lateral thoracic translation posture) for the treatment of low back pain: A CBP® case report. Journal of Physical Therapy Science. 2018;**30**(9):1202-1205

[17] Harrison DD, Janik TJ, Troyanovich SJ, Holland B. Comparisons of lordotic cervical spine curvatures to a theoretical ideal model of the static sagittal cervical spine. Spine. 1996;**21**(6):667-675

[18] Harrison DD, Janik TJ, Troyanovich SJ, Harrison DE, Colloca CJ. Evaluations of the assumptions used to derive an ideal normal cervical spine model. Journal of Manipulative and Physiological Therapeutics. 1997;**20**(4):246-256

[19] Harrison DD, Harrison DE, Janik TJ, Cailliet R, Haas JW, Ferrantelli J, et al. Modeling of the sagittal cervical spine as a method to discriminate hypolordosis: Results of elliptical and circular modeling in 72 asymptomatic subjects, 52 acute neck pain subjects, and 70 chronic neck pain subjects. Spine. 2004;**29**:2485-2492

[20] Harrison DE, Janik TJ, Harrison DD, Cailliet R, Harmon S. Can the thoracic kyphosis be modeled with a simple geometric shape? The results of circular and elliptical modeling in 80 asymptomatic subjects. Journal of Spinal Disorders. 2002;**15**(3):213-220

[21] Harrison DE, Harrison DD, Janik TJ, Cailliet R, Haas JW. Do alterations in vertebral and disc dimensions affect an elliptical model of the thoracic kyphosis? Spine. 2003;**28**(5):463-469

[22] Troyanovich SJ, Cailliet R, Janik TJ, Harrison DD, Harrison DE. Radiographic mensuration characteristics of the sagittal lumbar spine from a normal population with a method to synthesize prior studies of lordosis. Journal of Spinal Disorders. 1997;**10**(5):380-386

[23] Janik TJ, Harrison DD, Cailliet R, Troyanovich SJ, Harrison DE. Can the sagittal lumbar curvature be closely approximated by an ellipse? Journal of Orthopaedic Research. 1998;**16**(6): 766-770

[24] Harrison DD, Cailliet R, Janik TJ, Troyanovich SJ, Harrison DE, Holland B. Elliptical modeling of the sagittal lumbar lordosis and segmental rotation angles as a method to discriminate between normal and low back pain subjects. Journal of Spinal Disorders. 1998;**11**(5):430-439

[25] Harrison DE, Harrison DD, Cailliet R, et al. Cobb method or Harrison posterior tangent method: which to choose for lateral cervical radiographic analysis. Spine. 2000;**25**:2072-2078

[26] Harrison DE, Cailliet R, Harrison DD, et al. Reliability of centroid, Cobb, and Harrison posterior tangent methods: Which to choose for analysis of thoracic kyphosis. Spine. 2001;**26**:E227-E234

[27] Harrison DE, Harrison DD, Cailliet R, et al. Radiographic analysis of lumbar lordosis: Centroid, Cobb, TRALL, and Harrison posterior tangent methods. Spine. 2001;**26**:E235-E242

[28] Harrison DE, Holland B, Harrison DD, et al. Further reliability analysis of the Harrison radiographic line drawing methods: Crossed ICCs for lateral posterior tangents and AP modified-Risser Ferguson. Journal of Manipulative and Physiological Therapeutics. 2002;**25**:93-98

[29] McAviney J, Schulz D, Bock R, Harrison DE, Holland B. Determining the relationship between cervical lordosis and neck complaints. Journal of Manipulative and Physiological Therapeutics. 2005;**28**(3):187-193

[30] Keller TS, Colloca CJ, Harrison DE, Harrison DD, Janik TJ. Influence of spine morphology on intervertebral disc loads and stresses in asymptomatic adults: Implications for the ideal spine. The Spine Journal. 2005;**5**(3):297-309

[31] Harrison DE, Colloca CJ, Harrison DD, Janik TJ, Haas JW, Keller TS. Anterior thoracic posture increases thoracolumbar disc loading. European Spine Journal. 2005;**14**(3): 234-242

[32] Keller TS, Harrison DE, Colloca CJ, Harrison DD, Janik TJ. Prediction of osteoporotic spinal deformity. Spine. 2003;**28**(5):455-462

[33] Harrison DE, Harrison DD, Janik TJ, William Jones E, Cailliet R, Normand M. Comparison of axial and flexural stresses in lordosis and three buckled configurations of the cervical spine. Clinical Biomechanics. 2001;**16**(4): 276-284

[34] Harrison DE, Jones EW, Janik TJ, Harrison DD. Evaluation of axial and flexural stresses in the vertebral body cortex and trabecular bone in lordosis and two sagittal cervical translation configurations with an elliptical shell model. Journal of Manipulative and Physiological Therapeutics. 2002;**25**(6): 391-401

[35] Harrison DE, Harrison DD, Cailliet R, Janik TJ, Troyanovich SJ. Cervical coupling during lateral head translations creates an S-configuration. Clinical Biomechanics (Bristol, Avon). 2000;**15**(6):436-440

[36] Harrison DE, Cailliet R, Harrison DD, Janik TJ, Troyanovich SJ, Coleman RR. Lumbar coupling during lateral translations of the thoracic cage relative to a fixed pelvis. Clinical Biomechanics (Bristol, Avon). 1999;**14**(10):704-709

[37] Harrison DE, Cailliet R, Harrison DD, Janik TJ. How do anterior/ posterior translations of the thoracic cage affect the sagittal lumbar spine, pelvic tilt, and thoracic kyphosis? European Spine Journal. 2002;**11**(3): 287-293

[38] Harrison DE, Harrison DD, Haas JW, Oakley PA. Spinal Biomechanics for Clinicians. Vol. I. Evanston, WY: Harrison Chiropractic Biophysics Seminars, Inc.; 2003

[39] Oakley PA, Cuttler JM, Harrison DE. X-ray imaging is essential for contemporary chiropractic and manual therapy spinal rehabilitation: Radiography increases benefits and reduces risks. Dose-Response. 2018;**16**(2):1559325818781437

[40] Harrison DE, Oakley PA. Scoliosis deformity reduction in adults: A CBP® Mirror image® case series incorporating the 'non-commutative property of finite rotation angles under addition' in five patients with lumbar and thoraco-lumbar scoliosis. Journal of Physical Therapy Science. 2017;**29**(11):2044-2050

[41] Haggard JS, Haggard JB, Oakley PA, Harrison DE. Reduction of progressive thoracolumbar adolescent idiopathic scoliosis by chiropractic biophysics® (CBP®) mirror image® methods following failed traditional chiropractic treatment: A case report. Journal of Physical Therapy Science. 2017;**29**(11): 2062-2067

[42] Harrison DE, Cailliet R, Betz J, Haas JW, Harrison DD, Janik TJ, et al. Conservative methods for reducing lateral translation postures of the head: A nonrandomized clinical control trial. Journal of Rehabilitation Research and Development. 2004;**41**(4):631-639

[43] Moustafa IM, Diab AA, Hegazy F, Harrison DE. Demonstration of central conduction time and neuroplastic changes after cervical lordosis rehabilitation in asymptomatic subjects: A randomized, placebo-controlled trial. Scientific Reports. 2021;**11**(1):15379

[44] Moustafa IM, Diab A, Shousha T, Harrison DE. Does restoration of sagittal cervical alignment improve cervicogenic headache pain and disability: A 2-year pilot randomized controlled trial. Heliyon. 2021;**7**(3): e06467

[45] Moustafa I, Youssef ASA, Ahbouch A, Harrison DE. Demonstration of autonomic nervous function and cervical sensorimotor control after cervical lordosis rehabilitation: A randomized controlled trial. Journal of Athletic Training. 2021;**56**(3):10

[46] Moustafa IM, Diab AA, Hegazy F, Harrison DE. Does improvement towards a normal cervical sagittal configuration aid in the management of cervical myofascial pain syndrome: A 1-year randomized controlled trial. BMC Musculoskeletal Disorders. 2018;**19**(1):396

[47] Moustafa IM, Diab AA, Harrison DE. The effect of normalizing the sagittal cervical configuration on dizziness, neck pain, and cervicocephalic kinesthetic sensibility: A 1-year randomized controlled study. European Journal of Physical and Rehabilitation Medicine. 2017;**53**(1):57-71

[48] Moustafa IM, Diab AAM, Hegazy FA, Harrison DE. Does rehabilitation of cervical lordosis influence sagittal cervical spine flexion extension kinematics in cervical spondylotic radiculopathy subjects? Journal of Back and Musculoskeletal Rehabilitation. 2017;**30**(4):937-941

[49] Moustafa IM, Diab AA, Taha S, Harrison DE. Addition of a sagittal cervical posture corrective orthotic device to a multimodal rehabilitation program improves short- and long-term outcomes in patients with discogenic cervical radiculopathy. Archives of Physical Medicine and Rehabilitation. 2016;**97**(12):2034-2044

[50] Moustafa IM. Does improvement towards a normal cervical configuration aid in the management of fibromyalgia. A randomized controlled trial. Bulletin of Faculty of Pharmacy, Cairo University. 2013;**18**(2):29-41

[51] Moustafa IM, Diab AM, Ahmed A, Harrison DE. The efficacy of cervical lordosis rehabilitation for nerve root function, pain, and segmental motion in cervical spondylotic radiculopathy. Physiotherapy. 2011;**97**(supplment): 846-847

[52] Moustafa IM, Walton LM, Raigangir V, Shousha TM, Harrison D. Reduction of posture hyperkyphosis improves short- and long-term outcomes in patients with neck pain. Abstract: International Journal of Orthopaedic & Sports Physical Therapy. 2020;**50**(1):CSM143

[53] Diab AAM, Moustafa IM. The efficacy of lumbar extension traction for sagittal alignment in mechanical low back pain: A randomized trial. Journal of Back and Musculoskeletal Rehabilitation. 2013;**26**(2):213-220

[54] Moustafa IM, Diab AA. Extension traction treatment for patients with discogenic lumbosacral radiculopathy: A randomized controlled trial. Clinical Rehabilitation. 2012;**27**(1):51-62

[55] Diab AA, Moustafa IM. Lumbar lordosis rehabilitation for pain and lumbar segmental motion in chronic mechanical low back pain: A randomized trial. Journal of Manipulative and Physiological Therapeutics. 2012;**35**(4):246-253

[56] Oakley PA, Ehsani NN, Moustafa IM, Harrison DE. Restoring

lumbar lordosis: A systematic review of controlled trials utilizing Chiropractic Bio Physics® (CBP®) non-surgical approach to increasing lumbar lordosis in the treatment of low back disorders. Journal of Physical Therapy Science. 2020;**32**(9):601-610

[57] Oakley PA, Ehsani NN, Moustafa IM, Harrison DE. Restoring cervical lordosis by cervical extension traction methods in the treatment of cervical spine disorders: A systematic review of controlled trials. Journal of Physical Therapy Science. 2021;**33**(10):784-794.

[58] Haas JW, Oakley PA, Harrison DE. Cervical pseudo-scoliosis reduction and alleviation of dystonia symptoms using chiropractic BioPhysics® (CBP®) technique: A case report with a 1.5-year follow-up. The Journal of Contemporary Chiropractic. 2019;2:131-137

[59] Jaeger JO, Oakley PA, Moore RR, Ruggeroli EP, Harrison DE. Resolution of temporomandibular joint dysfunction (TMJD) by correcting a lateral head translation posture following previous failed traditional chiropractic therapy: A CBP® case report. Journal of Physical Therapy Science. 2018;**30**(1):103-107

[60] Oakley PA, Harrison DE. Alleviation of pain and disability in a post-surgical C4-C7 total fusion patient after reducing a lateral head translation (side shift) posture: A CBP® case report with a 14 year follow-up. Journal of Physical Therapy Science. 2018;**30**(7):952-957

[61] Berry RH, Oakley P, Harrison D. Alleviation of radiculopathy by structural rehabilitation of the cervical spine by correcting a lateral head translation posture (-TxH) using Berry translation traction as a part of CBP methods: A case report. The Chiropractic Journal of Australia. 2017;**45**(1):63-72

[62] Berry RH, Oakley PA, Harrison DE. Alleviation of chronic headaches by correcting lateral head translation posture (-TxH) using Chiropractic Biophysics & Berry Translation Traction. Annals of Vertebral Subluxation Research. 2017;(1-2):87-92.

[63] Oakley PA, Berry RH, Harrison DE. A structural approach to the postsurgical laminectomy case. Journal of Vertebral Subluxation Research. 2007;(March 19):1-7.

[64] Nuckols TK, Lim YW, Wynn BO, et al. Rigorous development does not ensure that guidelines are acceptable to a panel of knowledgeable providers. Journal of General Internal Medicine. 2008;**23**(1):37-44

[65] Rome P, Waterhouse JD. An evidence-based narrative of the evidence-base *concept*. Asia-Pacific Chiropractic Journal. 2020;**1**:004. https://doi.org/10.46323/2021004

[66] Ebrall P, Doyle M. The value of case reports as clinical evidence. The Chiropractic Journal of Australia. 2020;**47**(1):29-43

[67] Fedorchuk C, Lightstone DF, McRae C, Kaczor D. Correction of grade 2 spondylolisthesis following a non-surgical structural spinal rehabilitation protocol using lumbar traction: A case study and selective review of literature. Journal of Radiology Case Reports. 2017;**11**(5):13-26

[68] Oakley PA, Harrison DE. Correction of multilevel lumbar retrolistheses by non-surgical extension traction procedures in a patient with congenital fusion of L5-S1: A CBP® case report with a 13-month follow-up. The Journal of Contemporary Chiropractic. 2020;**3**(1):137-142

[69] Fedorchuk C, Haugen H. Reduction in three levels of lumbar degenerative spondylolisthesis following chiropractic care: A case report & review of the literature. Annals of Vertebral Subluxation Research. 2020;(Dec. 3):165-170.

[70] Fedorchuk CA, Lightstone DF, Oakley PA, Harrison DE. Correction of a double spondylolisthesis of the lumbar spine utilizing chiropractic biophysics® technique: A case report with 1-year follow-up. Journal of Physical Therapy Science. 2021;**33**(1):89-93

[71] Fedorchuk C, Lightstone DF, DeVon CR, Katz E, Wilcox J. Improvements in cervical spinal canal diameter and neck disability following correction of cervical lordosis and cervical spondylolistheses using chiropractic BioPhysics technique: A case series. Journal of Radiology Case Reports. 2020;**14**(4):21-37

[72] Fedorchuk C, Lightstone D. Reduction in cervical anterolisthesis & pain in a 52-year-old female using chiropractic biophysics® technique: A case study and selective review of literature. Annals of Vertebral Subluxation Research. 2016;**3**:118-124

[73] Oakley PA, Harrison DE. Reducing thoracic Hyperkyphosis subluxation deformity: A systematic review of chiropractic BioPhysics® methods employed in its structural improvement. The Journal of Contemporary Chiropractic. 2018;**1**(1):59-66

[74] Fortner MO, Oakley PA, Harrison DE. Alleviation of chronic spine pain and headaches by reducing forward head posture and thoracic hyperkyphosis: A CBP® case report. Journal of Physical Therapy Science. 2018;**30**(8):1117-1123

[75] Oakley PA, Jaeger JO, Brown JE, Polatis TA, Clarke JG, Whittler CD, et al. The CBP® mirror image® approach to reducing thoracic hyperkyphosis: A retrospective case series of 10 patients. Journal of Physical Therapy Science. 2018;**30**(8):1039-1045

[76] Fortner MO, Oakley PA, Harrison DE. Treating 'slouchy' (hyperkyphosis) posture with chiropractic biophysics®: A case report utilizing a multimodal mirror image® rehabilitation program. Journal of Physical Therapy Science. 2017;**29**(8): 1475-1480

[77] Miller JE, Oakley PA, Levin SB, Harrison DE. Reversing thoracic hyperkyphosis: A case report featuring mirror image® thoracic extension rehabilitation. Journal of Physical Therapy Science. 2017;**29**(7):1264-1267

[78] Fedorchuk C, Snow E. Reduction in thoracic hyperkyphosis with increased peak expiratory flow (PEF), forced expiratory volume (FEV) and SF-36 scores following CBP protocols in asymptomatic patients: A case series. Annals of Vertebral Subluxation Research. 2017;(Oct. 12):189-200.

[79] Jaeger JO, Oakley PA, Colloca CJ, et al. Non-surgical reduction of thoracic hyper-kyphosis in a 24-year old music teacher utilizing chiropractic biophysics® technique. British Journal of Medicine and Medical Research. 2016;**11**:1-9

[80] Gubbels CM, Werner JT, Oakley PA, Harrison DE. Reduction of thoraco-lumbar junctional kyphosis, posterior sagittal balance, and increase of lumbar lordosis and sacral inclination by chiropractic BioPhysics® methods in an adolescent with back pain: A case report. Journal of Physical Therapy Science. 2019;**31**(10):839-843

[81] Fortner MO, Oakley PA, Harrison DE. Chiropractic biophysics management of straight back syndrome and exertional dyspnea: A case report with follow-up. The Journal of Contemporary Chiropractic. 2019;**2**:115-122

[82] Betz JW, Oakley PA, Harrison DE. Relief of exertional dyspnea and spinal pains by increasing the thoracic kyphosis in straight back syndrome (thoracic hypo-kyphosis) using CBP® methods: A case report with long-term

follow-up. Journal of Physical Therapy Science. 2018;**30**(1):185-189

[83] Fedorchuk C, Lightstone DF, Comer RD, Weiner MT, McCoy M. Improved glycosylated hemoglobin, hyperglycemia, and quality of life following thoracic hypokyphosis vertebral subluxation correction using Chiropractic BioPhysics®: A prospective case report. Journal of Diabetes & Metabolism. 2018;**9**(10):1-10

[84] Mitchell JR, Oakley PA, Harrison DE. Nonsurgical correction of straight back syndrome (thoracic hypokyphosis), increased lung capacity and resolution of exertional dyspnea by thoracic hyperkyphosis mirror image® traction: A CBP® case report. Journal of Physical Therapy Science. 2017;**29**(11):2058-2061

[85] Haas JW, Harrison DE, Oakley PA. Non-surgical reduction in anterior sagittal balance subluxation and improvement in overall posture in a geriatric suffering from low back pain and sciatica: A CBP® case report. The Journal of Contemporary Chiropractic. 2020;**3**(1):45-50

[86] Anderson JM, Oakley PA, Harrison DE. Improving posture to reduce the symptoms of Parkinson's: A CBP® case report with a 21 month follow-up. Journal of Physical Therapy Science. 2019;**31**(2):153-158

[87] Harrison DE, Oakley PA. Non-operative correction of flat back syndrome using lumbar extension traction: A CBP® case series of two. Journal of Physical Therapy Science. 2018;**30**(8):1131-1137

[88] Oakley PA, Ehsani NN, Harrison DE. Non-surgical reduction of lumbar hyperlordosis, forward sagittal balance and sacral tilt to relieve low back pain by Chiropractic BioPhysics® methods: A case report. Journal of Physical Therapy Science. 2019;**31**(10): 860-864

[89] Harrison DE, Oakley PA, Betz JW. Anterior head translation following cervical fusion-a probable cause of post-surgical pain and impairment: A CBP® case report. Journal of Physical Therapy Science. 2018;**30**(2):271-276

[90] Fedorchuk C, Lightstone DF, Andino H. Failed neck surgery: Improvement in neck pain, migraines, energy levels, and performance of activities of daily living following subluxation correction using Chiropractic Biophysics® Technique: A case study. Annals of Vertebral Subluxation Research. 2017;(May 18):93-100

[91] Calabrese EJ. Cancer risk assessment foundation unraveling: New historical evidence reveals that the US National Academy of Sciences (US NAS), biological effects of atomic radiation (BEAR) committee genetics panel falsified the research record to promote acceptance of the LNT. Archives of Toxicology. 2015;**89**(4):649-650

[92] Calabrese EJ. An abuse of risk assessment: How regulatory agencies improperly adopted LNT for cancer risk assessment. Archives of Toxicology. 2015;**89**(4):647-648

[93] Calabrese EJ. On the origins of the linear no-threshold (LNT) dogma by means of untruths, artful dodges and blind faith. Environmental Research. 2015;**142**:432-442

[94] Scott BR, Sanders CL, Mitchel REJ, Boreham DR. CT scans may reduce rather than increase risk of cancer. The Journal of the American Physicians and Surgeons. 2008;**13**(1):8-11

[95] Lemon JA, Phan N, Boreham DR. Single CT scan prolongs survival by extending cancer latency in Trp53 heterozygous mice. Radiation Research. 2017;**188**(4.2):505-511

[96] Lemon JA, Phan N, Boreham DR. Multiple CT scans extend lifespan by

delaying cancer progression in cancer-prone mice. Radiation Research. 2017;**188**(4.2):495-504

[97] Cuttler JM. Application of low doses of ionizing radiation in medical therapies. Dose-Response. 2020;**18**(1):1559325819895739

[98] Calabrese EJ, Dhawan G, Kapoor R, Kozumbo WJ. Radiotherapy treatment of human inflammatory diseases and conditions: Optimal dose. Human & Experimental Toxicology. 2019;**38**(8): 888-898

[99] Pollycove M, Feinendegen LE. Radiation-induced versus endogenous DNA damage: Possible effect of inducible protective responses in mitigating endogenous damage. Human and Experimental Toxicology. 2003;**22**(6):290-306

[100] Pollycove M. Radiobiological basis of low-dose irradiation in prevention and therapy of cancer. Dose-Response. 2006;**5**(1):26-38

[101] Feinendegen LE, Cuttler JM. Biological effects from low doses and dose rates of ionizing radiation: Science in the service of protecting humans, a synopsis. Health Physics. 2018;**114**(6): 623-626

Chapter 9

Complementary Treatment for Women with Breast Cancer: A Psychomotor Therapy Approach

Guida Veiga and Graça Duarte Santos

Abstract

Women with breast cancer face a diversity of physical, psychological, and social changes that affect their health and well-being across the different stages of the cancer journey, including treatment and survival. Moreover, breast cancer often results in greater distress than any other neoplasm, challenging women's body, identity, and quality of life. Given the multiplicity of mind–body related problems that may confront women with breast cancer, psychomotor therapy is a valuable therapeutic approach for these women. This chapter presents a framework based on psychological and neurobiological research to understand how a mind–body approach as psychomotor therapy improves cancer-related symptoms, readjusts body schema, body image and identity, thus contributing to women with breast cancer's health and well-being. Two intervention programs, uniquely designed as a complementary approach of medical care for women in the treatment and survival phases, are also described. The impact of these programs on health and quality of life indicators of women with breast cancer are also presented.

Keywords: mind–body, oncology, psychomotricity, body image, health, quality of life

1. Introduction

Breast cancer is the most prevalent malignancy and is also the most common cause of death in women. In 2020 around 2.3 million cases were diagnosed, there were 7.8 million women alive with a breast cancer diagnosis made in the last 5 years and 685 thousand estimated deaths [1]. The rates of curative treatment and overall survival have also been increasing, and the prognosis has been improving [2]. Nevertheless, diagnosis and multiple treatments come with short- and long-term adverse physical and psychological effects that affect the quality of life of patients and survivors [3, 4].

Either present or absent, the breast is a significantly visual body part [5]. The breast is also a highly symbolic organ associated with motherhood, femininity, and self-image. These symbols evoke dimensions that range from nutrition to eroticism across multiple cultures [6]. Therefore, the diagnosis of breast cancer has a profound physical and psychosocial impact on women. That is, an attack on the integrity of the woman's breast is more than a physical attack, but also an attack to the femininity symbol, bearing a notable intimate, social and cultural significance [6] and impacting socio-emotional well-being [7].

Going through the entire post-diagnostic and therapeutic period often implies taking a transformative journey through a suspended femininity, lived in a different body. The concept of body goes beyond its physical dimension and should be replaced by the concept of corporeality, which is related to an existential perspective of the body, that encompasses multiple dimensions of the human being, such as the physical body, the mental and the spiritual dimension [8]. Merleau Ponty's model allows a perspective on the person beyond the 'biomedical' perspective or even the 'psychological' perspective. The body itself, the sick body in breast cancer, is considered a space of existence where many dynamics intersect and are experienced: internal and external, past and present, anticipated and bereaved, accompanied and lonely. Hence, breast cancer should be considered from a holistic perspective, enabling the connection of the different mind–body dimensions. Such an integrative approach will result in integrated interventions that allow women with breast cancer to rediscover and rebuild themselves in this new body throughout a transformative journey.

2. Breast cancer: a challenge to women's body, identity and quality of life

Breast cancer treatment often involves several long-term interventions. Typically, it involves a surgery (mastectomy or lumpectomy), followed by additional therapies that may include chemotherapy alone or in combination, radiotherapy and hormone therapy. These treatments lead to several side effects such as changes or loss of one or both breasts, visible scars, hair, eyebrows and eyelashes loss, lymphedema, increased body weight and difficulty getting used to prostheses [9, 10]. Therefore, the various dimensions of the body are affected in its functionality and shape (or disshape). Besides, the imminence of a terminus of that body is a constant. Henceforth, survivors tend to be hypervigilant of their bodily sensations, which is even more intense before the routine exams due to the fear of cancer recurrence [11]. All the treatments and associated effects significantly impact women with breast cancer's body schema and body image [3, 12, 13]. In breast cancer, all cognitive survival schemes and bodily schemes interact in a complex way throughout the process of adjustment to the disease and the survival phase [14].

Body image is considered as the mental image of the body, the subjective perception of one's physical and appearance, health status, normal bodily functioning and sexuality [15]. Body image is also related to other dynamic elements, such as the subjective perspective of one's opening or distancing to others, the dimensions of tension/relaxation, activity/passivity and to the perception of femininity/masculinity [16]. Considering the context of a potentially deadly disease and associated decreased vital energy, loss or change of body and role in family, social and professional milieus, breast cancer is, therefore, a real test to one's body image, which is itself the foundation of identity. In fact, research shows that 77% of women with breast cancer have body image disturbances that persist beyond cancer treatments and reconstructive surgeries [10]. These disturbances are even more significant in women undergoing more radical surgeries. For example, six months after a mastectomy, only 63% of the women feel comfortable when fully clothed, and 21% feel comfortable when unclothed [14].

The body image disturbances and the organic factors (e.g., decreased sexual desire) associated to breast cancer have a significant impact on intimate relationships [3] and sexuality itself [17]. It is important to note that sexuality goes beyond sexual activity but mostly to intimacy. It is related to the experience of an interiority expressed to the other in a corporeal dimension, involving the real body and the imaginary body. The surgery often brings psychological distress accompanied by a feeling of emotional rupture that extends to the intimate relationship with the partner. Moreover, the various effects of chemotherapy (e.g., fatigue, weight changes, alopecia) also impact sexual health and intimate relationships. Also, hormone therapy, which often extends throughout time (5 or 10 years), is responsible for profound changes in sexual desire. In fact, high rates of sexual disturbances have been reported in women's breast cancer: around 70% of sexual dysfunctions and 30% of other sexual complaints throughout the treatment and the survival phases [18].

Moreover, the uncertainty, fear, pain, fatigue, discomfort, sleep disturbances and cognitive impairment associated with a breast cancer diagnosis and treatment result in anxiety and depressive symptoms [19, 20]. These mental health symptoms are common at diagnosis and often become more intense with treatment burden and in the survival phase [21–23] and may affect the treatment, especially regarding compliance with treatment protocols, follow-up exams, and social and family routines [24].

In this pathway, it is also important to consider stress. From the diagnosis to the survival phase, stress is prevalent [25, 26]. Despite the low prevalence of post-traumatic stress disorder [27, 28], clinically significant symptoms are relatively common, and the diagnosis and the treatment are often experienced as traumatic [28, 29]. Although stress is an adaptive response of the body to internal or/and external challenges, prolonged exposure to stress conditions, such as a breast cancer diagnosis and/or associated treatment, leads to neuroendocrine dysregulations and immune dysfunctions [30]. Moreover, chronic stress can also affect behavioral processes and pathways involved in cancer progression [31] and block health-protective behaviors, such as adherence to treatments [22].

Finally, the adverse effects described above regarding physical and emotional wellbeing, along with the difficulties on social functioning [32], compromise the quality of life both in the treatment phase and in the survival phase [10, 33].

Either in the diagnosis, the treatment or the survival phase, the experience of a body limited by fatigue, pain, or even of a new/different/foreign body (i.e., with a prosthesis) involves mourning the previous body and readjusting the body scheme and the body image. Besides, all the changes associated with women's breast cancer are deeply rooted in a painful corporeality that embraces an interiority threatened by its continuity, visibility, and wellbeing. Therefore, dealing with breast cancer implies an internal and external recognition and readaptation to the new body and an internal symbolic reorganization of the female, intimate, and social identity [34].

3. The importance of body-oriented interventions for women with breast cancer

Treating women with breast cancer requires a multidimensional and continued approach throughout the various phases. In the first phase - the announcement of the diagnosis - it is essential to understand how the woman is experiencing her own body, helping her to locate vulnerabilities, disharmonies and difficult emotions and identify their origins. Therefore, a place for self-expression (verbal or non-verbal) supported and validated by a present and non-judgmental therapist is paramount. It is also crucial to support the discovery and the exploration of a new, more fragile, and less genitalized physical intimacy, preserving sensitive physical contact at the level of caresses and words. Besides, monitoring the maintenance of an adapted physical activity and encouraging relaxation and body care is also critical at this stressful phase [34, 35].

The second phase – treatments – is highly remarkable at the corporeal dimension. As mentioned before, in this phase, significant changes are felt at the experience of the real body (internal and external sensations) and the imaginary body (representations). Regarding the real body, it is important to minimize the impact of these physical (e.g., fatigue, physical discomfort) and esthetic changes. However, it is also essential to help them observe and relate to this "new" body, especially discovering good sensations in the body under attack. As in the previous phase, it is crucial to encourage and validate women's self-expression of the suffering and frustrations of this phase.

The perspective of being therapeutically supported should continue throughout the survival phase. In this phase, it is essential to support women to experience their bodies as autonomous, active, and relational, therefore fostering their self-esteem.

In all phases, it is essential to promote a positive experience of the body, so women with breast cancer can rediscover and reinvest in their bodies as a place of safety and pleasure. In this context, body-oriented interventions play a decisive role as they allow listening and observing bodily sensations as a starting and connecting point with the inner life.

The implementation of body-oriented interventions as complementary to cancer treatment has increased significantly, reflecting the growing interest in complementing medical treatment with other non-pharmacological approaches [36]. These interventions are reported to promote a better adaptation to the disease, the body and its new characteristics [37], contributing to symptoms' control and improving health status and quality of life [38].

Based on the body–mind relationship, psychomotor therapy is a body-oriented therapy that uses the body as the primary mediator to promote health and well-being. In psychomotor therapy, the body in movement and in relation supports sensory and psychic integration processes. Through various bodily mediations such as relaxation, therapeutic touch, play, body and artistic expression, psychomotor therapy helps the person feel, think, use and accommodate his/her body as a central platform of his/her emotions and inner life. This chapter focus two of these approaches implemented at different stages of breast cancer: psychomotor touch-massage regarding the treatment phase and psychomotor relaxation concerning the survival phase.

3.1 Psychomotor touch-massage

The therapeutic aims of psychomotor therapy go beyond bodily functionality and include developing the individual's bodily and psychic identity [39]. Therefore, psychomotor touch is more than a mechanical and segmented functional action, seeking to improve the body's functionality and relief physical pain. In psychomotor therapy, the physical, emotional, symbolic, and unconscious dimensions of touch are also considered. Hence, psychomotor touch also seeks to improve body schema and body image and relief emotional pain. The primary intention is, through touch, to communicate to the person that he/she is important, that his/her pain and fears are recognized and that there is a person, a therapist, who is interested in providing him/her sensations of relief and well-being. Thus, psychomotor touch offers an opportunity of feeling and integrating the pleasure of touch, the pleasure of being touched by someone who is interested (who invests) and who takes care of him/her [40].

Among a diversity of touch techniques, psychomotor touch-massage has proved to be an important complementary therapeutic approach to breast cancer treatment. The psychomotor massage-touch consists of a slow and gentle touch that conveys an embracing and structuring contact. The person is dressed, usually in a prone position with eyes closed. Touch is accompanied by passive mobilizations and micro-stretching of all body segments, emphasizing the extremities (finger and toes) and joints. Except for the erogenous zones, the whole body is mobilized, starting with the upper limbs, lower limbs, and the head. Respect for each person's body and personal space is a priority, and therefore the methodology is flexible. It is the method that adapts to the person and not the other way around. As the person relaxes, breathing and or stretching movements can be added, allowing for a more profound release of tension, and redirecting the person's attention to bodily sensations. Finally, a dialog about the sensory experience, the emotions and ideas derived during the psychomotor touch-massage is established [40].

As mentioned above, the treatment phase is a moment of suffering and loneliness, where the body is attacked from the outside and the inside. The gentil embracement and support provided by the psychomotor touch-massage is therefore particularly important in the treatment phase. It gives a pleasurable sensory experience, a pleasure experienced with another, and a communication, essentially on the non-verbal level, which secures and contains. The suffering body is thus supported, relieved, validated and revalued by the other. On the other hand, the support and balance provided by the touch provide a maternalization, as an internal momentum supported by the attentive, available and supporting presence of the therapist.

A program of psychomotor touch-massage was implemented with women with breast cancer during the treatment phase. The program involved two sessions per week for 8 weeks and was implemented at the oncology department of a Portuguese public hospital. At the end of the program, there were improvements in the quality of life of the women who participated in the program, compared to those who were part of the control group and, therefore, kept their usual routines [41]. Besides, qualitative analysis of interviews conducted at the end of the intervention revealed that all participants reported that touch-massage was helpful in their healing process. On the other hand, a large majority (84.62%) felt relief from the symptoms associated with the treatment, and reported to have changed the way they face their disease [42].

Other similar therapeutic approaches have also been shown to effectively improve perceived stress, cancer-related physical symptoms and mental health symptoms, including depression and anxiety [43–45]. Besides, similar touch-based approaches have also been shown to positively impact the neuroendocrine and immune systems of breast cancer patients and survivors, increasing dopamine and serotonin levels, NK cells and lymphocytes, and decreasing cortisol and beta-amylase concentrations [43, 44, 46].

3.2 Psychomotor relaxation

Psychomotor relaxation involves the regulation of the tonus and attention through several techniques, such as body awareness, muscular relaxation, or breathing techniques [47]. Through relaxation, the person can obtain neuromuscular relaxation in each part of the body, locating the tension and passivity in the different segments compared to the rest of the body and integrating what is felt in the tension and passivity phases. The therapist observes the tonic changes, facilitates the association between sensations, images and emotions and promotes reflection on the meaning of the tonic-emotional experience, thus facilitating the psychic elaboration of sensations [48]. Thus, the entire corporeality is mobilized, favoring a new experience of the body (real and imaginary). Psychomotor relaxation implies the presence of another, a therapist that recognizes, evaluates and values the person's intimate expression, as well as a relationship, a bond that stabilizes and provides the necessary security for the person's investment [49].

Unlike psychomotor touch-massage, relaxation sessions are characterized by the diversity of proposals and sensations experienced, which promote a progressive internal rediscovery of the body itself, as a source of pleasure, security, and possibility. This process is essential for the elaboration of the losses associated with breast cancer [50]. The woman discovers her body, an active and skilled body that she can use to feel better. Thus, while in the first sessions, relaxation is induced by the therapist, as the sessions progress the participants gain autonomy and actively relax their bodies and minds. This growing autonomy, supported by a continuous and secure therapeutic relationship, is fundamental in the survival phase, a phase in which treatments, consultations and social support suddenly cease, giving place to emptiness and an expected autonomy, often difficult to support.

Besides, the possibility of expressing the inner experience and incorporating such sensory and emotional experience in one's personal story and identity (past and present) is of paramount importance for women survivors of breast cancer, as it facilitates the literal and metaphorical communication of the experience and, therefore, its elaboration. When this communication and elaboration happens within a group, the therapeutic process becomes even more powerful. Indeed, the group context allows sharing experiences and the validation of one's feelings by similar others. In a group, members have an opportunity to see how others experience the same changes and emotions and cope with similar-or even worse -circumstances as themselves [51].

Participating in a therapeutic group also reduces social isolation and promotes social support. Social support can significantly impact stress management, adjustment to cancer, quality of life, and cancer-related symptoms [52, 53]. Support from other group members also generates a need to be available to support others and a sense of belonging and commitment to the group, which fosters a sense of meaning and increases the motivation for the session [37]. In fact, one of the main incentives for adherence to group intervention programs is the increase of social support and the decrease of social isolation provided by therapeutic groups for breast cancer survivors [54].

With the increase of cancer survivors and the associated need of improving their quality of life, some therapeutic relaxation programs have been developed. In particular, after an oncology department of a Portuguese public hospital identified the need to provide therapeutic support to breast cancer survivors, a psychomotor relaxation program was developed and implemented. Through movement, awareness, self-regulation and body expression, an affective and positive experience of the body, in a context of individual and collective construction, was provided to a group of women with breast cancer, aiming to improve their health, well-being and bodily and affective experience. The program involved group sessions of 45 minutes, twice a week, for 8 weeks. The sessions began with an initial dialog, in which the participants prepared for the session and could share their feelings. Then followed a moment of body centering and breathing regulation, in which exercises of body (and breathing) awareness and muscle relaxation were proposed. Then, a guided imagery moment enabled rediscovering the inner body and the pleasant sensations of calm, comfort, and satisfaction. Afterwards, body and attentional activation stretches were proposed. Finally, there was a moment for the expressive representation of the experienced sensations, which led to the final dialog, encouraging sharing emotions, difficulties, and life experiences [55].

The participants were always receptive and enthusiastic about the proposed activities throughout the program, becoming progressively autonomous. As the sessions progressed, they were increasingly able to focus attention on their bodies and particularly on bodily sensations and to regulate the moments of arousal, as well as to transpose the acquired skills to their daily life (e.g., relax in moments of greater anxiety, relax on sleepless nights to fall asleep). At the end of the program, significant improvements were revealed in physical (e.g., more vitality and less fatigue) and mental health, quality of life, body appreciation and interoceptive awareness [55].

In this study [55], variations in salivary cortisol concentrations between the beginning and the end of the session were analyzed. Although there were no significant changes at the beginning of the program, in the 15th session, there was a significant decrease from the beginning to the end of the session, indicating that the participants learned to self-regulate their stress levels effectively. Interestingly, the control group, which did not participate in the program, and kept their usual routines, faced a decrease in the health and quality of life indicators and affective experience of the body. These study showed that psychomotor relaxation effectively promotes the health and quality of life of women survivors of breast cancer. Not participating in relaxation sessions implies that health and quality of life indicators deteriorate throughout the survival phase [55].

Other studies have revealed that similar therapeutic approaches effectively decreased cancer-related symptoms (e.g., fatigue, pain, sleep) and inflammatory processes [54, 56, 57] and improved mental health symptoms [56–59]. Besides, other studies showed that therapeutic relaxation promotes social support, which results in increased social well-being [60].

4. Conclusions

Breast cancer is a significant challenge to women's body, identity and quality of life. All the changes associated with breast cancer are deeply rooted in a painful corporeality, threatened by its continuity, visibility and well-being. Therefore, either in the diagnosis, the treatment or the survival phase, the real body (internal and external) and the imaginary body must be carefully considered. Minimizing the impact of cancer on physical well-being is important. But mourning the previous body, rediscovering the pleasure and possibilities of the new body, and reorganizing the intimate and social identity is of paramount importance, bringing benefits for emotional and social well-being.

Psychomotor therapy is a beneficial, complementary approach to medical care for women with breast cancer. In the field of pain and psychosomatic changes, psychomotor therapy enables a unique experience of the body and a reconstruction of women's identity, which results in improved health and quality of life.

Acknowledgements

This work would not have been possible without the enthusiasm and involvement of Daniela Guerreiro, Joana Oliveira and Marta Fonseca, the psychomotor therapists who carried out the interventions described. We would also like to thank the women who participated in these programs, and the Oncology Department of the Hospital do Espírito Santo of Évora, especially Doctor Rui Dinis.

Author details

Guida Veiga[1,2]* and Graça Duarte Santos[1,2]

1 Departamento de Desporto e Saúde, Escola de Saúde e Desenvolvimento Humano, Universidade de Évora, Évora, Portugal

2 Comprehensive Health Research Centre, Universidade de Évora, Évora, Portugal

*Address all correspondence to: gveiga@uevora.pt

References

[1] World Health Organization. Breast cancer [Internet]. 2021. Available from: https://www.who.int/news-room/fact-sheets/detail/breast-cancer [Accessed: 2021-07-05]

[2] Siegel RL, Miller KD, Fuchs HE, Jemal A. Cancer statistics, 2021. CA: a cancer journal for clinicians. 2021;71:7-33. DOI: 10.3322/caac.21654

[3] Sebri V, Durosini I, Triberti S, Pravettoni G. The efficacy of psychological intervention on body image in breast cancer patients and survivors: A systematic-review and meta-analysis. Frontiers in Psychology. 2021;12:611954. DOI: 10.3389/fpsyg.2021.611954

[4] Von Ah D, Crouch AD, Monahan PO, Stump, TE, Unverzagt FW, Storey S, Coheen AA, Cella D, Champion VL. Association of cognitive impairment and breast cancer survivorship on quality of life in younger breast cancer survivors. Journal of Cancer Survivorship. 2021. DOI: 10.1007/s11764-021-01075-x

[5] Klein R, Siegers G, Woodman D. Erotic. Maternal. Cultural. Symbolic. Medical. What are breasts? How are they imagined? And who gets to decide? Imaginations: Revue d'Études Interculturelles de l'Image/ Imaginations: Journal of Cross-Cultural Image Studies. 2020;11:5-15. DOI: 10.17742/ IMAGE.BR.11.1.1

[6] Francequin G. Cancer du sein: une féminité à reconstruire. Toulouse: Éditions Érès; 2012. 268 p. DOI: 10.3917/eres.franc.2012.01

[7] Hanson Frost M, Suman VJ, Rummans TA, Dose AM, Taylor M, Novotny P, Johnson R, Evans RE. Physical, psychological and social well-being of women with breast cancer: the influence of disease phase. Psycho-Oncology: Journal of the Psychological, Social and Behavioral Dimensions of Cancer. 2000:9:221-231. DOI: 10.1002/1099-1611(200005/06)9:3<221::aid-pon456>3.0.co;2-t

[8] Merleau-Ponty M. Phénoménologie de la perception. Paris: Gallimard; 1976

[9] Rebelo V, Rolim L, Carqueja E, Ferreira S. Avaliação da qualidade de vida em mulheres com cancro da mama: um estudo exploratório com 60 mulheres portuguesas. Psicologia, Saúde & Doenças. 2007;8:13-32

[10] American Cancer Society. Cancer facts & figures 2019. Atlanta: American Cancer Society; 2019

[11] Yi J, Syrjala K. Anxiety and depression in cancer survivors. Medical Clinics Of North America. 2017;101:1099-1113. DOI: 10.1016/j.mcna.2017.06.005

[12] Cooling J. The Influence of body image on intervention with breast cancer patients [thesis]. Kentucky: Graduate School of Eastern Kentucky University; 2020

[13] Zhou K, Wang W, Li M, An J, Huo L, He X, Li J, Li X. Body image mediates the relationship between post-surgery needs and health-related quality of life among women with breast cancer: a cross-sectional study. Health and Quality of Life Outcomes. 2020;18:163. DOI: 10.1186/s12955-020-01400-5

[14] Moorey S. Breast cancer and body image. In: Nasser M, Baistow K., Treasure J, editors. The Female Body in Mind: The Interface Between The Female Body And Mental Health Routledge; 2007. p. 72-90. DOI: 10.4324/9780203939543

[15] Dolbeault S, Cayrou S, Brédart A, Viala A, Desclaux B, Saltel B,

Gauvain-Piquard A, Hardy P, Dickes P. The effectiveness of a psycho-educational group after early-stage breast cancer treatment: results of a randomized French study. Psycho-Oncology. 2009;18:647-656. DOI: 10.1002/pon.1440

[16] Bruchon-Schweitzer M. Une psychologie du corps. Paris: Presses Universitaires de France; 1990. 328 p. DOI: 10.3917/puf.bruch.1990.01

[17] Faria BM, Rodrigues IM, Marquez LV, Pires US, Oliveira SV. The impact of mastectomy on body image and sexuality in women with breast cancer: a systematic review. Psicooncología. 2021:18;91-115. DOI: 10.5209/psic.74534

[18] Rojas KE, Matthews N, Raker C, Clark MA, Onstad M, Stuckey A, Gass J. Body mass index (BMI), postoperative appearance satisfaction, and sexual function in breast cancer survivorship. Journal of Cancer Survivorship. 2018:12;127-133 DOI: 10.1007/s11764-017-0651-y

[19] Yousaf M, Farooq S, Rizwan B, Khalid S, Azhar S, Shahbaz A, Zubair R, Nasir H, Tariq T. Psychological consequences among female patients suffering from breast tumor. Journal of Humanities And Social Science. 2020:25;42-46. DOI: 10.9790/0837-2504034953

[20] Spiegel D, Riba M. Managing anxiety and depression during treatment. The Breast Journal. 2015:21;97-103. DOI: 10.1111/tbj.12355

[21] Conley C, Bishop B, Andersen B. Emotions and emotion regulation in breast cancer survivorship. Healthcare. 2016:4;56. DOI: 10.3390/healthcare4030056

[22] Ellis EM, Nelson WL, Ferrer RA. Trajectories of current and predicted satisfaction with one's life following a cancer diagnosis. Annals of Behavioral Medicine. 2019:53;158-168. DOI: 10.1093/abm/kay025

[23] Hack TF, Pickles T, Ruether JD, Weir L, Bultz BD, Mackey J, Degner LF. Predictors of distress and quality of life in patients undergoing cancer therapy: impact of treatment type and decisional role. Psychooncology. 2010:19;606-616. DOI: 10.1002/pon.1590

[24] Pais-Ribeiro J, Silva I, Ferreira T, Martins A, Meneses R, Baltar M. Validation study of a Portuguese version of the Hospital Anxiety and Depression Scale. Psychology, Health & Medicine. 2007:12;225-237. DOI: 10.1080/13548500500524088

[25] Gil F, Costa G, Hilker I, Benito. First anxiety, afterwards depression: psychological distress in cancer patients at diagnosis and after medical treatment. Stress and Health. 2012:28;362-367. DOI: 10.1002/smi.2445

[26] Riba MB, Donovan KA, Andersen B, Braun I, Breitbart WS, Brewer BW, Buchmann LO, Clark MM, Collins M, Corbett C, Fleishman S, Garcia S, Greenberg DB, Handzo RGF, Hoofring L, Huang CH, Lally R, Martin S, McGuffey L, Mitchell W, Morrison LJ, Pailler M., Palesh O, Parnes, F, Pazar JP, Ralston L, Salman J, Shannon-Dudley MM, Valentine AD, McMillian NR, Darlow SD. Distress management. Journal of the National Comprehensive Cancer Network. 2019:17;1229-1249. DOI: 10.6004/jnccn.2019.0048s

[27] Abbey G, Thompson SB, Hickish T, Heathcote D. A meta-analysis of prevalence rates and moderating factors for cancer-related post-traumatic stress disorder. Psychooncology. 2015: 24;371-381. DOI: 10.1002/pon.3654

[28] Parikh D, Ieso PD, Garvey G, Thachil T, Ramamoorthi R, Penniment M, Jayaraj R. Post-traumatic

stress disorder and post-traumatic growth in breast cancer patients-a systematic review. Asian Pacific Journal of Cancer Prevention. 2015:16; 641-646. DOI: 10.7314/APJCP.2015.16.2.641

[29] Mehnert A, Koch U. Prevalence of acute and post-traumatic stress disorder and comorbid mental disorders in breast cancer patients during primary cancer care: a prospective study. Psychooncology. 2007:16;181-188. DOI: 10.1002/ pon.1057

[30] Borgi M, Collacchi B, Ortona E, Cirulli F. Stress and coping in women with breast cancer: unravelling the mechanisms to improve resilience. Neuroscience & Biobehavioral Reviews. 2020:119;406-421. DOI: 10.1016/j. neubiorev.2020.10.011

[31] Antoni MH, Lutgendorf SK, Cole SW, Dhabhar FS, Sephton SE, McDonald PG, Stefanek M, Sood AK. The influence of bio-behavioural factors on tumour biology: pathways and mechanisms. Nature Reviews Cancer. 2006:6:240-248. DOI: 10.1038/nrc1820

[32] Sun L, Ang E, Ang W, Lopez V. Losing the breast: A meta-synthesis of the impact in women breast cancer survivors. Psycho-Oncology. 2017:27;376-385. DOI: 10.1002/pon.4460

[33] Holzner B, Kemmler G, Kopp M, Moschen R, Schweigkofler HR, Du Nser M, Margreiter R, Fleischhacker WW, Sperner-Unterweger, B. Quality of life in breast cancer patients—not enough attention for long-term survivors?. Psychosomatics. 2001:42;117-123. DOI: 10.1176/appi.psy.42.2.117

[34] Santos GD. Corporeidade, sexualidade e doença oncológica. In: Encontro de Profissionais de Saúde: Sexualidade na Doença Oncológica. 9 Novembro 2018. Portugal: Évora, 2018

[35] Manne S, Ostroff J. Coping with breast cancer - a couples-focused group intervention. Oxford University Press; 2008. 119 p. ISBN: 978-0195342901

[36] Nayeri ND, Bakhshi F, Khosravi A, Najafi Z. The effect of complementary and alternative medicines on quality of life in patients with breast cancer: A systematic review. Indian Journal of Palliative Care. 2020:26;95-104. DOI: 10.4103/IJPC.IJPC_183_19

[37] Servan-Schreiber D. Anticancro: Uma nova maneira de viver. Alfragide: Lua de Papel; 2008. 399 p. ISBN: 978-989-23-1744-1

[38] Deng G, Cassileth B. Complementary or alternative medicine in cancer care—myths and realities. Nature Reviews Clinical Oncology. 2013:10;656-664. DOI: 10.1038/ nrclinonc.2013.125

[39] Potel C. Psychomotricité: entre théorie et pratique. 3ème ed. Paris: Press Éditions; 2008. 350 p. ISBN: 978-2-84835-190-2

[40] Veiga G, Hillenbrand A. Pereira C. O toque terapêutico no envelhecimento. In: F Mendes, C Pereira, J Bravo, editores. Envelhecer em segurança no Alentejo - Compreender para agir. Évora: Universidade de Évora; 2019. p. 329-345. ISBN: 978-989-99122-9-8.

[41] Oliveira JP. Relaxação e toque terapêutico em mulheres com cancro da mama: impacto de uma intervenção psicomotora na ansiedade, dor e qualidade de vida [tese]. Évora: Universidade de Évora. 2019

[42] Oliveira JP, Fonseca M, Santos GD. Relaxação e toque terapêutico em mulheres com cancro da mama: Impacto de uma intervenção psicomotora na ansiedade, depressão e qualidade de vida. in prep

[43] Hernandez-Reif M, Field T, Ironson G, Beutler J, Vera Y, Hurley J, Fletcher MA, Schanberg S, Kuhn C,

Fraser M. Natural killer cells and lymphocytes increase in women with breast cancer following massage therapy. The International Journal of Neuroscience. 2005:115; 495-510. DOI: 10.1080/00207450590523080

[44] Listing M, Krohn M, Liezmann C, Kim I, Reisshauer A, Peters E, Klapp BF, Rauchfuss M. The efficacy of classical massage on stress perception and cortisol following primary treatment of breast cancer. Archives of Women's Mental Health. 2010:13; 165-173. DOI: 10.1007/s00737-009-0143-9

[45] Listing M, Reisshauer A, Krohn M, Voigt B, Tjahono G, Becker J, Klapp BF, Rauchfuss M. Massage therapy reduces physical discomfort and improves mood disturbances in women with breast cancer. Psychooncology. 2009:18;1290-1299. DOI: 10.1002/pon.1508

[46] Billhult A, Lindholm C, Gunnarsson R, Stener-Victorin E. The effect of massage on immune function and stress in women with breast cancer - A randomized controlled trial. Autonomic Neuroscience: Basic and Clinical. 2009:150; 111-115. DOI: 10.1016/j.autneu.2008.03.006

[47] Veiga G, Marmeleira J. Regulação emocional: Contributos das técnicas de relaxação. In: A Candeias, A Portelada, C Vaz Velho, E Galindo, E Pires, L Borralho, L Grácio, N Costa, K Reschke, E Witruk, editors. Multiple approaches to the study and intervention in stress. Proceedings of the International Seminar. Évora: Universidade de Évora; 2018. p. 52-66. ISBN: 978-989-8550-67-5

[48] Martins R. A relaxação terapêutica no contexto da saúde mental – o corpo como ponte entre a emoção e a razão. In: V Fonseca, M Martins, editors. Progressos em psicomotricidade. Cruz Quebrada: FMH Edições; 2001. p. 95-108. ISBN: 972-735-081-X

[49] Veiga G. Corpo e Emoção: A importância das intervenções de mediação corporal no funcionamento emocional. In AR Mira, J Fernandes, G Veiga, J Marmeleira, editores. Prática psicomotora: reflexões, contextos e mediadores. Évora: Universidade de Évora; in prep.

[50] Coly-Layani S. Une approche psychomotrice en service d'oncologie: expérience de la relaxation auprès de patientes atteintes d'un cancer du sein [these]. Paris: Universite de Bordeaux; 2014

[51] Spira J, Reed G. Group psychotherapy for women with breast cancer. American Psychological Association; 2003. 210 p. DOI: 10.1037/10461-000

[52] Leung J, Pachana NA, McLaughlin D. Social support and health-related quality of life in women with breast cancer: a longitudinal study. Psychooncology. 2014:23;1014-1020. DOI: 10.1002/pon.3523

[53] Ozdemir D, Tas Arslan F. An investigation of the relationship between social support and coping with stress in women with breast cancer. Psychooncology. 2018:27;2214-2219. DOI: 10.1002/pon.4798

[54] Elkins G, Fisher W, Johnson A. Mind–body therapies in integrative oncology. Current Treatment Options In Oncology. 2010:11;128-140. DOI: 10.1007/s11864-010-0129-x

[55] Guerreiro, D. Efeitos de um programa de intervenção psicomotora nos indicadores de saúde e bem-estar de mulheres sobreviventes de cancro da mama [tese]. Évora: Universidade de Évora. 2021

[56] Bower JE, Crosswell AD, Stanton AL, Crespi CM, Winston D, Arevalo J, Ma J, Cole SW, Ganz PA. Mindfulness meditation for younger breast cancer survivors: A randomized controlled trial. Cancer. 2014:121;1231-1240. DOI: 10.1002/cncr.29194

[57] Rabin C, Pinto B, Fava J. Randomized trial of a physical activity and meditation intervention for young adult cancer survivors. Journal of Adolescent and Young Adult Oncology. 2015:5;41-47. DOI: 10.1089/jayao.2015.0033

[58] Carlson, LE, Tamagawa R, Stephen J, Doll R, Faris P, Dirkse D, Speca M. Tailoring mind-body therapies to individual needs: patients' program preference and psychological traits as moderators of the effects of mindfulness-based cancer recovery and supportive-expressive therapy in distressed breast cancer survivors. Journal of the National Cancer Institute Monographs. 2014:50;308-314. DOI: 10.1093/jncimonographs/lgu034

[59] Lipschitz DL, Kuhn R, Kinney AY, Donaldson GW, Nakamura Y. Reduction in salivary α-amylase levels following a mind–body intervention in cancer survivors—an exploratory study. Psychoneuroendocrinology. 2013:38;1521-1531. DOI: 10.1016/j.psyneuen.2012.12.021

[60] Browning K, Kue J, Lyons F, Overcash J. Feasibility of mind–body movement programs for cancer survivors. Oncology Nursing Forum. 2017:44;446-456. DOI: 10.1188/17.onf.446-456

Section 4

Complementary Therapies, Technologic and Science Perspectives

Chapter 10

The Role of Complementary and Alternative Medicines in the Treatment and Management of COVID-19

Bhagawati Saxena

Abstract

Interception of coronavirus disease 2019 (COVID-19) into our life and its rapid global expansion, humanity has succumbed to a vulnerable position. COVID-19 is proclaiming millions of lives, underscores the urgent need for more effective therapeutic interventions. This disease created catastrophe and developments of new drugs and vaccines take a long duration. Hence, scientists and medical society turned their heads towards different approaches of treatment, referred to as complementary and alternative medicine (CAM) for eradicating the deadly virus. Ayurveda, herbal medicines, nutritional supplements, naturopathy, and yoga are some of the CAMs which have emerged as a ray of hope in these times. The understanding of the COVID-19 pathogenesis and its impact on immunity will progress the effective management of this lethal infectious disease. The host immune response has an elementary function of defense against the majority of infectious diseases including COVID-19. This chapter focuses on the utilization of various CAMs (Ayurveda, yoga, herbs, phytochemicals and nutritional supplements) in COVID-19 treatment. An additional attempt has been made in this chapter on the potential of CAMs to assist in improving immunological reactions against infections and thus may be an efficient approach in the prevention and/or management of severe acute respiratory syndrome coronavirus 2 infections.

Keywords: COVID-19, SARS-CoV-2, Complementary and Alternative Medicines, Innate immunity, Adaptive immunity, Micronutirents

1. Introduction

The coronavirus disease 2019 (COVID-19) proclaiming millions of lives, is an infectious respiratory disease affecting the lungs. COVID-19 is devastating mainly in patients of old age and with co-morbidities like obesity, cardiovascular complications etc. COVID-19 is caused by recently recognized coronavirus termed as severe acute respiratory syndrome coronavirus 2 (SARS-CoV-2) [1]. COVID-19 outbreak was instigated in December 2019 from the Wuhan city of China, which is rapidly spreading worldwide and badly impacted the entire world [2]. The COVID-19 pandemic is currently the prevalent world health crisis and a daily large number of new cases is reported around the world [3, 4]. By June 24, 2021, the mortality rates raised to 3.9 million among 180 million confirmed cases of COVID-19. Currently, the world healthcare system is in severe crisis due to the constant and varied challenges created by COVID-19. Initially, due to the lack of understanding regarding novel coronavirus and vaccines or any treatment for the COVID-19, governments officials globally implemented various non-pharmaceutical interventions (NPIs), such as the utilization of masks, social distancing, hand-washing, remote working, closures of schools and colleges, restrictions on public gatherings, fourteen days quarantines, for the slow transmission of the disease [5]. These measures are found to be effective in mitigating the number of cases [6, 7], however, they lead to a considerable impact on the social, economic [8] and psychological wellbeing of the society [9].

Government's professionals, pharmaceutical companies and professionals in the health care system are taking great efforts to manage and combat the disease across the world. To alleviate the burden on society, a massive effort is being made by health care professionals worldwide to develop and get access to different vaccines [10, 11]. Vaccination has been started around the globe after a year of the first reported cases of COVID-19 [12]. Vaccines were developed and have been found successful in decreasing the number of patients affected with COVID-19 as well as the severity of the disease, however, it is not completely avoiding the risk of being affected with COVID-19. Additionally, new strains of coronavirus are also gradually identified. Recently it is found that novel coronavirus is having various mutations. This means that there are slight changes in the genetic composition of the virus. The Delta-plus variant is a mutated version of the Delta variant (the virus that wreaked havoc in the second wave). Delta plus is considered highly infectious. The virus can potentially dodge immune response, vaccines and antibody therapies. However, more research has to be done in this context. Few cases have been recorded in some states of India. The Government official has classified it as a Variant of Concern (VOC). There is no certainty regarding delta plus and the current numbers cannot determine any particular trend. Certain vaccines work against the Delta Plus variant, but they show 3 to 8 times less efficacy as compared to other variants. There are no conclusive reports about these variants but we should not keep our guards down [13, 14]. The United States Food and Drug Administration (U.S. FDA) approved the antiviral drug, remdesivir (Veklury), for treating COVID-19 affected patients requiring hospitalization. Remdesivir approved to be administered in the health care setting or hospital that is efficient enough of affording acute care comparable to inpatient hospital care. This approval of using remdesivir for treating COVID-19 does not include the entire population rather it is only approved for hospitalized patients who are adults and pediatric ($\geq$12 years of age) with a bodyweight of at least 40 kilograms [15]. Moreover, health care systems are facing huge difficulties in combating the enormous demands of medicines and vaccines. Thus, providing additional therapies for preventing and curing the disease is an important step in combating this pandemic. Currently, the worldwide impetus is unabated, and a third wave is also predicted.

India and China are known for their rich history of traditional medicine [16]. Indian households are being considered as a hub of natural products, consisting of a plethora of pharmacologically active ingredients inspired by the traditional medication system (Ayurveda) [16]. Complementary and alternative medicines (CAMs) have emerged as a ray of hope in these times [17]. The following book chapter focuses on 'the role of CAMs in the prevention, treatment and management of COVID-19'.

2. Pathogenesis of COVID-19

The recently identified SARS-CoV-2 is a new member added into the family of β-coronavirus with earlier known members like Severe Acute Respiratory Syndrome

Coronavirus (SARS-CoV) and the Middle East Respiratory Syndrome Coronavirus (MERS-CoV), which results in severe pulmonary pneumonia and potentially deadly acute respiratory distress syndrome (ARDS). The large population of COVID-19 patients is asymptomatic. Six prominent symptoms include dry cough, malaise, fatigue, fever, dyspnea, secretion or sputum among various clinical manifestations noticed in patients infected with SARS-CoV-2. The gastrointestinal symptoms consist of vomiting, anorexia, and diarrhea in the patients affected with COVID-19. Pathogenesis of COVID-19 is classified into three discrete clinical phases based on the cells/tissue being infected. These three phases include asymptomatic state, upper and conducting airway response and hypoxia, ground-glass infiltrates and progression to ARDS. In Phase, I of asymptomatic state inhaled SARS-CoV-2, bind to the receptor present on the epithelial cells i.e., angiotensin-converting enzyme-2 (ACE-2) on the nasal cavity and begin reproducing [18]. There is local propagation of the COVID-19 virus and an inadequate innate immunity in the asymptomatic stage. In phase II, there is an occurrence of the upper airway and conducting airway infection. In this phase or stage, there is a robust immune response when the virus migrates and propagates down the conducting duct and along the respiratory tract. Epithelium of the upper and conducting airway infected virally results in the release of cytokines [19]. During this phase, clinical manifestations are observed. Predictions and monitoring of the subsequent course of the disease may be improved by determining the host immune responses. In most of the patients infected with SARS-CoV-2, the infection will be mild and mostly limited to the upper and conducting airways [20]. These patients do not require hospitalization and may be monitoring of patients at home with conventional symptomatic treatment will be adequate [19]. In the third stage or phase III, there will be ground-glass infiltrates, hypoxia and progression to ARDS. Typically, around 20% of the patients infected with SARS-CoV-2 advance to the severe stage and develop pulmonary infiltrates and ARDS. In this stage, the virus reaches and infects the gas exchange unit of the lungs i.e., alveolar type II cells mainly in the subpleural region of lungs [21]. Once the virus reaches the type II alveolar cells self-replicating pulmonary toxins are released and it results in apoptosis and cell death [22]. This in turn causes diffuse alveolar injury, with a few multinucleated large cells and a fibrin membrane rich in hyaline [23, 24]. Extensive scarring, fibrosis, and various kinds of ARDS may occur from aberrant wound healing. Improvement requires epithelial cells regeneration and robust innate and adaptive immune responses. Patients with older age or co-morbidities are at greater risk due to weakened capacity to repair the damaged epithelium and deteriorated immune response against the virus. In the elderly, the mucociliary clearance is also reduced and this allows propagation and rapid spread into the gas exchange unit of the lungs [25].

3. Interaction of virus with the immune system

Manifestations of COVID-19 is extremely heterogeneous, with a wide clinical spectrum varying from asymptomatic infection through mild upper respiratory and conducting airways infection, to severe pneumonia leading to fatality [24, 26]. Recognizing the machinery for the virus invasion into the host body and its interaction with the host immunity will facilitate the prevention and treatment of the COVID-19. Infection with SARS-CoV-2 has two distinct clinical phases: primary and secondary inflammatory phases. The primary phase involves the invasion of viral in the host and its replication and the inflammatory phase involves exaggerated host immune response towards the virus. Augmented host immune response eventually results in fast and uncontrolled deterioration and worsening of respiration and ultimately emerges the need for hospitalization [27, 28]. SARS-CoV-2 is a lower respiratory tract virus and enters the host through a specific receptor i.e., ACE-2, resulting in pneumonia in severe cases. It chiefly consists of four structural proteins including nucleocapsid polymer, small envelope glycoprotein, membrane glycoprotein and spike polymer, as well as numerous accessory proteins. Spike protein projected from the surface of the virus is responsible for the attachment with ACE-2 assists the invasion of viruses into the host cells [29]. ACE2 is mainly expressed on the lung, kidney, intestine and epithelial cells of blood vessels. It is worth mentioning that spike protein is considered as the potential target in the vaccination against COVID-19. The innate and the adaptive immunity pathways are two pieces of machinery of the host immune system against foreign pathogens [30]. To effectively deal with and rapidly control the spread of viral infection, the innate immunity activates and concomitantly stimulates the adaptive immunological reactions. The innate system is the first-line defense against the pathogen which comprises of external defense mechanism (e.g. epithelial cells or the mucous membranes in the nasopharynx, lung, gut, periodontium and skin), nonspecific phagocytic leukocytes (macrophages and neutrophils) as well as serum proteins [30, 31]. Adaptive immune build up in a long time includes a specific response i.e., production of protein molecules known as antibodies that react with the antigens of infectious agents to eradicate the virus and to forbid progression of the disease to severe stages [32]. The host immune system via frequently interacting innate and adaptive mechanisms defends against external pathogens. Better management and prevention of disease requires timely identification of disease as well as its influence on the immune system. The disease complexity is further noticeable when it is reported variability in susceptibility to severe infection and mortality in certain sections of the population. However, earlier literature reported that the viral infection alerts immune system operations and influences immunoglobulin levels, antibody generation, phagocytosis, lymphocyte transformation etc. [33]. Similarly, SARS-CoV-2 also impacted the innate and adaptive immunity of the host.

3.1 Impact of SARS-CoV-2 on innate immunity

It has been reported in numerous studies that interleukin-6 (IL-6) is upregulated in patients affected with SARS-CoV-2 [24]. IL-6 is chiefly produced by monocytes or macrophages. IL-6 employs immune mediators and results in the cytokine storm, which cause tissue damage and uncontrolled systemic inflammation [34]. Moreover, inflammatory cytokines including chemokines, interferon-gamma (IFN-γ), IFN-γ induced protein 10 (IP-10), tumor necrosis factor (TNF-α), interleukin-10 (IL-10) and monocyte chemoattractant protein-1 (MCP-1) are observed to be augmented in patients affected with COVID-19 [24]. Lactate dehydrogenase is a marker of pyroptosis and is also found to be augmented in patients affected with COVID-19, and is considered to be correlated with the severity of the disease as well as the rate of mortality. Innate immune response was observed to be activated in COVID-19 patients, but unsuccessful to commence robust interferon (IFN) responses. The deficient of IFN responses could probably result in insufficiency in confining the viral load and viral infection at the initial stage of disease progression [34]. There is limited literature regarding the mechanisms underlying the SARS-CoV-2 induced mitigation of IFN responses. Macrophages play important role in immune responses against viral infection. ACE2 receptors are found to be expressed on the surface of macrophages [35]. This leads to increased susceptibility of macrophages to SARS-CoV-2 infection. This signifies that macrophages may serve as a possible reservoir of the COVID-19 virus [36].

3.2 Impact of SARS-CoV-2 on adaptive immunity

Stimulation of the innate immunity subsequently activates the adaptive immunity. Thymus cells (T cells) and bone marrow- or bursa-derived cells (B cells) are key players in adaptive immunity. Effector T cells mediate cellular response against the virus by either directly killing the cells infected with the virus or by discharging regulatory and pro-inflammatory mediators. B cells mediate the humoral responses by producing neutralizing antibodies (NAbs). The released NAbs in turn obstruct the interaction between the spike protein of SARS-CoV-2 and ACE2 expressed on the surface of the cell membrane and thus block the invasion of the virus into the host cell. On the contrary, the virus-specific antibodies interact with complementary receptors expressed on the exterior of the host cell and thus assist the entrance of the virus into the host cells. This is termed antibody-dependent enhancement (ADE) [37]. The NAbs titer is reported to be associated with disease severity [38]. However, there is a range of levels of NAbs among various patients, demonstrating the individual variation in immune responses towards viral infection. Cellular immunity is another intend of the adaptive immune system is against viral infections including the cluster of differentiation 4 (CD4) and the cluster of differentiation 8 (CD8) positive T cells. CD4 and CD8 are glycoproteins that serve as a co-receptor for the T-cell receptor (TCR). CD4+ T releases cytokines, which help cytotoxic T cells and B cells. On the other hand, the CD8+ T cells after being activated eradicate the infected cells. Depletion as well as the exhaustion of peripheral CD4+ and CD8+ T cells are reported in COVID-19 patients [39]. This depletion and exhaustion of T cells may be due to the augmented level of IL-6 in COVID-19 patients [40].

4. Management of COVID-19 with the use of complementary and alternative medicines (CAMs) endorsement

Complementary and Alternative Medicine (CAM) is an umbrella term for a broad range of substances and treatments which consist of a cluster of a variety of medic and health care supplies, orders, and actions not characterized under the conceptual framework of medicines. The definition of CAM throughout the literature is not consistent. However, the National Centre for Complementary and Alternative Medicines (NCCAM) of the National Institute of Health (NIH) defines CAM as "a group of diverse medical and health care systems, products, and practices that are not currently fall under the category of conventional medicine"(NCCAM, 2002) [41]. CAM is utilized either as an alternative or adjuvant therapy of conventional treatments.

The inclination towards using CAM in and around the world, both in terms of prophylactic as well as therapeutic strategies against problems related to health, has been augmented recently [42]. CAM is an extremely broad area that consists of all health beliefs, values, practices, as well as methods exterior to the streamlined present health care system [43]. These are further classified into five important categories by National Center for Complementary and Integrative Health (NCCIH). The first category includes alternative medical systems/whole medical systems (homeopathy, traditional Chinese medicine, ayurvedic medicine), the second category includes biologically-based therapies (probiotics, minerals, vitamins, phytochemicals, whole diets and functional foods, animal-derived extracts, amino acids, proteins and fatty acids), the third category includes manipulative and body-based methods (chiropractic, osteopathic manipulation, reflexology and massage), the fourth category includes mind–body therapies; healing techniques based on mind–body therapies (art, praying, meditation, dance, music) and finally the fifth category includes energy-oriented treatments or energy therapies or (therapeutic touch, Qi gong, healing touch) [44].

Greater than 80% of the population around the globe utilizes CAMs. The foundation of the National CAM-Center leads to a significantly augmented number of CAM-related basic research and clinical trials based on CAM therapies. Approximately 30% of the adult population of the U.S. [45] and 10–40% of Europe [46] use CAM. It is predicted that the market per annum for herbal remedies, consisting of raw materials and herbal products will expand by 15% and 5% respectively. The global market for the herbal drug is projected to be $62 billion, which is likely to rise to $5 trillion by 2050 [47]. Herbal remedies for boosting the immune system are consumed in several countries across the globe to uplift health, endorse the body's defense against various infectious as well as prohibit and cure several infectious diseases [48]. In this section, several examples of CAMs projected for preventing and curing diseases are elaborated.

4.1 Methodology

Databases such as PubMed, Scopus, Embase, Google Scholar, Web of Science, and Cochrane were searched without time limitation to find relevant articles exploring the impact of CAM in COVID-19. The terms and words searched included "COVID-19", "SARS-CoV-2", "CAM", "micronutrients", "phytochemical", "Ayurveda", "extract", "essential oil", "herbal medicines", "In vitro", "In vivo", "clinical trial" etc.

4.2 Ayurveda and yoga as the prophylactic and adjuvant therapy of COVID-19

To develop a preventive and curative intervention for COVID-19, the Ministry of Ayurveda, Yoga, and Naturopathy, Unani, Siddha, and Homeopathy (AYUSH), Government of India (GoI), formulated an interdisciplinary AYUSH research and development task force and guidelines for initiating, monitoring, coordinating efforts and conducting clinical studies of diverse traditional medicines against COVID-19 [49].

Visualizing the severity and infectivity of COVID-19, the Ministry of AYUSH, GoI recommended certain immunity boosters like lukewarm water, Kadha, (an ayurvedic preparations containing curcumin, ginger, cumin seeds, fennel seeds, cloves and honey) and homeopathic medicine 'Arsenic Album 30C' [50]. Ayurveda defined NPIs in addition to pharmacological as preventive measures in combating COVID-19. NPIs recommended by the Ministry of AYUSH include sadvritta (Sad means 'good' and vritta means 'regimen'), healthy lifestyles, enough sleep, adequate physical activity, avoidance and isolation from infected persons [51]. Certain medicines suggested by Ayurveda include turmeric (*Curcuma longa*), garlic (*Allium sativum*), Ajwain or Carom (*Trachyspermum Ammi*) as a disinfectant for the prevention of COVID-19 [52].

The nose, mouth and eyes, are the main entry portals for the droplets consisting of the virus, SARS-CoV-2. Before reaching and final attack on the lungs, the virus stays in the nose and throat region for hours. The virus is coated with fatty acid which helps in adhering the virus to the moist mucosal layers and thus facilitates its entrance into the host cells by attaching to definite receptors [53]. Ayurveda mentioned various interventions that interfere in these entry portals [54] for virus invasion to the lungs by improving the innate immunologic response of the mucus membranes. These measures work as "physiological masks" or "local prophylaxis" for obstructing the viral invasion. The common recommendation for respiratory diseases written in Ayurvedic texts [55] includes consumption of hot food, hot water, steam inhalation, gargling, local applications and herbal decoctions with medicated water. These may be useful for relief in mild cases [53]. Ayurveda recommended drinking hot and warm water for improving the digestion of Ama. Ama is a pro-inflammatory mediator of weaken metabolic disorders and is associated with augmented susceptibility to infections [56].

Warm oils and liquids are employed as mouth rinses (Kavala) or gargles (gandusha) to thoroughly clean the mouth and throat [57]. The oily decoctions coat the mucosa as biofilm as well as rinse the oral cavity, tonsillar area, and pharynx. These decoctions also have supplementary benefits of antioxidant, immunomodulatory, and antimicrobial [58]. It is well known that host mucosal immunity plays a vital role in controlling infectious agents [59]. Literature regarding Yoga advocates Jala neti which implies rinsing of the nasal passage with saline water [60]. Randomized controlled trials (RCTs) reported the effectiveness of saline water in upper respiratory infections [61].

4.3 Herb/phytochemicals

Herbal products are consumed in various countries across the globe. Literature suggests immune-boosting properties of these herbal materials which endorse the normal resistance ability of the body against infectious pathogens and to raise health, and as well as to cure and to prohibit diverse infectious diseases [48]. Curcumin, a polyphenolic compound isolated from turmeric, which is a commonly used food colorant and spice [62], can augment the antibody reaction even if it is consumed at reduced doses [63]. Additionally, literature shows that curcumin has a promising affinity for protein binding towards SARS-CoV-2 and thus directly inhibit the invasion of SARS-CoV-2 into target cells [64]. The ability of curcumin in improving various disease conditions is attributed partially to its capability to modulate the immune responses [63]. Numerous reports show that curcumin can alter the proliferation as well as the activation of T cells [65, 66]. Additionally, curcumin has the potential of regulating the response and growth of various immune cells like natural killer (NK) cells, B cells, T cells, dendritic cells (DCs), macrophages and neutrophils [63]. Glycyrrhizin, an active phytochemical moiety found in liquorice was observed to be efficient in comparison to commonly used anti-virals in mitigating the replication of SARS-CoV as well as inhibiting its adsorption and penetration [67]. A recent in-vitro study also showed that glycyrrhizin is a potential inhibitor of SARS-CoV-2 replication by hindering the viral main protease (Mpro) [68]. Molecular docking study showed two phytoconstituents Somniferine and Withanoside V from Ashwagandha (*Withania somnifera*) [69, 70], Tinocordiside [70] and berberine [71] from Giloy (Tinospora cordifolia) and three active ingredients i.e., Vicenin, Ursolic acid and Isorientin 4'-O-glucoside 2″-O-p-hydroxybenzoagte isolated from Tulsi (*Ocimum sanctum*) [70] may have an antiviral effect against novel coronavirus via potentially inhibiting Mpro of SARS-CoV-2.

4.4 Nutritional supplements

Recently conducted studies show that suboptimal intake of micronutrients and inadequate nutritional status can lead to poor immunity and consequently affect the severity of infections. Nutritional supplements emerge to reinforce the immune system. Micronutrients consisting of a variety of vitamins (A, D, C, E, B6, B12, folate) and minerals (iron, zinc, selenium and copper) are engaged in various stages of the immune responses against foreign pathogens. A study conducted in the United Arab Emirates (UAE) confirmed the association of low levels of vitamin

D3 (25(OH)D3) (<12 ng/mL) with severity and death due to COVID-19 [72]. Another study shows that hospitalized COVID-19 patients receiving vitamin D3 (calcifediol) in contrast with those not consuming vitamin D3, was significantly linked with a lesser rate of mortality during the initial thirty days of hospitalization [73]. Supplementation with vitamin D at high-dose may be well-tolerated, effective, and readily accessible for the management of COVID-19 [74]. One report showed that intake of a high dose of vitamin D has significantly reduced the inflammatory markers (neutrophil/lymphocyte ratio, ferritin, C-reactive protein (CRP), lactate dehydrogenase (LDH), IL-6 associated with COVID-19 without any side effects [75]. A study confirmed that deficiency of vitamin D is correlated with severe lung injury, disease prolongation and risk of mortality, in COVID-19 patients [76]. Another study shows that combination therapy of vitamin D with vitamin B12 and magnesium in geriatric patients with COVID-19 was correlated with a considerable decline in the proportion of patients with clinical deterioration and requiring intensive care support and oxygen support [77]. Vitamin D was found to modulate innate and adaptive immune systems [78, 79]. It augments the innate immune responses while attenuates the adaptive immune responses [78]. Vitamin D metabolites directly target the adaptive immune cells [80] and it is an important part of intricate features that control the immune response against infection [81]. These findings necessitate examining the level of vitamin D in pediatric as well as geriatric persons to maintain it at optimum levels for the prevention of SARS-CoV-2 infection.

In addition to the consumption of higher doses of vitamin D3, previously it was also stated that coronavirus pandemic can be considerably controlled by the utilization of high amounts of vitamin C. Significantly low levels of vitamin C in patients affected with COVID-19 were found and daily supplementation of 100 mg/kg is highly recommended [82]. A high dose of intravenous vitamin C might repress cytokine storms associated with COVID-19, and facilitate improving pulmonary function and lessen the risk of ARDS associated with COVID-19 [83]. As SARS-CoV-2 was found to affect the host immune system, it seems crucial to boost the natural immunity and antioxidant capacity to lessen the effect of any virus infection. Vitamin C is known for its ability to activate the immune system. Therefore it seems promising to administered vitamin C concomitantly with other medications to cure the infection in acute conditions. The ingestion of vitamin C orally up to the daily threshold of bowel tolerance seems to be effective for the majority of persons. However, intravenous administration of vitamin C is suggested for serious cases. On the other side, there are certain reports, claiming that the overstimulation of immune cells in COVID-19 leads to cytokine storm which ultimately causes lung injury following pneumonia. Certain clinical investigations also suggested that intravenous administration of vitamin C in high-dose can be a safe and effective choice for the management of COVID-19 infection in its early stages. Even though previous literature recognized and approved the antiviral activity of vitamin C, but its impact has not been studied widely and, limited information is available on its effect on coronavirus. Moreover, some studies show that adjunctive intravenous administration of vitamin C for the treatment of infection in critically ill COVID-19 patients was unable to reduce the rate of mortality, ventilator settings, the requirement of vasopressor, etc. [84]. Therefore although vitamin C is vital for lessening the inflammatory response and assists in boosting the immune system of the host, there is a lack of substance to support that utilization of vitamin C at a high dose can be successful in the prevention or management of COVID-19. Moreover, as Therapeutic Goods Administration (TGA) [85] declared that more studies are required for any recommendation for utilizing intravenous vitamin C in the management of COVID-19. In addition to vitamin C and vitamin D3, it was reported that vitamin K antagonist regular use was correlated with augmented mortality in hospitalized elderly patients affected with COVID-19 [86].

Studies show that treatment with zinc as adjuvant therapy was appeared to be feasible and safe for the management of COVID-19. However, the infusion of zinc causes limited infusion site irritation on the periphery [87]. Zinc supplement was found to be efficiently clear the SARS-CoV-2 from the nasopharynx in a lesser time than other symptomatic therapy [88]. Zinc cation (Zn^{2+}) coupled with zinc ionophores pyrithione and found to inhibit RNA polymerase of coronavirus and thus block the replication of the virus [89]. Additionally, zinc also mitigates the invasion of the virus by escalating the cell membrane stability as well as stimulate interferon-alpha (IFN-α) and IFN-γ formation and attenuate tumor necrosis factor (TNF) and mononuclear cells [90]. Apart from zinc, iron also plays a vital component of enzymes involved in the stimulation of immune cells, lower levels of iron was found to influence severe symptoms associated with COVID-19. Selenium contributes to adaptive immunity by boosting the production and development of antibodies. Lack of selenium can lessen antibody production, compromised cellular immunity, attenuated the cytotoxicity of NK cells, and decreased response to vaccination. Oxidative stresses alter the viral genome from a mildly pathogenic form to a highly virulent form of the virus in the host. Selenium is a known anti-oxidant. Hence selenium with vitamin E and a cluster of certain enzymes scavenges the free radicals and lessens the oxidative stress and thus as a result, the adjuvant therapy of selenium may be considered for the treatment of COVID-19 infection [91].

5. Limitations

Literature shows that people who either have positive attitudes towards CAM or those who consume CAM are unwilling to comply with conventional therapy, most prominently the vaccinations and to follow the official COVID-19 guidelines [92–98]. It has been reported that the optimistic attitudes towards CAM are correlated with negative attitudes towards vaccination is not evidence-based but because of an underlying outlook on health or perhaps a reluctance to stick to conventional therapy [93–95]. Those who utilize CAM perceived CAM as a natural, safe approach to improve the host immunity, while vaccines are considered as a risky option [94]. Additionally, both anti-vaccination attitudes and higher utilization of CAM are correlated to the poor trust of individuals towards the healthcare system or medical authorities [92].

6. Summary/conclusion

It is apparent from the above findings, that the understanding of the COVID-19 pathogenesis and its impact on immunity will progress the management of this lethal infectious disease. As per the earlier studies, the host immune response has an elementary function of defense against the majority of infectious diseases including COVID-19. In this chapter specifically attempt has been made on the utilization of various NPIs, herbs, phytochemicals and micronutrients which has the potential to assist in the prevention and/or management of SARS-CoV-2 infection. Thus utilization of CAMs may be an efficient approach in improving immunological reactions against infections. Moreover, the consumption of vitamins and minerals was observed to be favorable in improving the immune system and its function. Although, certain clinical studies reported the success of CAMs in the treatment, prevention and management of COVID-19, additional studies through clinical analysis as well as consumers' experience on CAMs are essential to draw strong conclusions in the success of utilization of CAMs for treatment, prevention and management of COVID-19.

Conflict of interest

"The authors declare no conflict of interest."

Abbreviations

ACE-2	Angiotensin-converting enzyme-2
ADE	Antibody-dependent enhancement
ARDS	Acute respiratory distress syndrome
AYUSH	Ayurveda, Yoga, and Naturopathy, Unani, Siddha, and Homeopathy
B cells	Bone marrow- or bursa-derived cells
CAM	Complementary and Alternative Medicine
CD4	Cluster of differentiation 4
CD8	Cluster of differentiation 8
COVID-19	Coronavirus Disease 2019
CRP	C - reactive protein
IFN	Interferon
IFN-α	Interferon alpha
IFN-γ	Interferon-gamma
IL-6	Interleukin 6
IL-10	Interleukin-10
IP-10	IFN-γ induced protein 10
LDH	Lactate dehydrogenase
MCP-1	Monocyte chemoattractant protein-1
MERS-CoV	Middle East Respiratory Syndrome Coronaviruses
Nabs	Neutralizing antibodies
NCCAM	National Centre for Complementary and Alternative medicines
NCCIH	National Center for Complementary and Integrative Health
NIH	National Institute of Health
NPIs	Non-pharmaceutical interventions
SARS-CoV	Severe Acute Respiratory Syndrome Coronavirus
SARS-CoV-2	Severe Acute Respiratory Syndrome Coronavirus 2
T cells	Thymus cells
TGA	Therapeutic Goods Administration
TNF	Tumor necrosis factor
TNF-α	Tumor necrosis factor alpha
U.S. FDA	United States Food and Drug Administration
VOC	Variant of Concern

Author details

Bhagawati Saxena
Department of Pharmacology, Institute of Pharmacy, Nirma University, Ahmedabad, Gujarat, India

*Address all correspondence to: bhagawati.saxena@nirmauni.ac.in; bsaxenapharm@gmail.com

References

[1] Singhal T. A review of coronavirus disease-2019 (COVID-19). Indian J Pediatr. 2020;87(4): 281-286. doi:10.1007/s12098-020-03263-6.

[2] Lai CC, Shih TP, Ko WC, Tang HJ, Hsueh PR. Severe acute respiratory syndrome coronavirus 2 (SARS-CoV-2) and coronavirus disease-2019 (COVID-19): The epidemic and the challenges. Int J Antimicrob Agents. 2020;55(3): 105924. doi: 10.1016/j.ijantimicag.2020.105924.

[3] Pollard CA, Morran MP, Nestor-Kalinoski AL. The COVID-19 pandemic: a global health crisis. Physiol Genomics. 2020;52(11):549-557. doi: 10.1152/physiolgenomics.00089.2020.

[4] Wang C, Horby PW, Hayden FG, Gao GF. A novel coronavirus outbreak of global health concern. Lancet. 2020;395(10223):470-473. doi: 10.1016/S0140-6736(20)30185-9.

[5] Desvars-Larrive A, Dervic E, Haug N, Niederkrotenthaler T, Chen J, Di Natale A, Lasser J, Gliga DS, Roux A, Sorger J, Chakraborty A, Ten A, Dervic A, Pacheco A, Jurczak A, Cserjan D, Lederhilger D, Bulska D, Berishaj D, Tames EF, Álvarez FS, Takriti H, Korbel J, Reddish J, Grzymała-Moszczyńska J, Stangl J, Hadziavdic L, Stoeger L, Gooriah L, Geyrhofer L, Ferreira MR, Bartoszek M, Vierlinger R, Holder S, Haberfellner S, Ahne V, Reisch V, Servedio VDP, Chen X, Pocasangre-Orellana XM, Garncarek Z, Garcia D, Thurner S. A structured open dataset of government interventions in response to COVID-19. Sci Data. 2020;7(1):285. doi: 10.1038/s41597-020-00609-9.

[6] Brauner JM, Mindermann S, Sharma M, Stephenson AB, Gavenčiak T, Johnston D, Salvatier J, Gavenciak T, Stephenson AB, Leech G, Altman G, Mikulik V, Norman A J, Monrad J T , Besiroglu T, Ge H, Hartwick M A, Teh Y W, Chindelevitch L, Gal Y, Kulveitet J. The effectiveness of eight nonpharmxutical interventions against COVID-19 in 41 countries. https://doi.org/10.1101/2020.05.28.20116129 (2020).

[7] Flaxman S, Mishra S, Gandy A, Unwin HJT, Mellan TA, Coupland H, Whittaker C, Zhu H, Berah T, Eaton JW, Monod M, Imperial College COVID-19 Response Team, Ghani AC, Donnelly CA, Riley S, Vollmer MAC, Ferguson NM, Okell LC, Bhatt S. Estimating the effects of non-pharmaceutical interventions on COVID-19 in Europe. Nature. 2020;584(7820):257-261. doi: 10.1038/s41586-020-2405-7.

[8] Nicola M, Alsafi Z, Sohrabi C, Kerwan A, Al-Jabir A, Iosifidis C, Agha M, Agha R. The socio-economic implications of the coronavirus pandemic (COVID-19): A review. Int J Surg. 2020;78:185-193. doi: 10.1016/j.ijsu.2020.04.018.

[9] Brooks SK, Webster RK, Smith LE, Woodland L, Wessely S, Greenberg N, Rubin GJ. The psychological impact of quarantine and how to reduce it: rapid review of the evidence. Lancet. 2020;395(10227):912-920. doi: 10.1016/S0140-6736(20)30460-8.

[10] WHO. 172 countries and multiple candidate vaccines engaged in COVID-19 vaccine Global access facility. 2020 [cited 2020 Sep 17]. Available from: https://www.who.int/news-room/detail/24-08-2020-172-countries-and-multiple-candidate-vaccines-engaged-in-covid-19-vaccine-global-access-facility

[11] Gavi. Why is no one safe until everyone is safe during a pandemic? Gavi, the Vaccine Alliance. 2020 [cited 2020 Sep 17]. Available from: https://

www.gavi.org/vaccineswork/why-no-one-safe-until-everyone-safe-during-pandemic

[12] Our World in Data. Coronavirus (COVID-19) Vaccinations. [cited 2021 Feb 15]. Available from https://ourworldindata.org/covid-vaccinations.

[13] https://www.who.int/news-room/feature-stories/detail/the-effects-of-virus-variants-on-covid-19-vaccines.

[14] https://www.who.int/en/activities/tracking-SARS-CoV-2-variants/ (Accessed on 6.7.21)

[15] Lotfi F, Akbarzadeh-Khiavi M, Lotfi Z, Rahbarnia L, Safary A, Zarredar H, Baghbanzadeh A, Naghili B, Baradaran B. Micronutrient therapy and effective immune response: a promising approach for management of COVID-19. Infection. 2021:1-15. doi: 10.1007/s15010-021-01644-3.

[16] Charan J, Bhardwaj P, Dutta S, Kaur R, Bist SK, Detha MD, Kanchan T, Yadav D, Mitra P, Sharma P. Use of Complementary and Alternative Medicine (CAM) and Home Remedies by COVID-19 Patients: A Telephonic Survey. Indian J Clin Biochem. 2020;36(1):1-4. doi: 10.1007/s12291-020-00931-4.

[17] Shankar A, Dubey A, Saini D, Prasad CP. Role of Complementary and Alternative Medicine in Prevention and Treatment of COVID-19: An Overhyped Hope. Chin J Integr Med. 2020 (8):565-567. doi: 10.1007/s11655-020-2851-y.

[18] Hoffmann M, Kleine-Weber H, Schroeder S, Krüger N, Herrler T, Erichsen S, Schiergens TS, Herrler G, Wu NH, Nitsche A, Müller MA, Drosten C, Pöhlmann S. SARS-CoV-2 Cell Entry Depends on ACE2 and TMPRSS2 and Is Blocked by a Clinically Proven Protease Inhibitor. Cell. 2020;181(2):271-280.e8. doi: 10.1016/j.cell.2020.02.052.

[19] Mason RJ. Pathogenesis of COVID-19 from a cell biology perspective. Eur Respir J. 2020;55(4):2000607. doi: 10.1183/13993003.00607-2020.

[20] Wu Z, McGoogan JM. Characteristics of and Important Lessons from the coronavirus disease 2019 (COVID-19) outbreak in China: summary of a report of 72 314 cases from the Chinese Center for Disease Control and Prevention. JAMA. 2020;323(13):1239-1242. doi: 10.1001/jama.2020.2648.

[21] Mossel EC, Wang J, Jeffers S, Edeen KE, Wang S, Cosgrove GP, Funk CJ, Manzer R, Miura TA, Pearson LD, Holmes KV, Mason RJ. SARS-CoV replicates in primary human alveolar type II cell cultures but not in type I-like cells. Virology. 2008;372(1):127-135. doi: 10.1016/j.virol.2007.09.045.

[22] Qian Z, Travanty EA, Oko L, Edeen K, Berglund A, Wang J, Ito Y, Holmes KV, Mason RJ. Innate immune response of human alveolar type II cells infected with severe acute respiratory syndrome-coronavirus. Am J Respir Cell Mol Biol. 2013;48(6):742-748. doi: 10.1165/rcmb.2012-0339OC.

[23] Gu J, Korteweg C. Pathology and pathogenesis of severe acute respiratory syndrome. Am J Pathol. 2007;170(4):1136-1147. doi: 10.2353/ajpath.2007.061088.

[24] Huang C, Wang Y, Li X, Ren L, Zhao J, Hu Y, Zhang L, Fan G, Xu J, Gu X, Cheng Z, Yu T, Xia J, Wei Y, Wu W, Xie X, Yin W, Li H, Liu M, Xiao Y, Gao H, Guo L, Xie J, Wang G, Jiang R, Gao Z, Jin Q, Wang J, Cao B. Clinical features of patients infected with 2019 novel coronavirus in Wuhan, China. Lancet. 2020;395(10223):497-506. doi: 10.1016/S0140-6736(20)30183-5.

[25] Ho JC, Chan KN, Hu WH, Lam WK, Zheng L, Tipoe GL, Sun J, Leung R,

Tsang KW. The effect of aging on nasal mucociliary clearance, beat frequency, and ultrastructure of respiratory cilia. Am J Respir Crit Care Med. 2001;163(4):983-988. doi: 10.1164/ajrccm.163.4.9909121.

[26] Guan WJ, Ni ZY, Hu Y, Liang WH, Ou CQ, He JX, Liu L, Shan H, Lei CL, Hui DSC, Du B, Li LJ, Zeng G, Yuen KY, Chen RC, Tang CL, Wang T, Chen PY, Xiang J, Li SY, Wang JL, Liang ZJ, Peng YX, Wei L, Liu Y, Hu YH, Peng P, Wang JM, Liu JY, Chen Z, Li G, Zheng ZJ, Qiu SQ, Luo J, Ye CJ, Zhu SY, Zhong NS; China Medical Treatment Expert Group for Covid-19. Clinical Characteristics of Coronavirus Disease 2019 in China. N Engl J Med. 2020;382(18):1708-1720. doi: 10.1056/NEJMoa2002032.

[27] Ruan Q, Yang K, Wang W, Jiang L, Song J. Clinical predictors of mortality due to COVID-19 based on an analysis of data of 150 patients from Wuhan, China. Intensive Care Med. 2020;46(5):846-848. doi: 10.1007/s00134-020-05991-x.

[28] Mehta P, McAuley DF, Brown M, Sanchez E, Tattersall RS, Manson JJ; HLH Across Speciality Collaboration, UK. COVID-19: consider cytokine storm syndromes and immunosuppression. Lancet. 2020;395(10229):1033-1034. doi: 10.1016/S0140-6736(20)30628-0.

[29] Astuti I, Ysrafil. Severe Acute Respiratory Syndrome Coronavirus 2 (SARS-CoV-2): An overview of viral structure and host response. Diabetes Metab Syndr. 2020;14(4): 407-412. doi: 10.1016/j.dsx.2020.04.020.

[30] Simon HB. The immunology of exercise. A brief review. JAMA. 1984;252(19):2735-2738.

[31] Fitzgerald L. Exercise and the immune system. Immunol Today. 1988;9(11):337-339. doi: 10.1016/0167-5699(88)91332-1.

[32] Shi Y, Wang Y, Shao C, Huang J, Gan J, Huang X, Bucci E, Piacentini M, Ippolito G, Melino G. COVID-19 infection: the perspectives on immune responses. Cell Death Differ. 2020 May;27(5):1451-1454. doi: 10.1038/s41418-020-0530-3.

[33] Notkins AL, Mergenhagen SE, Howard RJ. Effect of virus infections on the function of the immune system. Annu Rev Microbiol. 1970;24:525-538. doi: 10.1146/annurev.mi.24.100170.002521.

[34] Zhang C, Wu Z, Li JW, Zhao H, Wang GQ. Cytokine release syndrome in severe COVID-19: interleukin-6 receptor antagonist tocilizumab may be the key to reduce mortality. Int J Antimicrob Agents. 2020;55(5):105954. doi: 10.1016/j.ijantimicag.2020.105954.

[35] Keidar S, Strizevsky A, Raz A, Gamliel-Lazarovich A. ACE2 activity is increased in monocyte-derived macrophages from prehypertensive subjects. Nephrol Dial Transplant. 2007;22(2):597-601. doi: 10.1093/ndt/gfl632.

[36] Park MD. Macrophages: a Trojan horse in COVID-19? Nat Rev Immunol. 2020; 20(6): 351. doi: 10.1038/s41577-020-0317-2.

[37] Wang C, Zhou X, Wang M, Chen X. The Impact of SARS-CoV-2 on the Human Immune System and Microbiome. Infectious Microbes & Diseases. 2020;3(1):14-21. doi: 10.1097/IM9.0000000000000045.

[38] Choe PG, Kang CK, Suh HJ, Jung J, Kang E, Lee SY, Song KH, Kim HB, Kim NJ, Park WB, Kim ES, Oh MD. Antibody Responses to SARS-CoV-2 at 8 Weeks Postinfection in Asymptomatic Patients. Emerg Infect Dis. 2020;26(10):2484-2487. doi: 10.3201/eid2610.202211.

[39] He Z, Zhao C, Dong Q, Zhuang H, Song S, Peng G, Dwyer DE. Effects of

severe acute respiratory syndrome (SARS) coronavirus infection on peripheral blood lymphocytes and their subsets. Int J Infect Dis. 2005 Nov;9(6):323-330. doi: 10.1016/j.ijid.2004.07.014.

[40] Zheng HY, Zhang M, Yang CX, Zhang N, Wang XC, Yang XP, Dong XQ, Zheng YT. Elevated exhaustion levels and reduced functional diversity of T cells in peripheral blood may predict severe progression in COVID-19 patients. Cell Mol Immunol. 2020;17(5):541-543. doi: 10.1038/s41423-020-0401-3.

[41] NCCAM. What Is Complementary and Alternative Medicine (CAM)? 2002. [June 10, 2004]. [Online]. Available: http://nccam.nih.gov/health/whatiscam/index.htm.

[42] Biçer ˙I, Yalçın Balçık P. Geleneksel ve tamamlayıcı tıp: Türkiye ve seçilen ülkelerinin incelenmesi. Hacettepe Sa˘glık ˙Idaresi Dergisi. 2019;22(1):245-257.

[43] Ali A, Katz DL. Disease Prevention and Health Promotion: How Integrative Medicine Fits. Am J Prev Med. 2015;49(5 Suppl 3):S230-S240. doi: 10.1016/j.amepre.2015.07.019.

[44] Koithan M. Introducing complementary and alternative therapies. J Nurse Pract. 2009;5(1):18-20. https://doi.org/10.1016/j.nurpra.2008.10.012.

[45] Clarke TC, Black LI, Stussman BJ, Barnes PM, Nahin RL. Trends in the use of complementary health approaches among adults: United States 2002-2012. Natl Health Stat Report. 2015;79:1-16. PMID: 25671660; PMCID: PMC4573565.

[46] Kemppainen LM, Kemppainen TT, Reippainen JA, Salmenniemi ST, Vuolanto PH. Use of complementary and alternative medicine in Europe: healthrelated and sociodemographic determinants. Scand J Public Health. 2018;46(4):448-455. https://doi.org/10.1177/1403494817733869.

[47] Nilashi M, Samad S, Yusuf SYM, Akbari E. Can complementary and alternative medicines be beneficial in the treatment of COVID-19 through improving immune system function? J Infect Public Health. 2020;13(6):893-896. doi: 10.1016/j.jiph.2020.05.009.

[48] Devasagayam TP, Sainis KB. Immune system and antioxidants, especially those derived from Indian medicinal plants. Indian J Exp Biol. 2002;40(6):639-655.

[49] Interdisciplinary AYUSH Research & Development Task Force. Ministry of AYUSH, Government of India. https://www.ayush. gov.in/docs/clinical-protocol-guideline.pdf. Accessed 16 Sep 2020.

[50] Advisory for Corona virus from AYUSH Ministry [cited 2020 May 11]. Available from: https://pib.gov.in/PressReleasePage.aspx?PRID=1600895#.

[51] P DN, ey. Seven shields of ayurveda between health and diseases. Annals Ayurvedic Med 2019;8:6-10.

[52] Bhatwalkar SB, Shukla P, Srivastava RK, Mondal R, Anupam R. Validation of environmental disinfection efficiency of traditional Ayurvedic fumigation practices. J Ayurveda Integr Med. 2019;10(3):203-206. doi: 10.1016/j.jaim.2019.05.002.

[53] Tillu G, Chaturvedi S, Chopra A, Patwardhan B. Public Health Approach of Ayurveda and Yoga for COVID-19 Prophylaxis. J Altern Complement Med. 2020;26(5):360-364. doi: 10.1089/acm.2020.0129.

[54] Paradkar H ed. Ashtanga Hrudaya of Vagbhata. Varanasi, India:

Chaukhambha Surbharati Prakashan, 2003:287-294.

[55] Acharya YT, ed. Shri Dalhanacharaya Nibandhasamgraha commentary of Sushruta Samhita. Varanasi, India: Chaukumba Sanskrit Sansthan, 2003:761-765.

[56] Sumantran VN, Tillu G. Cancer, inflammation, and insights from Ayurveda. Evid Based Complement Alternat Med. 2012;2012:306346. doi: 10.1155/2012/306346.

[57] Amruthesh S. Dentistry and Ayurveda - IV: classification and management of common oral diseases. Indian J Dent Res. 2008;19(1):52-61. doi: 10.4103/0970-9290.38933.

[58] Shanbhag VK. Oil pulling for maintaining oral hygiene - A review. J Tradit Complement Med. 2016;7(1):106-109. doi:10.1016/j.jtcme.2016.05.004

[59] Novak N, Haberstok J, Bieber T, Allam JP. The immune privilege of the oral mucosa. Trends Mol Med. 2008;14(5):191-198. doi: 10.1016/j.molmed.2008.03.001.

[60] Muktibodhananda S. Hatha Yogo Pradipika. Light on Hatha Yoga. 4th ed. Munger, India: Bihar School of Yoga, 2012:202-205.

[61] King D, Mitchell B, Williams CP, Spurling GK. Saline nasal irrigation for acute upper respiratory tract infections. Cochrane Database Syst Rev. 2015;(4):CD006821. doi: 10.1002/14651858.CD006821.pub3.

[62] Richart SM, Li YL, Mizushina Y, Chang YY, Chung TY, Chen GH, Tzen JT, Shia KS, Hsu WL. Synergic effect of curcumin and its structural analogue (Monoacetylcurcumin) on anti-influenza virus infection. J Food Drug Anal. 2018;26(3):1015-1023. doi: 10.1016/j.jfda.2017.12.006.

[63] Jagetia GC, Aggarwal BB. "Spicing up" of the immune system by curcumin. J Clin Immunol. 2007;27(1):19-35. doi: 10.1007/s10875-006-9066-7.

[64] Suravajhala R, Parashar A, Malik B, Nagaraj AV, Padmanaban G, Kavi Kishor P, Polavarapu R, Suravajhala P. Comparative Docking Studies on Curcumin with COVID-19 Proteins. Preprints. 2020;2020050439. doi: 10.20944/preprints202005.0439.v1.

[65] Ranjan D, Chen C, Johnston TD, Jeon H, Nagabhushan M. Curcumin inhibits mitogen stimulated lymphocyte proliferation, NFkappaB activation, and IL-2 signaling. J Surg Res. 2004;121(2):171-177. doi: 10.1016/j.jss.2004.04.004.

[66] Ranjan D, Johnston TD, Wu G, Elliott L, Bondada S, Nagabhushan M. Curcumin blocks cyclosporine A-resistant CD28 costimulatory pathway of human T-cell proliferation. J Surg Res. 1998;77(2):174-178. doi: 10.1006/jsre.1998.5374.

[67] Cinatl J, Morgenstern B, Bauer G, Chandra P, Rabenau H, Doerr HW. Glycyrrhizin, an active component of liquorice roots, and replication of SARS-associated coronavirus. Lancet. 2003;361(9374):2045-2046. doi: 10.1016/s0140-6736(03)13615-x.

[68] van de Sand L, Bormann M, Alt M, Schipper L, Heilingloh CS, Steinmann E, Todt D, Dittmer U, Elsner C, Witzke O, Krawczyk A. Glycyrrhizin Effectively Inhibits SARS-CoV-2 Replication by Inhibiting the Viral Main Protease. Viruses. 2021;13(4):609. doi: 10.3390/v13040609.

[69] Tripathi MK, Singh P, Sharma S, Singh TP, Ethayathulla AS, Kaur P. Identification of bioactive molecule from Withania somnifera (Ashwagandha) as SARS-CoV-2 main protease inhibitor. J Biomol Struct Dyn. 2020:1-14. doi:10.1080/07391102.2020.1790425.

[70] Shree P, Mishra P, Selvaraj C, Singh SK, Chaube R, Garg N, Tripathi YB. Targeting COVID-19 (SARS-CoV-2) main protease through active phytochemicals of ayurvedic medicinal plants - Withania somnifera (Ashwagandha), Tinospora cordifolia (Giloy) and Ocimum sanctum (Tulsi) - a molecular docking study. J Biomol Struct Dyn. 2020:1-14. doi: 10.1080/07391102.2020.1810778.

[71] Chowbdhury P. In silico investigation of phytoconstituents from Indian medicinal herb 'Tinospora cordifolia (giloy)' against SARS-CoV-2 (COVID-19) by molecular dynamics approach. J Biomol Struct Dyn. 2020:1-18. doi: 10.1080/07391102.2020.1803968.

[72] AlSafar H, Grant WB, Hijazi R, Uddin M, Alkaabi N, Tay G, Mahboub B, Al Anouti F. COVID-19 Disease Severity and Death in Relation to Vitamin D Status among SARS-CoV-2-Positive UAE Residents. Nutrients. 2021;13(5):1714. doi: 10.3390/nu13051714.

[73] Alcala-Diaz JF, Limia-Perez L, Gomez-Huelgas R, Martin-Escalante MD, Cortes-Rodriguez B, Zambrana-Garcia JL, Entrenas-Castillo M, Perez-Caballero AI, López-Carmona MD, Garcia-Alegria J, Lozano Rodríguez-Mancheño A, Arenas-de Larriva MDS, Pérez-Belmonte LM, Jungreis I, Bouillon R, Quesada-Gomez JM, Lopez-Miranda J. Calcifediol Treatment and Hospital Mortality Due to COVID-19: A Cohort Study. Nutrients. 2021;13(6):1760. doi: 10.3390/nu13061760.

[74] Annweiler C, Beaudenon M, Gautier J, Simon R, Dubée V, Gonsard J, Parot-Schinkel E; COVIT-TRIAL study group. COvid-19 and high-dose VITamin D supplementation TRIAL in high-risk older patients (COVIT-TRIAL): study protocol for a randomized controlled trial. Trials. 2020;21(1):1031. doi: 10.1186/s13063-020-04928-5.

[75] Lakkireddy M, Gadiga SG, Malathi RD, Karra ML, Raju ISSVPM, Ragini, Chinapaka S, Baba KSSS, Kandakatla M. Impact of daily high dose oral vitamin D therapy on the inflammatory markers in patients with COVID 19 disease. Sci Rep. 2021;11(1):10641. doi: 10.1038/s41598-021-90189-4.

[76] Sulli A, Gotelli E, Casabella A, Paolino S, Pizzorni C, Alessandri E, Grosso M, Ferone D, Smith V, Cutolo M. Vitamin D and Lung Outcomes in Elderly COVID-19 Patients. Nutrients. 2021 Feb 24;13(3):717. doi: 10.3390/nu13030717.

[77] Tan CW, Ho LP, Kalimuddin S, Cherng BPZ, Teh YE, Thien SY, Wong HM, Tern PJW, Chandran M, Chay JWM, Nagarajan C, Sultana R, Low JGH, Ng HJ. Cohort study to evaluate the effect of vitamin D, magnesium, and vitamin B12 in combination on progression to severe outcomes in older patients with coronavirus (COVID-19). Nutrition. 2020;79-80:111017. doi: 10.1016/j.nut.2020.111017.

[78] Bikle DD. Vitamin D and the immune system: role in protection against bacterial infection. Curr Opin Nephrol Hypertens. 2008;17(4):348-352. doi: 10.1097/MNH.0b013e3282ff64a3.

[79] Kempinska-Podhorodecka A, Milkiewicz M, Wasik U, Ligocka J, Zawadzki M, Krawczyk M, Milkiewicz P. Decreased Expression of Vitamin D Receptor Affects an Immune Response in Primary Biliary Cholangitis via the VDR-miRNA155-SOCS1 Pathway. Int J Mol Sci. 2017;18(2):289. doi: 10.3390/ijms18020289.

[80] Peelen E, Knippenberg S, Muris AH, Thewissen M, Smolders J, Tervaert JW, Hupperts R, Damoiseaux J.

Effects of vitamin D on the peripheral adaptive immune system: a review. Autoimmun Rev. 2011;10(12):733-743. doi: 10.1016/j.autrev.2011.05.002.

[81] Gruber-Bzura BM. Vitamin D and Influenza-Prevention or Therapy? Int J Mol Sci. 2018;19(8):2419. doi: 10.3390/ijms19082419.

[82] Xing Y, Zhao B, Yin L, Guo M, Shi H, Zhu Z, Zhang L, He J, Ling Y, Gao M, Lu H, Mao E, Zhang L. Vitamin C supplementation is necessary for patients with coronavirus disease: An ultra-high-performance liquid chromatography-tandem mass spectrometry finding. J Pharm Biomed Anal. 2021;196:113927. doi: 10.1016/j.jpba.2021.113927.

[83] Liu F, Zhu Y, Zhang J, Li Y, Peng Z. Intravenous high-dose vitamin C for the treatment of severe COVID-19: study protocol for a multicentre randomised controlled trial. BMJ Open. 2020 Jul 8;10(7):e039519. doi: 10.1136/bmjopen-2020-039519.

[84] Li M, Ching TH, Hipple C, Lopez R, Sahibzada A, Rahman H. Use of Intravenous Vitamin C in Critically Ill Patients With COVID-19 Infection. J Pharm Pract. 2021:8971900211015052. doi: 10.1177/08971900211015052.

[85] Administration, T.G. No evidence to support intravenous high-dose vita-min C in the management of COVID-19; 2020. Retrieved on 21 April,2020 from https://www.tga.gov.au/alert/no-evidence-support-intravenous-high-dose-vitamin-c-management-covid-19.

[86] Ménager P, Brière O, Gautier J, Riou J, Sacco G, Brangier A, Annweiler C, Geria-Covid Study Group OBOT. Regular Use of VKA Prior to COVID-19 Associated with Lower 7-Day Survival in Hospitalized Frail Elderly COVID-19 Patients: The GERIA-COVID Cohort Study. Nutrients. 2020;13(1):39. doi: 10.3390/nu13010039.

[87] Patel O, Chinni V, El-Khoury J, Perera M, Neto AS, McDonald C, See E, Jones D, Bolton D, Bellomo R, Trubiano J, Ischia J. A pilot double-blind safety and feasibility randomized controlled trial of high-dose intravenous zinc in hospitalized COVID-19 patients. J Med Virol. 2021 May;93(5):3261-3267. doi: 10.1002/jmv.26895.

[88] Elalfy H, Besheer T, El-Mesery A, El-Gilany AH, Soliman MA, Alhawarey A, Alegezy M, Elhadidy T, Hewidy AA, Zaghloul H, Neamatallah MAM, Raafat D, El-Emshaty WM, Abo El Kheir NY, El-Bendary M. Effect of a combination of nitazoxanide, ribavirin, and ivermectin plus zinc supplement (MANS.NRIZ study) on the clearance of mild COVID-19. J Med Virol. 2021;93(5):3176-3183. doi: 10.1002/jmv.26880.

[89] Te Velthuis AJ, van den Worm SH, Sims AC, Baric RS, Snijder EJ, van Hemert MJ. Zn(2+) inhibits coronavirus and arterivirus RNA polymerase activity in vitro and zinc ionophores block the replication of these viruses in cell culture. PLoS Pathog. 2010;6(11):e1001176. doi: 10.1371/journal.ppat.1001176.

[90] Pasternak CA. A novel form of host defense: membrane protection by Ca2+ and Zn2+. Biosci Rep. 1987;7(2):81-91. doi: 10.1007/BF01121871.

[91] Tomo S, Saikiran G, Banerjee M, Paul S. Selenium to selenoproteins - role in COVID-19. EXCLI J. 2021 Apr 16;20:781-791. doi: 10.17179/excli2021-3530.

[92] Soveri A, Karlsson LC, Maki O, Antfolk J, Waris O, Karlsson H, Karlsson L, Lindfelt M, Lewandowsky S. Trait reactance and trust in doctors as predictors of vaccination behavior, vaccine attitudes, and use of complementary and alternative medicine in parents of young children.

PLoS One. 2020;15(7):e0236527. doi: 10.1371/journal.pone.0236527.

[93] Browne M, Thomson P, Rockloff MJ, Pennycook G. Going against the herd: Psychological and cultural factors underlying the "vaccination confidence gap". PLoS One. 2015;10(9):e0132562. doi: 10.1371/journal.pone.0132562.

[94] Attwell K, Ward PR, Meyer SB, Rokkas PJ, Leask J. "Do-it-yourself": vaccine rejection and complementary and alternative medicine (CAM). Soc Sci Med. 2018 Jan;196:106-114. doi:10.1016/j.socscimed.2017.11.022.

[95] Bryden GM, Browne M, Rockloff M, Unsworth C. Anti-vaccination and pro-CAM attitudes both reflect magical beliefs about health. Vaccine. 2018;36(9):1227-1234. https://doi.org/10.1016/j.vaccine.2017.12.068.

[96] Hornsey MJ, Lobera J, Díaz-Catalán C. Vaccine hesitancy is strongly associated with distrust of conventional medicine, and only weakly associated with trust in alternative medicine. Soc Sci Med. 2020;255:113019. doi: 10.1016/j.socscimed.2020.113019.

[97] Hadjipanayis A, van Esso D, Del Torso S, Dornbusch HJ, Michailidou K, Minicuci N, Pancheva R, Mujkic A, Geitmann K, Syridou G, Altorjai P, Pasinato A, Valiulis A, Soler P, Cirstea O, Illy K, Mollema L, Mazur A, Neves A, Zavrsnik J, Lapii F, Efstathiou E, Kamphuis M, Grossman Z. Vaccine confidence among parents: Large scale study in eighteen European countries. Vaccine. 2020;38(6):1505-1512. doi: 10.1016/j.vaccine.2019.11.068.

[98] Lewandowsky S, Woike JK, Oberauer K. Genesis or Evolution of Gender Differences? Worldview-Based Dilemmas in the Processing of Scientific Information. J Cogn. 2020;3(1):9. doi: 10.5334/joc.99.

Chapter 11

The Use of Evidence-Based Acupuncture: Current Evidence

Dedi Ardinata

Abstract

Evidence-based medicine (EBM), which emphasizes that medical decisions must be based on the most recent best evidence, is gaining popularity. Individual clinical expertise is combined with the best available external clinical evidence derived from systematic research in the practice of EBM. The key and core of EBM is the hierarchical system for categorizing evidence. The Grading of Recommendations, Assessment, Development and Evaluations (GRADE) system divides evidence quality into four categories: high, moderate, low, and very low. GRADE is based on the lowest quality of evidence for any of the outcomes that are critical to making a decision, reducing the risk of mislabeling the overall evidence quality, when evidence for a critical outcome is lacking. This principle is also used in acupuncture as a complementary and integrative treatment modality, but incorporating scientific evidence is more difficult due to a number of factors. The goal of this chapter is to discuss how to establish a clinical evidence system for acupuncture, with a focus on the current quality of evidence for a variety of conditions or diseases.

Keywords: acupuncture, evidence-based medicine, GRADE, quality of evidence, meta-analysis

1. Introduction

Gordon Guyatt coined the term "evidence-based medicine (EBM)" in 1990 in an unpublished program description, and it was first published in 1992 [1]. This was the first time that an evidence-based practice has been formally established (EBP). Evidence-based practice requires making health care decisions based on the most up-to-date, valid, and relevant evidence. These decisions should be made by those receiving care, with the explicit and tacit knowledge of those providing care, and within the constraints of the available resources [2]. Clinical decision making is the culmination of a process that began with clinical reasoning, problem solving, and an awareness of the patient and health care environment [3]. Pursuing evidence-based acupuncture paves the way for the acupuncture field to fully integrate with modern health care, but there are obstacles. Acupuncture is actually classified as a complementary and alternative medicine modality but is only very rarely included in standard care guidelines, despite overwhelming evidence that it is more effective than the current guideline-based interventions for a variety of conditions [4].

2. The quality of evidence

While it is critical for acupuncture practitioners to understand the effects of acupuncture, they frequently have concerns about which conditions (diseases) acupuncture therapy has had the most evidence of benefit and the least risk to their patients. Guidelines were already being published at a higher rate than before. Acupuncturists should understand how guidelines are developed to make effective choices concerning health care. The GRADE approach has been adopted by national and international organizations that develop guidelines for acupuncture practitioners. GRADE is a system for assessing the quality of available evidence that supports acupuncture therapy for patients with a variety of conditions. The evidence was categorized as being of high, moderate, low, or very low quality [5]. The study design is critical in determining the quality of the evidence. Randomized controlled trials (RCTs) are initially given a higher grade due to their generally lower susceptibility to bias [6] than observational studies [7]. RCTs will be degraded since they have a bias that can be identified [8]. When multiple high-quality studies show consistent results, observational studies can be upgraded [9]. Factors that can lead to downgrading the quality of evidence: risk of bias: a lack of randomization, allocation concealment, and blinding biases; inconsistency: the results of different trials show significant and unexplained variation; indirectness of evidence: a comparison of a population, outcome, or intervention that is not direct; imprecision: wide confidence intervals reduce the data's quality; publication bias: studies with "negative" results are not published. Factors that can lead to an upgrade: large effect: the effect is so large that common biases in observational studies cannot possibly explain the result; dose-response relationship: the outcome is proportional to the amount of exposure. All plausible biases only reduce an apparent treatment effect: all possible confounders would only serve to dilute the effect that was observed [10]. GRADE levels do not always imply a recommendation, and the GRADE process is differentiated from the recommendation process. Although a high level of evidence is more likely to result

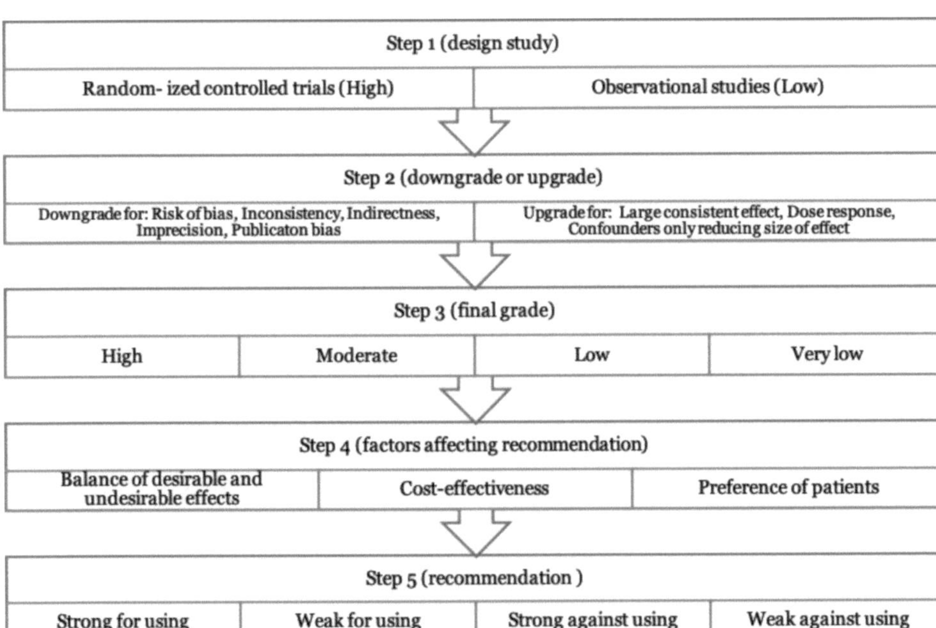

Figure 1.
Recommendation steps using the GRADE method.

in a recommendation, in some cases, a low or very low level of evidence can lead to a strong recommendation [11]. Other factors, such as cost, clinical judgment, and patient preference, must be considered in the development of recommendations, in addition to the quality of evidence [12]. Acupuncture practitioners will be able to make better clinical decisions if they understand the GRADE method [5]. There are five steps to the GRADE process, which we explain with examples in **Figure 1**.

3. Methods

The published systematic reviews/meta-analyses (SRs/MAs) were retrieved using Google Scholar with the following search terms: "systematic review" AND "meta-analysis" AND "(selected conditions)" AND "GRADE" AND "acupuncture". The literature search was carried out from January 2018 to July 2021.

3.1 Inclusion and exclusion criteria for literature selection

3.1.1 Inclusion criteria

1. Systematic reviews and meta-analyses

2. The main treatments for migraine prophylaxis, headache (chronic tension type and chronic episodic), low back pain, knee osteoarthritis pain, allergic rhinitis (seasonal and perennial/persistent), chemotherapy-induced nausea, and vomiting (CINV), postoperative nausea and vomiting (PONV), and postoperative pain

3. Using Recommendations Assessment, Development, and Evaluation (GRADE) to assess the quality of evidence

4. Language is restricted to English.

3.1.2 Exclusion criteria

1. A protocol for systematic review and meta-analysis

2. Animal studies

3. Incomplete literature

We determined eight conditions, such as migraine prophylaxis, headache (chronic tension type and chronic episodic), low back pain, knee osteoarthritis pain, allergic rhinitis (seasonal and perennial/persistent), chemotherapy-induced nausea, and vomiting (CINV), postoperative nausea and vomiting (PONV), and postoperative pain, based on results and strong evidence from The Acupuncture Evidence Project: A Comparative Literature Review (Revised edition), 2017th [11].

4. Results of the search

A total of 1286 articles related to eight conditions were searched (**Table 1**). After reviewing the abstract and full text of the article, 17 systematic reviews and meta-analyses of the six conditions that met the inclusion criteria were finally

Conditions	Total articles	Article selected	Year of publication
Migraine prophylaxis	286	5	2018; 2019; 2020
Headache (chronic tension type and chronic episodic)	33	2	2020; 2021
Low back pain	436	3	2018; 2020
Knee osteoarthritis	201	2	2019; 2020
Allergic rhinitis	35	0	—
Chemotherapy-induced nausea and vomiting (CINV)	34	0	—
Postoperative nausea and vomiting (PONV)	79	2	2020; 2021
Postoperative pain	182	3	2020; 2021
Total	1286	17	

Table 1.
Total articles and articles selected.

included [13–29], and articles related to allergic rhinitis and chemotherapy-induced nausea and vomiting (CINV) did not meet the criteria for inclusion (**Table 1**).

5. The quality of evidence for each condition

5.1 Migraine prophylaxis

Migraine is characterized by recurrent, pulsating headaches, and increased intracranial blood flow, which are caused by vasomotor and cerebrocortical dysfunction, vasospasm, and excessive stress. Stimuli such as light, sound, or physical activity can set it off [30]. Pharmacological treatment, which includes propranolol, sodium valproate, topiramate, flunarizine, and metoprolol, has been proven to be effective for migraine prophylaxis. However, all of these treatments have significant and often intolerable adverse effects [31, 32]. Because of these adverse effects, people are becoming more interested in and using complementary health approaches to treat migraines, and because of its measurable effects on the duration and frequency of migraine attacks, acupuncture has received increasing attention as a worthy adjunct to migraine therapeutic interventions [33].

5.1.1 Previous quality of evidence

Migraine frequency can be reduced with acupuncture. Acupuncture is superior to sham and may be as effective as prophylactic drugs, according to evidence of moderate quality [34]. Acupuncture appears to be at least as effective as conventional migraine preventative medication, and it's also safer, lasts longer, and expenses less – (A narrative review of high-quality RCTs with a large sample size) [35]. Acupuncture is superior to sham in terms of effectiveness and risk of recurrence, according to moderate to high-quality evidence [36].

5.1.2 Current quality of evidence

Even though there are some inconsistencies in the results of current RCTs comparing the efficacy of acupuncture vs. sham or no treatment or western medicine, the most recent evidence shows that acupuncture improves migraine patients significantly. Xu et al. conducted 14 RCTs for migraine without aura that met all inclusion criteria and data standards of quality from 1467 studies based on an electronic database and found that when acupuncture therapy was compared to medical therapy, the evidence supporting the difference in migraine frequency was very low, whereas the evidence supporting the difference in migraine days, effective rate, and VAS scores was low. Because of the risk of bias, inconsistency, and inaccuracy, the quality of evidence supporting the primary outcome is low (to very low) [13]. At three months of follow-up, moderate evidence suggests that acupuncture is "at least non-inferior" to the now-proven, conventional treatment for reducing headache frequency, when compared to placebo [15]. Giovanardi et al. concluded that acupuncture was more effective and safer than medication or sham acupuncture in the treatment of migraines based on high-quality evidence [16]. Furthermore, acupuncture has benefits in terms of pain management and safety for acute migraine treatment and prevention, but the quality of evidence for SR/MA acupuncture for migraine even now needs to be improved [14].

5.1.3 Conclusion

Despite some limitations to acupuncture therapy, the quality of recent evidence from the SRs/MAs suggests that acupuncture is more effective and safer than medication or sham acupuncture for migraine prophylaxis in reducing headache frequency.

5.2 Headache (chronic tension type and chronic episodic)

The most common type of primary headache in the general population is the tension-type headache (TTH) [37]. Chronic tension-type headache (CTTH) is a disorder that arises from episodic tension-type headaches, with daily or highly frequent headache bouts lasting hours or days [38]. Simple analgesics and nonsteroidal anti-inflammatory drugs are the drugs of choice for episodic treatment, with combination analgesics containing caffeine showing their effect in seconds; however, nonpharmacological care should always be attempted despite a lack of scientific evidence [39]. Psychotherapy, behavior therapy, physical therapy, and acupuncture therapy are common nonpharmacological treatments that are frequently used in conjunction with other pharmacological treatments, and their efficacy has been proven [40]. In previous investigations, acupuncture support for tension-type headaches was shown to be insufficient. However, the Cochrane review has identified it as a beneficial, non-pharmacologic therapy for episodic-type and chronic stress–type headaches, based on newly added data [41].

5.2.1 Previous quality of evidence

Linde et al. have looked at 12 trials with a total of 2349 individuals and found that the GRADE quality of evidence is moderate to low, owing to the lack of blinding and varying effect sizes, but suggested that acupuncture is effective in treating episodic-type or chronic tension-type headaches [42]. Acupuncture can improve the intensity, frequency, and disability associated with headaches in the workplace. However, the evidence seems to be of low quality [43].

5.2.2 Current quality of evidence

Acupuncture has been shown to be more effective than other treatments for some THH outcomes, according to Huang et al. and Kolokotsios et al., who conducted investigations and assessed the quality of evidence in RCTs on the effectiveness of acupuncture over sham acupuncture, non-acupuncture therapy, Chinese patent medicine, nonsteroidal anti-inflammatory drugs, and drug therapy for some THH outcomes. In this study, Huang et al. assessed the methodological quality, reliability, and outcome measures of SRs/MAs on the use of acupuncture for TTH [18]. The GRADE results revealed that 69.4% of the results provided low- or very-low-quality evidence, 11.1% provided moderate-quality evidence, and 19.4% provided high-quality evidence, further recommending that acupuncture appears to be an effective treatment modality for TTH, but the credibility of the results is limited due to the methodological quality and generally low quality of evidence [18]. The results of four studies with 557 participants found that the acupuncture group had lower quality evidence in terms of headache frequency and visual analog scale (VAS) scores when compared to the control group after their last treatment, whereas Kolokotsios et al. found low-quality evidence in terms of headache frequency and VAS scores when compared to the control group after their last treatment. Both the severity and the frequency of headaches were reduced over the long term, with the results being statistically significant only in the case of the pain intensity reduction [19].

5.2.3 Conclusion

Acupuncture treatment is useful for patients suffering from tension-type headaches, with both the intensity and the frequency of their headaches decreasing over time. Consequently, additional research should be undertaken on this topic to determine its usefulness in reducing the frequency and intensity of headaches.

5.3 Low back pain

The term "low back pain (LBP)" refers to pain, muscle tension, or stiffness that occurs below the costal border and above the inferior gluteal folds, and maybe associated with or without sciatica (pain traveling down the leg from the lower back) [44]. Even though many patients with back pain recover within a year, some will develop a chronic illness characterized by fluctuating or persistent pain of low or medium severity that is punctuated by periods of no pain or painful exacerbation [45]. Non-specific low back pain (NSLBP) is the most common type of LBP. When the pathoanatomical source of the pain cannot be ascertained, this term is used [46]. The underlying pathophysiology of NSLBP is, by definition, unknown. Therefore, treatment is primarily focused on alleviating pain symptoms, and a variety of pharmacological and non-pharmacological intervention modalities are utilized in clinical practice to achieve this goal [47]. Various pharmacological treatments for low back pain are associated with low to moderate, primarily short-term effects on pain. According to new research, acetaminophen is ineffective for acute low back pain, while duloxetine has only the modest effects on chronic low back pain [48]. Acupuncture, stretching, heat application, massage, and manual spinal manipulation are among the non-pharmacological treatments recommended by the American College of Physicians for acute and chronic non-radicular low back pain (non-radicular LBP) in their clinical practice recommendations [45].

5.3.1 Previous quality of evidence

Liang et al. examined the research situation and trends pertaining to the global use of acupuncture for low back pain during the past 20 years (1997–2016) and concluded that according to clinical practice guidelines from the United States, acupuncture for LBP was only weakly suggested in 2007. However, moderate-quality evidence was reported in 2017, which demonstrated that acupuncture has been widely utilized to treat LBP [49]. Acupuncture has high-quality evidence whereas acupressure, on the other hand, offers moderate-quality evidence for the treatment of low back pain, according to Wellington et al. [50]. In the short term, acupuncture alone or as an addition to standard care improved pain and function in people with LBP, evidence ranging from low to high quality, and it should be recommended in ordinary clinical practice [51]. According to the findings of another study, acupuncture had moderate-quality evidence for pain and function in chronic low back pain but low-quality evidence for pain and function in acute low back pain [52].

5.3.2 *Current quality of evidence*

A large number of acupuncture randomized controlled trials have indicated that the treatment is ineffective. These findings are based on acupuncture randomized controlled trials in which a real acupuncture group was compared to a sham acupuncture (SA) or placebo acupuncture (PA) group. The argument over placebo effects presents a conundrum for those working in the field of acupuncture. Xiang et al. reviewed seven meta-analyses of SA or PA for LBP and found statistically significant differences in post-intervention pain reduction between SA or PA and routine or waiting list care, with moderate and high quality of evidence, but low in disability [20]. Procedures that are comparable to real acupuncture may be used in clinical trials, which may cause the results to be biased [51]. After reviewing 14 trials (2110 participants) comparing the efficacy of acupuncture to that of sham therapy or placebo for NSLBP, Xiang et al. reported statistically significant differences in pain reduction between acupuncture and sham therapy or placebo. The GRADE findings indicate that post-intervention and follow-up pain intensity in both acute/subacute and chronic LBP are of moderate quality of evidence [21]. Mu et al. assessed the effectiveness of acupuncture with a sham intervention, no therapy, or usual care in the treatment of chronic nonspecific low back pain. Acupuncture may not be more effective than sham treatment in alleviating pain immediately after treatment, did not appear to be significantly more effective in alleviating pain immediately after treatment, did not appear to be more effective in improving function immediately after treatment, and did not appear to improve the quality of life in the short term when compared to usual care. Acupuncture was found to be more effective than no treatment in terms of pain alleviation and functional improvement right after treatment. There maybe no difference in adverse event rates between acupuncture and sham. The evidence's certainty ranged from low to moderate. Problems with masking acupuncturists or participants were found in many experiments. A small sample size resulted in inconsistent and imprecise results [22]. Although the Cochrane systematic review (CSR) is regarded as the highest level of evidence, it cannot be ruled out that the CSR in acupuncture may have methodological flaws [53].

5.3.3 *Conclusion*

Acupuncture had a significant effect on pain intensity but not on function in patients with (sub)acute and chronic nonspecific LBP when compared to sham acupuncture or placebo. Acupuncture, on the other hand, is more effective in the short run than no treatment at improving pain and function. Acupuncture as a treatment for chronic low back pain is a popular choice. The availability, cost, and patient preference may all influence the guidelines for evaluating SA or PA control procedures to establish the specific effect of acupuncture on placebo pain.

5.4 Knee osteoarthritis

Knee osteoarthritis (OA) is a complex, degenerative joint disease marked by chronic pain and functional impairment [54]. The pathophysiology of osteoarthritis is complicated, involving mechanical, inflammatory, and metabolic processes that eventually contribute to structural destruction and synovial joint failure [55]. Knee OA pain is usually intermittent and primarily weight bearing (mechanical) in origin. Intermittent pain is frequently predictable, but when it gets more severe, more frequent, or unpredictable, patients are more certain to describe it as unacceptable [56]. The major goals of treatment have been to alleviate pain, restore function, and delay the disease's progression [57]. Recently, there has been no consensus on the optimal treatment for knee OA symptoms. In individuals with knee OA, standard pharmacological treatment always begins with analgesics and nonsteroidal anti-inflammatory drugs (NSAIDs). However, it frequently results in noticeable deleterious consequences, such as gastrointestinal problems, hepatorenal toxicity, and adverse events associated with an increased risk of cardiovascular disease [58, 59]. Apart from the aforementioned therapies, acupuncture has emerged as a viable option for treating knee OA as a complementary therapy. Additionally, several randomized controlled trials have shown acupuncture's efficacy in treating knee OA. Acupuncture has been widely used as a complementary and alternative therapy for patients with knee OA due to its high safety and lack of side effects [60]. Although numerous trials have examined the usefulness of acupuncture for knee OA, its efficacy remains debatable. Emerging concerns about blinding, the validity of sham controls, sample size, effect size, and expectations have arisen [61]. Evidence from non-Cochrane reviews indicates that acupuncture may be beneficial in relieving symptomatic pain associated with knee OA.

5.4.1 Previous quality of evidence

Acupuncture, similar to balneotherapy, is superior to sham acupuncture, muscle-strengthening exercises, Tai Chi, weight loss, standard care, and aerobic exercise for knee OA (in order of rank). According to a sub-analysis of moderate- to high-quality studies, acupuncture is superior to routine care and muscle-strengthening exercises [62].

5.4.2 Current quality of evidence

The GRADE results suggest that acupuncture has a higher overall effective rate, short-term effective rate, and fewer adverse reactions than Western medicine as a treatment for knee OA. In 2019, an overview of non-Cochrane SRs, which included a meta-analysis, concluded that acupuncture was beneficial for alleviating pain associated with knee OA. Due to the following constraints, evidence was reduced to "medium" or "low" quality: Most results were produced by a limited sample size and were based on imprecision. Because of the insufficient literature search, some of the results had a significant potential for publication bias, which could not be ruled out [23]. Regarding patients with knee OA, Zhang et al. compared the therapeutic efficacy of acupuncture + hyaluronic acid injection to hyaluronic acid injection alone. These studies, which were all published between 2012 and 2018, found that the combined therapy was more effective than hyaluronic acid injections alone in reducing pain. According to the GRADE system, the evidence quality for the key outcomes ranged from very low to low [24].

5.4.3 Conclusion

Acupuncture may have some advantages in the management of knee OA, and it is more effective in pain alleviation when combined with a hyaluronic acid injection. However, due to the low quality of evidence, small sample size, and high risk of the studies, rigorously conducted randomized controlled trials with large sample numbers are required to confirm the findings. Thus, improved methodological quality is required.

5.5 Postoperative nausea and vomiting

One of the most prevalent adverse events following surgery is postoperative nausea and vomiting (PONV). It is unpleasant for patients, raises the possibility of additional adverse consequences, including readmission, and increases the costs, the health care facility revenue [63]. Nausea indicates a feeling of upcoming vomiting, while vomiting defines the reflux of gastrointestinal contents [64]. A number of factors, including the patient's demographics and the surgery type, influence the risk of PONV. Some surgeries, such as gynecologic, breast, and open-heart surgery, have been associated with an increased risk of PONV [65], whereas patient risk factors include female gender, nonsmoking, a history of PONV, and motion nausea [66]. Weibel et al. evaluated the quality of evidence for the effectiveness and safety of single-antiemetic drugs and combinations of antiemetic drugs used to prevent postoperative nausea and vomiting in adults following general anesthesia [67] and discovered high-certainty evidence of clinical efficacy compared to placebo for aprepitant, ramosetron, granisetron, dexamethasone, and ondansetron; moderate certainty evidence of. However, more studies are needed to investigate the drugs' possible side effects as well as patient populations with comorbidities (e.g., individuals with diabetes and heart disease) [67]. Hypnosis, relaxation imagery, music therapy, aromatherapy, acupressure, acupuncture, and electroacupuncture have all been included in recent studies and publications as complementary and alternative medicine interventions for PONV [68]. Numerous studies were placebo-controlled clinical trials, which effectively eliminated the placebo effect. Acupuncture appears to be more successful at controlling nausea than vomiting [69–71]. The PC6 acupoint is one of the most commonly utilized and studied acupoints for the prevention and treatment of PONV. Cheong et al. showed that using a single point of PC6 alone or in combination with other acupoints and alternative acupoints could help in the prevention and treatment of PONV [72]. The mechanism underlying acupuncture's effectiveness to reduce PONV is still under investigation. Serotonin transmission and beta-endorphin release may be affected [73–75].

5.5.1 Previous quality of evidence

Lee et al. found low-quality evidence supporting the use of PC6 acupoint stimulation over sham (compared to the last update in 2009) and moderate-quality evidence showing no difference between PC6 acupoint stimulation and antiemetic drugs to prevent PONV. There was inconclusive evidence supporting the use of a combined strategy of PC6 acupoint stimulation and antiemetic drugs over drug prophylaxis, and further high-quality trials are needed [76].

5.5.2 Current quality of evidence

A growing number of studies have demonstrated the effectiveness of acupuncture in preventing and treating postoperative nausea and vomiting [26]. Fu et al.

reviewed 50 RCTs published from 1997 to 2020 with 5980 patients. Both single therapy-electroacupuncture, acupressure, transcutaneous electrical nerve stimulation (TENS), acupoint plaster, acupoint injection, and 5-hydroxytryptamine (5HTRA) receptor antagonists- and combination therapy (TENS + 5HTRA, acupressure + 5HTRA) had a better clinical effectiveness rate than placebo. However, the quality of evidence for acupuncture therapy in preventing PONV is moderate, low, and very low. None of the acupuncture therapy was regarded as high-quality evidence [25]. The results indicated that acupuncture was effective in reducing postoperative vomiting, both during the first 4 h (low quality) and within 24 h postoperatively (low quality); acupuncture was effective in reducing the first 4-h (moderate quality) and 0–24-h postoperative vomiting (moderate quality) when performed before and during anesthesia, respectively. Acupuncture was also effective in treating 0–24-h postoperative nausea (moderate quality) and in reducing the utilization of remedies during the first 4 h (moderate quality).

5.5.3 Conclusion

In adults, TENS + 5HTRA may be the best treatment, while in children, acupuncture reduces the incidence of PONV as well as the use of antiemetics, particularly during the first few hours after surgery. Future work should determine the best technique or combination of techniques for acupuncture and also explore the use of acupuncture as a part of the complementary and integrative treatment of PONV.

5.6 Postoperative pain

Postoperative pain is acute pain that occurs following tissue injury associated with surgery and should resolve during the healing process. This normally takes up to 3 months, after which the pain is considered to be chronic or persistent [77]. Armstrong et al. found a significant correlation between increased preoperative and postoperative pain scores and anxiety, current smoking, psychological conditions, and current opioid use. Additionally, Armstrong et al. recommended for a multimodal approach to postoperative pain management and developed a pain sequence to help providers [78]. Multimodal analgesia is an essential component of such care. Further, there has been a recent renewal of interest in non-opioid alternatives or adjuncts in controlling postoperative pain, often in the context of multimodal analgesia [79]. Intravenous acetaminophen, non-steroidal anti-inflammatory drugs (NSAIDs), magnesium, ketamine, dexmedetomidine, liposomal bupivacaine, and newer neuraxial and peripheral regional techniques, as well as patient-controlled modalities, are gaining importance. Acupuncture and transcutaneous electrical nerve stimulation may be useful as adjuncts in multimodal analgesia packages [79]. Acupuncture is a well-known and widely used treatment for pain and other conditions. There have been increasing numbers of clinical trials evaluating the efficacy of acupuncture and related techniques for postoperative analgesia. Sun et al. [80] evaluated 15 studies on the efficacy of acupuncture and related techniques for acute postoperative pain management in surgery: abdominal, maxillofacial, knee, hemorrhoidectomy, back, thoracotomy, hip arthroplasty, and molar extraction. They suggested that perioperative administration of acupuncture might be useful as an adjunct to postoperative analgesia [80].

5.6.1 Previous quality of evidence

Barlow et al. [81] found that acupressure reduced pain and acupuncture did not reduce pain but resulted in reduced use of ibuprofen (low-quality evidence). Chen et al. [82] found acupuncture superior to sham in post-operative fentanyl use, time to the first request for fentanyl, and pain intensity (low-quality evidence). Wu et al. [77] found that some forms of acupuncture (acupuncture, electroacupuncture (EA), and transcutaneous electrical acupoint stimulation (TEAS)) improved pain on day 1 after surgery and reduced opioid use; subgroup analysis showed that acupuncture and TEAS were superior to EA (moderate-quality evidence).

5.6.2 Current quality of evidence

Yin et al. [27] found that acupuncture in combination with conventional treatment showed no statistical difference in pain reduction in Postcholecystectomy syndrome. The quality of the evidence for the overall outcomes was acceptable. The results showed that there was 7.7% of outcomes with very low-quality evidence, 46.15% with low-quality evidence, 46.15% with moderate-quality evidence, and none with high-quality evidence. However, it is difficult for therapists and patients to use blinding for acupuncture [27]. Qin et al. (2020) assessed the effectiveness of acupuncture and related techniques for postoperative pain after hemorrhoidectomy. They found that auricular acupressure plus acupuncture, acupuncture, other acupuncture techniques, and auricular acupressure were significantly superior over usual care, and auricular acupressure plus acupuncture ranked the most effective when analyzed for pain intensity, but the findings were limited by the quality of the evidence. Park et al. [29] assessed the quality of evidence in RCTs comparing pain scores between the EA and the sham groups, finding low cumulative evidence certainty across all studies. A low rating was given because there was inconsistency and a high risk of bias across all studies. However, according to data synthesized from previous studies, EA demonstrated the possibility of reducing pain for patients after thoracotomy with lower amounts of opioid analgesics [29].

5.6.3 Conclusion

Acupuncture may improve the overall symptoms of Postcholecystic Syndrome. Acupuncture plus auricular acupressure is effective at reducing pain after postoperative hemorrhoidectomy, and electroacupuncture has the possibility of reducing pain for patients after thoracotomy.

Conflict of interest

The authors declare no conflict of interest.

Author details

Dedi Ardinata
Faculty of Medicine, Department of Physiology, Universitas Sumatera Utara, Sumatera Utara, Indonesia

*Address all correspondence to: dedi1@usu.ac.id

References

[1] Guyatt G, Cairns J, Churchill D, Cook D, Haynes B, Hirsh J, et al. Evidence-based medicine: A New approach to teaching the practice of medicine. JAMA: The Journal of the American Medical Association. 1992;**268**:2420-2425. DOI: 10.1001/jama.1992.03490170092032

[2] Dawes M, Summerskill W, Glasziou P, Cartabellotta A, Martin J, Hopayian K, et al. Sicily statement on evidence-based practice. BMC Medical Education. 2005;**5**:1-7. DOI: 10.1186/1472-6920-5-1

[3] Maudsley G, Strivens J. "Science", "critical thinking" and "competence" for Tomorrow's Doctors. A review of terms and concepts. Medical Education. 2000;**34**:53-60. DOI: 10.1046/j.1365-2923.2000.00428.x

[4] Godwin J. Rising to the challenges of evidence-based medicine: A way forward for acupuncture. Journal of Alternative and Complementary Medicine. 2014;**20**:805-809. DOI: 10.1089/acm.2014.0213

[5] Austin TM, Richter RR, Sebelski CA. Introduction to the GRADE approach for guideline development: Considerations for physical therapist practice. Physical Therapy. 2014;**94**:1652-1659

[6] Odgaard-Jensen J, Vist GE, Timmer A, Kunz R, Akl EA, Schünemann H, et al. Randomisation to protect against selection bias in healthcare trials. Cochrane Database of Systematic Reviews. 2011;**2011**:1-49. DOI: 10.1002/14651858.MR000012.pub3

[7] Lu CY. Observational studies: A review of study designs, challenges and strategies to reduce confounding. International Journal of Clinical Practice. 2009;**63**:691-697. DOI: 10.1111/j.1742-1241.2009.02056.x

[8] Ioannidis JPA. Why Most Published Research Findings are False. PLoS Medicine. 2005;**2**:696-701.DOI: 10.1371/journal.pmed.0020124

[9] Rogozinska E, Gargon E, Olmedo-Requena R, Asour A, Cooper NAM, Vale CL, et al. Methods used to assess outcome consistency in clinical studies: A literature-based evaluation. PLoS One. 2020;**15**:1-12. DOI: 10.1371/journal.pone.0235485

[10] Goldet G, Howick J. Understanding GRADE: An introduction. Journal of Evidence-Based Medicine. 2013;**6**:50-54. DOI: 10.1111/jebm.12018

[11] McDonald J, Janz S. The Acupuncture Evidence Project: A Comparative Literature Review (Revised Edition). 2017th ed. Brisbane, Australian Acupuncture and Chinese Medicine Association Ltd; 2017, 2017. Available from: http://www.acupuncture.org.au

[12] Balshem H, Helfand M, Schünemann HJ, Oxman AD, Kunz R, Brozek J, et al. GRADE guidelines: 3. Rating the quality of evidence. Journal of Clinical Epidemiology. 2011;**64**: 401-406. DOI: 10.1016/j.jclinepi.2010.07.015

[13] Xu J, Qing ZF, Pei J, Ji J. Acupuncture for migraine without aura: A systematic review and meta-analysis. Journal of Integrative Medicine. 2018;**16**:312-321. DOI: 10.1016/j.joim.2018.06.002

[14] Zhang XT, Li XY, Zhao C, Hu YY, Lin YY, Chen HQ, et al. An overview of systematic reviews of randomized controlled trials on acupuncture treating migraine. Pain Research and Management. 2019;**2019**:1-12. DOI: 10.1155/2019/5930627

[15] Li YX, Xiao XL, Zhong DL, Luo LJ, Yang H, Zhou J, et al. Effectiveness and

safety of acupuncture for migraine: An overview of systematic reviews. Pain Research and Management. 2020;**2020**: 1-14. DOI: 10.1155/2020/3825617

[16] Giovanardi CM, Cinquini M, Aguggia M, Allais G, Campesato M, Cevoli S, et al. Acupuncture vs. pharmacological prophylaxis of migraine: A systematic review of randomized controlled trials. Frontiers in Neurology. 2020;**11**:1-15. DOI: 10.3389/fneur.2020.576272

[17] Trinh KV, Diep D, Chen KJQ. Systematic review of episodic migraine prophylaxis: Efficacy of conventional treatments used in comparisons with acupuncture. Medical Acupuncture. 2019;**31**:85-97. DOI: 10.1089/acu.2019.1337

[18] Huang J, Shen M, Qin X, Guo W, Li H. Acupuncture for the treatment of tension-type headache: An overview of systematic reviews. Evidence-based Complementary and Alternative Medicine. 2020;**2020**:1-10. DOI: 10.1155/2020/4262910

[19] Kolokotsios S, Stamouli A, Koukoulithras I, Plexousakis M, Drousia G. The effectiveness of acupuncture on headache intensity and frequency in patients with tension-type headache: A systematic review and meta-analysis. Cureus. 2021;**13**:1-14. DOI: 10.7759/cureus.14237

[20] Xiang Y, He J, Li R. Appropriateness of sham or placebo acupuncture for randomized controlled trials of acupuncture for nonspecific low back pain: A systematic review and meta-analysis. Journal of Pain Research. 2018;**11**:83-94. DOI: 10.2147/JPR.S152743

[21] Xiang Y, He JY, Tian HH, Cao BY, Li R. Evidence of efficacy of acupuncture in the management of low back pain: A systematic review and meta-analysis of randomised placebo- or sham-controlled trials. Acupuncture in Medicine. 2020;**38**: 15-24. DOI: 10.1136/acupmed-2017-011445

[22] Mu J, Furlan AD, Lam WY, Hsu MY, Ning Z, Lao L. Acupuncture for chronic nonspecific low back pain. Cochrane Database of Systematic Reviews. 2020;**2020**:1-171. DOI: 10.1002/14651858.CD013814

[23] Li J, Li YX, Luo LJ, Ye J, Zhong DL, Xiao QW, et al. The effectiveness and safety of acupuncture for knee osteoarthritis: An overview of systematic reviews. Medicine (United States). 2019;**98**:1-9. DOI: 10.1097/MD.0000000000016301

[24] Zheng Y, Duan X, Qi S, Hu H, Wang M, Ren C, et al. Acupuncture therapy plus hyaluronic acid injection for knee osteoarthritis: A meta-analysis of randomized controlled trials. Evidence-based Complementary and Alternative Medicine. 2020;**2020**:1-10. DOI: 10.1155/2020/4034105

[25] Fu C-W, Shu Q, Jiao Y, Wu T, Song A-Q, Zhu Q-C, et al. Acupuncture in preventing postoperative nausea and vomiting: A systematic review and Bayesian network meta-analysis. TMR Non-Drug Therapy. 2021;**4**:1-9. DOI: 10.12032/TMRND20210525030

[26] Zhang Y, Zhang C, Yan M, Wang N, Liu J, Wu A. The effectiveness of PC6 acupuncture in the prevention of postoperative nausea and vomiting in children: A systematic review and meta-analysis. Paediatric Anaesthesia. 2020;**30**:552-563. DOI: 10.1111/pan.13860

[27] Yin Z, Xiao Q, Xu G, Cheng Y, Yang H, Zhou J, et al. Acupuncture for the postcholecystectomy syndrome: A systematic review and meta-analysis. Evidence-based Complementary and Alternative Medicine. 2020;**2020**:1-19. DOI: 10.1155/2020/7509481.

[28] Zhang Y, Zhang C, Yan M, Wang N, Liu J, Wu A. Acupuncture and related techniques for postoperative pain after hemorrhoidectomy: A systematic review and meta-analysis. Paediatric Anaesthesia. 2020;**30**:552-563. DOI: 10.1111/pan.13860

[29] Park S, Lyu YR, Park SJ, Oh MS, Jung IC, Lee E-J. Electroacupuncture for post-thoracotomy pain: A systematic review and meta-analysis. PLoS One. 2021;**16**:e0254093. DOI: 10.1371/journal.pone.0254093

[30] Hayne DP, Martin PR. Relating photophobia, visual aura, and visual triggers of headache and migraine. Headache. 2019;**59**:430-442. DOI: 10.1111/head.13486

[31] Carville S, Padhi S, Reason T, Underwood M. Diagnosis and management of headaches in young people and adults: Summary of NICE guidance. BMJ (Online). 2012;**345**:1-5. DOI: 10.1136/bmj.e5765

[32] Carsten P. Evidence-based guideline update: Pharmacologic treatment for episodic migraine prevention in adults: Report of the quality standards subcommittee of the American academy of neurology and the American headache society. Neurology. 2013;**80**:869-870. DOI: 10.1212/01.wnl.0000427909.23467.39

[33] Urits I, Patel M, Putz ME, Monteferrante N, Nguyen D, An D, et al. Acupuncture and its role in the treatment of migraine headaches. Neurology and Therapy. n.d.;**9**:375-394. DOI: 10.6084/m9.figshare.12981695

[34] Linde K, Allais G, Brinkhaus B, Fei Y, Mehring M, Vertosick EA, et al. Acupuncture for the prevention of episodic migraine. Cochrane Database of Systematic Reviews. 2016;**2016**:1-148. DOI: 10.1002/14651858.CD001218.pub3

[35] da Silva AN. Acupuncture for migraine prevention. Headache: The Journal of Head and Face Pain. 2015;**55**: 470-473. DOI: 10.1111/head.12525

[36] Yang Y, Que Q, Ye X, Zheng GH. Verum versus sham manual acupuncture for migraine: A systematic review of randomised controlled trials. Acupuncture in Medicine. 2016;**34**:76-83. DOI: 10.1136/acupmed-2015-010903

[37] Jensen RH. Tension-type headache—The normal and most prevalent headache. Headache. 2018;**58**:339-345. DOI: 10.1111/head.13067

[38] Olesen J, Bes A, Kunkel R, Lance JW, Nappi G, Pfaffenrath V, et al. The international classification of headache disorders, 3rd edition (beta version). Cephalalgia. 2013;**33**:629-808. DOI: 10.1177/0333102413485658

[39] Bendtsen L, Evers S, Linde M, Mitsikostas DD, Sandrini G, Schoenen J. EFNS guideline on the treatment of tension-type headache—Report of an EFNS task force. European Journal of Neurology. 2010;**17**:1318-1325. DOI: 10.1111/j.1468-1331.2010.03070.x

[40] Smitherman TA, Penzien DB, Rains JC. Challenges of nonpharmacologic interventions in chronic tension-type headache. Current Pain and Headache Reports. 2007;**11**: 471-477

[41] Linde K, Allais G, Brinkhaus B, Manheimer E, Vickers A, White AR. Acupuncture for tension-type headache. Cochrane Database of Systematic Reviews. 2009:1-3. DOI: 10.1002/14651858.CD007587

[42] Linde K, Allais G, Brinkhaus B, Fei Y, Mehring M, Shin BC, et al. Acupuncture for the prevention of tension-type headache. Cochrane Database of Systematic Reviews. 2016;**2016**:1-54. DOI: 10.1002/14651858.CD007587.pub2

[43] Lardon A, Girard MP, Zaïm C, Lemeunier N, Descarreaux M, Marchand AA. Effectiveness of preventive and treatment interventions for primary headaches in the workplace: A systematic review of the literature. Cephalalgia. 2017;**37**:64-73. DOI: 10.1177/0333102416636096

[44] Vlaeyen JWS, Maher CG, Wiech K, van Zundert J, Meloto CB, Diatchenko L, et al. Low back pain. Nature Reviews Disease Primers. 2018;**4**:1-18. DOI: 10.1038/s41572-018-0052-1

[45] Qaseem A, Wilt TJ, McLean RM, Forciea MA. Noninvasive treatments for acute, subacute, and chronic low back pain: A clinical practice guideline from the American College of Physicians. Annals of Internal Medicine. 2017;**166**:514-530. DOI: 10.7326/M16-2367

[46] Kongsted A, Kent P, Axen I, Downie AS, Dunn KM. What have we learned from ten years of trajectory research in low back pain? BMC Musculoskeletal Disorders. 2016;**17**:1-11. DOI: 10.1186/s12891-016-1071-2

[47] Maher C, Underwood M, Buchbinder R. Non-specific low back pain. The Lancet. 2017;**389**:736-747. DOI: 10.1016/S0140-6736(16)30970-9

[48] Chou R, Deyo R, Friedly J, Skelly A, Weimer M, Fu R, et al. Systemic pharmacologic therapies for low back pain: A systematic review for an American College of physicians clinical practice guideline. Annals of Internal Medicine. 2017;**166**:480-492. DOI: 10.7326/M16-2458

[49] Oliveira CB, Maher CG, Pinto RZ, Traeger AC, Lin CWC, Chenot JF, et al. Clinical practice guidelines for the management of non-specific low back pain in primary care: An updated overview. European Spine Journal. 2018;**27**:2791-2803. DOI: 10.1007/s00586-018-5673-2

[50] Wellington J. Noninvasive and alternative management of chronic low back pain (efficacy and outcomes). Neuromodulation. 2014;**17**:24-30. DOI: 10.1111/ner.12078

[51] Appleyard I, Lundeberg T, Robinson N. Should systematic reviews assess the risk of bias from sham-placebo acupuncture control procedures? European Journal of Integrative Medicine. 2014;**6**:234-243. DOI: 10.1016/j.eujim.2014.03.004

[52] Roger C, Richard D, Janna F, Andrea S, Robin H, Melissa W, et al. Noninvasive Treatments for Low Back Pain. Comparative Effectiveness Review No. 169. Rockville:Agency for Healthcare Research and Quality; 2016

[53] Li R, Jiang Y, Hu R, He X, Fang J. Effectiveness and safety of tenosynovitis of the long head of the biceps brachii with acupuncture: A protocol for a systematic review and meta-analysis. Trials. 2020;**21**:1-7. DOI: 10.1186/s13063-020-04800-6

[54] Hunter DJ, Bierma-Zeinstra S. Osteoarthritis. The Lancet. 2019;**393**:1745-1759. DOI: 10.1016/S0140-6736(19)30417-9

[55] Fu K, Robbins SR, McDougall JJ. Osteoarthritis: The genesis of pain. Rheumatology (United Kingdom). 2018;**57**:iv43-iv50. DOI: 10.1093/rheumatology/kex419

[56] Liu A, Kendzerska T, Stanaitis I, Hawker G. The relationship between knee pain characteristics and symptom state acceptability in people with knee osteoarthritis. Osteoarthritis and Cartilage. 2014;**22**:178-183. DOI: 10.1016/j.joca.2013.11.012

[57] Zhang W, Moskowitz RW, Nuki G, Abramson S, Altman RD, Arden N, et al.

OARSI recommendations for the management of hip and knee osteoarthritis, Part II: OARSI evidence-based, expert consensus guidelines. Osteoarthritis and Cartilage. 2008;**16**:137-162. DOI: 10.1016/j.joca.2007.12.013

[58] Baigent C, Bhala N, Emberson J, Merhi A, Abramson S, Arber N, et al. Vascular and upper gastrointestinal effects of non-steroidal anti-inflammatory drugs: Meta-analyses of individual participant data from randomised trials. The Lancet. 2013;**382**:769-779. DOI: 10.1016/S0140-6736(13)60900-9

[59] Bensman A. Non-steroidal anti-inflammatory drugs (NSAIDs) systemic use: The risk of renal failure. Frontiers in Pediatrics. 2020;7:1-2. DOI: 10.3389/fped.2019.00517

[60] Li R, Sun J, Hu H, Zhang Q, Sun R, Zhou S, et al. Research trends of acupuncture therapy on knee osteoarthritis from 2010 to 2019: A bibliometric analysis. Journal of Pain Research. 2020;**13**:1901-1913. DOI: 10.2147/JPR.S258739

[61] Kolasinski SL, Neogi T, Hochberg MC, Oatis C, Guyatt G, Block J, et al. 2019 American College of Rheumatology/Arthritis Foundation Guideline for the management of osteoarthritis of the hand, hip, and knee. Arthritis and Rheumatology. 2020;**72**:220-233. DOI: 10.1002/art.41142

[62] Corbett MS, Rice SJC, Madurasinghe V, Slack R, Fayter DA, Harden M, et al. Acupuncture and other physical treatments for the relief of pain due to osteoarthritis of the knee: Network meta-analysis. Osteoarthritis and Cartilage. 2013;**21**:1290-1298. DOI: 10.1016/j.joca.2013.05.007

[63] Gan TJ, Diemunsch P, Habib AS, Kovac A, Kranke P, Meyer TA, et al. Consensus guidelines for the management of postoperative nausea and vomiting. Anesthesia and Analgesia. 2014;**118**:85-113. DOI: 10.1213/ANE.0000000000000002

[64] Becker DE. Nausea, vomiting, and hiccups: A review of mechanisms and treatment. Anesthesia Progress. 2010;**57**:150-156; quiz 157. DOI: 10.2344/0003-3006-57.4.150

[65] Tateosian V, Gan TJ. Another quest for the holy grail of abolishing post operative nausea and vomiting. Journal of Clinical Anesthesia. 2017;**41**:58-59. DOI: 10.1016/j.jclinane.2017.06.007

[66] Jin Z, Gan TJ, Bergese SD. Prevention and treatment of postoperative nausea and vomiting (Ponv): A review of current recommendations and emerging therapies. Therapeutics and Clinical Risk Management. 2020;**16**:1305-1317. DOI: 10.2147/TCRM.S256234

[67] Weibel S, Schaefer MS, Raj D, Rücker G, Pace NL, Schlesinger T, et al. Drugs for preventing postoperative nausea and vomiting in adults after general anaesthesia: An abridged Cochrane network meta-analysis. Anaesthesia. 2021;**76**:962-973. DOI: 10.1111/anae.15295

[68] Stoicea N, Gan TJ, Joseph N, Uribe A, Pandya J, Dalal R, et al. Alternative therapies for the prevention of postoperative nausea and vomiting. Frontiers in Medicine. 2015;**2**:1-5. DOI: 10.3389/fmed.2015.00087

[69] Gan TJ, Jiao KR, Zenn M, Georgiade G. A randomized controlled comparison of electro-acupoint stimulation or ondansetron versus placebo for the prevention of postoperative nausea and vomiting. Anesthesia & Analgesia. 2004;**99**: 1070-1075

[70] Alizadeh R, Esmaeili S, Shoar S, Bagheri-Hariri S, Shoar N. Acupuncture

in preventing postoperative nausea and vomiting: Efficacy of two acupuncture points versus a single one. JAMS Journal of Acupuncture and Meridian Studies. 2014;7:71-75. DOI: 10.1016/j.jams.2013.04.005

[71] Smith C, Crowther C. The placebo response and effect of time in a trial of acupuncture to treat nausea and vomiting in early pregnancy. Complementary Therapies in Medicine. 2002;**10**:210-216. DOI: 10.1016/S0965-2299(02)00072-9

[72] Cheong KB, Zhang JP, Huang Y, Zhang ZJ. The effectiveness of acupuncture in prevention and treatment of postoperative nausea and vomiting—A systematic review and meta-analysis. PLoS One. 2013;**8**:1-17. DOI: 10.1371/journal.pone.0082474

[73] Lee EJ, Warden S. The effects of acupuncture on serotonin metabolism. European Journal of Integrative Medicine. 2016;**8**:355-367. DOI: 10.1016/j.eujim.2016.06.022

[74] Liu JL, Chen SP, Gao YH, Meng FY, Bin WS, Wang JY. Effects of repeated electroacupuncture on β-endorphin and adrencorticotropic hormone levels in the hypothalamus and pituitary in rats with chronic pain and ovariectomy. Chinese Journal of Integrative Medicine. 2010;**16**:315-323. DOI: 10.1007/s11655-010-0503-3

[75] Ma S-X. Neurobiology of acupuncture: Toward CAM. Evidence-based Complementary and Alternative Medicine. 2004;**1**:41-47

[76] Lee A, Chan SKKC, Fan LTYT. Stimulation of the wrist acupuncture point PC6 for preventing postoperative nausea and vomiting. The Cochrane Database of Systematic Reviews. 2015;**11**:1-164. DOI: 10.1002/14651858.CD003281.pub4

[77] Wu MS, Chen KH, Chen IF, Huang SK, Tzeng PC, Yeh ML, et al. The efficacy of acupuncture in post-operative pain management: A systematic review and meta-analysis. PLoS One. 2016;**11**:1-12. DOI: 10.1371/journal.pone.0150367

[78] Schug SA, Lavand'Homme P, Barke A, Korwisi B, Rief W, Treede RD. The IASP classification of chronic pain for ICD-11: Chronic postsurgical or posttraumatic pain. Pain. 2019;**160**:45-52. DOI: 10.1097/j.pain.0000000000001413

[79] Mitra S, Carlyle D, Kodumudi G, Kodumudi V, Vadivelu N. New advances in acute postoperative pain management. Current Pain and Headache Reports. 2018;**22**:1-11. DOI: 10.1007/s11916-018-0690-8

[80] Sun Y, Gan TJ, Dubose JW, Habib AS. Acupuncture and related techniques for postoperative pain: A systematic review of randomized controlled trials. British Journal of Anaesthesia. 2008;**101**:151-160. DOI: 10.1093/bja/aen146

[81] Barlow T, Downham C, Barlow D. The effect of complementary therapies on post-operative pain control in ambulatory knee surgery: A systematic review. Complementary Therapies in Medicine. 2013;**21**:529-534. DOI: 10.1016/j.ctim.2013.06.008

[82] Chen CC, Yang CC, Hu CC, Shih HN, Chang YH, Hsieh PH. Acupuncture for pain relief after total knee arthroplasty: A randomized controlled trial. Regional Anesthesia and Pain Medicine. 2015;**40**:31-36. DOI: 10.1097/AAP.0000000000000138

Chapter 12

Vibration Therapy for Health Promotion

Danúbia da Cunha de Sá-Caputo, Adérito Seixas, Redha Taiar and Mario Bernardo-Filho

Abstract

Vibration therapy has been used as a clinical intervention, in which mechanical vibration is transmitted to a part or to the whole body of the individual. It is very important to point out that mechanical vibration is a natural stimulus that is part of the daily life of all living beings and is periodically added to the organism due to a movement of the body. When, for several reasons, the person cannot add mechanical vibration to the body, the mechanical vibration generated by a device can be transmitted to the person in contact with it. When the intervention aims to treat a complaint referring to a specific anatomical segment, it is called local or segmental vibration therapy. However, when mechanical vibration is transmitted to the whole person's body, aiming for an improvement in the performance, or as a clinical intervention, the procedure is called Systemic vibration therapy. The biological effects would be due to the mechano-transduction mechanism by which cells convert mechanical stimulus into biological activity, releasing various hormones and other substances. This form of mechano-transduction is important to physiological processes in the body, including proprioception, effects on bone mineral density, muscle, balance, and functionality, promoting the modulation of biological effects through specific signaling pathways. In this chapter, the use of mechanical vibration as an intervention aiming to improve and optimize daily life is discussed, either as a local or systemic application, targeting a specific part of the body or the whole body, respectively.

Keywords: whole-body vibration exercise, local vibration therapy, systemic vibration therapy, Mechano-biomodulation, daily life

1. Introduction

Technological development in different areas of knowledge has led to the emergence of new procedures that have been progressively incorporated into professional activities in different sectors, including in health sciences. As a consequence, everyone must be prepared to be challenged and use what technological advances have to offer, providing better living conditions for all people who need help to improve their health condition and quality of life. Knowledge about potential benefits and limitations will guide the best way to take advantage of new technologies [1–3]. Thus, the establishment of safety-related criteria that must be followed together with the update in the level of evidence of related publications will guide the effectiveness of the procedure with the safe use of the technique without adverse events [4–7].

Particularly, in the health sector, these challenges have a special dimension. Health professionals must be able to critically analyze the available information to choose the safest and most beneficial interventions, incorporating scientific evidence, clinical expertise, patient preferences and values to make decisions. This is the basis for evidence-informed practice, which allows patients to have the maximum benefits from these new technologies without being subjected to unnecessary risks [5–7]. Vibration therapy, is an example of a technological intervention, supported by research findings and with neglectable risks for the patients [8–10].

The exposition of the body to mechanical vibration, as a clinical intervention, is not recent, but the use of mechanical vibration in the context of health promotion (in different conditions), with well-defined criteria started in 6th decade of the last century. Vibration therapy has been used as a clinical intervention, in which mechanical vibration is transmitted to the part [10] or whole body [11, 12] of the individual. Specific biomechanical parameters, position of the individual, exposition and rest time, and periodicity are established according to the condition to be treated and the desired effect. Whole-body vibration exercise is an exercise promoted on a vibrating platform, while mechanical vibration is being transmitted [8, 9, 12].

2. Mechanical vibration

2.1 General characteristics

Mechanical vibration is a physical agent of wave nature. It can be produced by different devices, such as a refrigerator engine, a motor vehicle engine, an air conditioner, and others. A vibrating platform is one of such examples. In all the examples provided, the device is outside the person's body, but if the person is in contact with it, the mechanical vibration is transmitted to the person [11, 12]. As shown in **Figure 1**, the waveforms of mechanical vibrations produced by different devices, can be deterministic (**Figure 1A**) or random in nature.

The mechanical vibration, that is generated in a vibrating platform [11, 12] or portable [10] devices, is characterized by the sinusoidal form, and this deterministic approach has particular interest for everything that will be covered in this book chapter on vibration therapy.

2.2 Mechanical vibration as a daily stimulus

It is very important to highlight that mechanical vibration is a natural stimulus that is part of the daily life of all living beings and is periodically added to the organism during movements [11, 12]. It is closely associated with the physiological responses of all organisms, including human being. The addition of mechanical vibration happens in a wide number of routine situations [11], such as walking, running, playing, being in a car or public transport, or doing a domestic activity, such as using a vacuum cleaner for cleaning or a fruit extractor while making a juice. Likewise, in professional activities such as driving a car, truck, train, or using dental equipment, mechanical vibration is transmitted to the individual that is in contact with the device that is producing the referred vibration [13, 14]. In addition, several structures of the human body naturally produce mechanical vibrations, such as the heart, digestive system, the shortening and stretching of muscle fibers, vessels of the vascular system, the vibrational energy of electrons in a chemical bond, or the vibration of molecules in the cellular metabolism. Likewise, many of the organic functions depend on mechanical vibrations at different levels of anatomical structures [12, 15, 16]. Of course, in general, this addition of mechanical vibration is

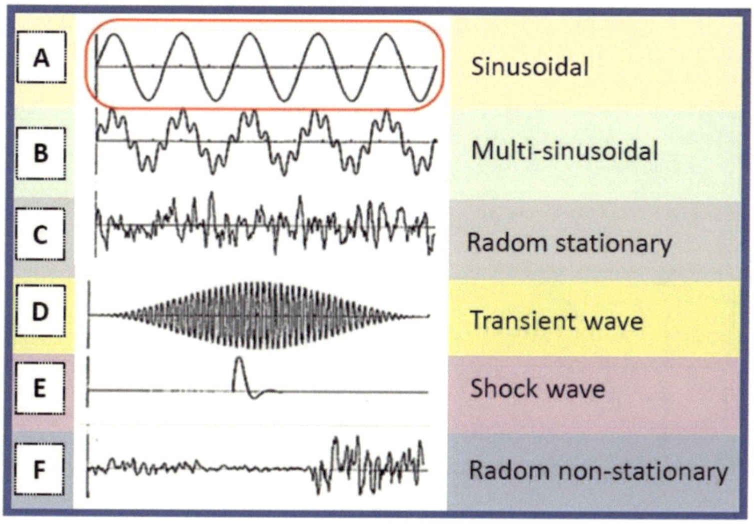

Figure 1.
Different waveforms related to mechanical vibration.

not fully perceived by the person, but when a movement is performed, mechanical vibration is added to the body. However, in some activities like walking or running, when the foot contacts the floor, mechanical vibration is more easily perceived. It may be relevant to consider that this addition of mechanical vibration would be the trigger for organic functions to take place and for the person to live with physical and mental health [12, 16].

When, for several reasons, the person cannot add mechanical vibration to the body, the mechanical vibration generated by a device can be transmitted to the person in contact with it. This procedure corresponds to a clinical intervention called vibration therapy [10–12].

2.3 Biomechanical characteristics of mechanical vibration

Vibration therapy, which is considered in this chapter, uses mechanical vibration, which is a physical agent that transports energy and is characterized by a displacement in relation to an equilibrium position with an oscillatory, sinusoidal, and deterministic movement, as shown in **Figure 2**.

In this case, biomechanical parameters such as frequency, amplitude, and peak-to-peak displacement can be conveniently adjusted depending on the outcome to be achieved and the individual's clinical conditions. These parameters need to be considered when designing a vibration therapy intervention protocol [8].

Frequency (f) is expressed in Hertz (Hz) and represents the number of cycles in one unit of time, for example, the second. Peak-to-peak displacement (D) is the measure of the perpendicular extension between the largest and smallest displacement of mechanical vibration expressed in millimeters (mm). The amplitude represents half the peak-to-peak displacement and is also expressed in mm. These parameters are represented in **Figure 3**. The path of the mechanical stimulus between the successive points Z1 and Z2, defines the cycle developed by the vibration. The number of cycles performed in the unit of time is the frequency [8, 11, 12]. An important observation is that at Z2, the stimulus begins again to have the same characteristics as point Z1.

The distance comprised by the straight-line segment between points Z1 and Z2, measured, for example, in mm, is defined as the wavelength of the mechanical

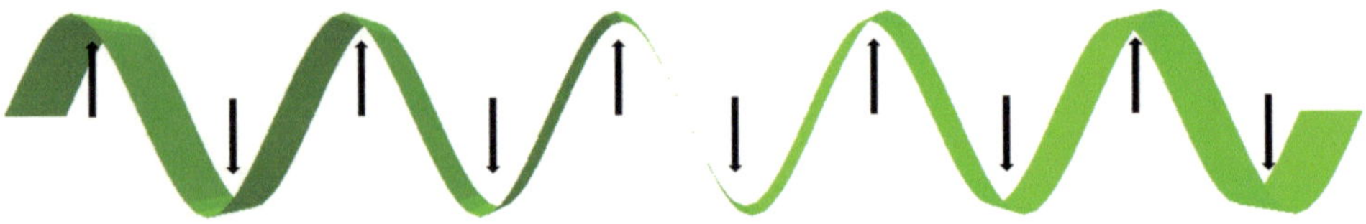

Figure 2.
Sinusoidal waveforms related to mechanical vibration.

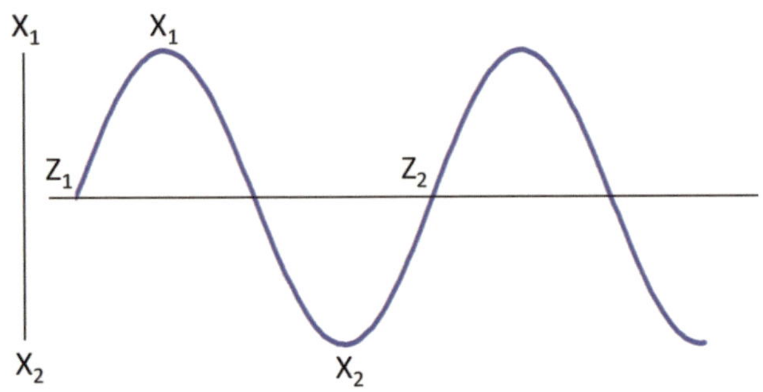

Figure 3.
Representation of a sinusoidal mechanical vibration.

stimulus. This corresponds to the projection of the entire cycle on the propagation plane. It is important to consider that in the International System of Measurements, the wavelength value would be expressed in meters. Considering the perpendicular measure between the highest point or the lowest point (x1) of the mechanical vibration and the propagation plane or the lowest point (x2) is the amplitude. The perpendicular of the point X1 up to the level of the x2 is the displacement peak-to-peak. The value of the displacement peak-to-peak corresponds to twice the amplitude [17].

The peak acceleration (Ap) of mechanical vibration depends on the frequency and the peak-to-peak displacement and is normally expressed in multiples of gravity (xg). The peak acceleration can be determined using accelerometers, or according to the equation Ap = 2 x π2 x f2 x D [17]. Peak acceleration allows defining the intensity or magnitude of mechanical vibration and of the vibration therapy.

Two mechanical vibrations, with the same frequency, with displacement with correspondences in points X1 and x2, are said to be in phase. On the other hand, when these coincidences do not occur, the two stimuli are out of phase. These considerations are relevant, in the same way, the stimulus generated in the platform has its own amplitude, the medium being crossed also presents mechanical vibration.

3. Mechanical vibration and vibration therapy

Throughout the history of humanity, it can be verified that through various procedures, mechanical vibration has been added to a person's body such as manipulation techniques, and others related to breathing, such as coughing and percussion [11, 18].

The addition of mechanical vibration can be through devices that transmit the mechanical vibration locally. When the intervention aims to treat a complaint referring to a specific anatomical segment, it is called local or segmental vibration therapy [10]. When mechanical vibration is transmitted to the whole person's body, aiming for an improvement in the physical performance, or as a clinical intervention, there is the generation of whole-body vibration exercises [8, 12] and, the procedure is called Systemic vibration therapy. As it is shown in **Figure 4**, the biological effects of mechanical vibrations would be due to the mechanotransduction mechanism by which cells (cellular structures and inner environment of the cell) convert mechanical stimulus into biological activity and there is the release of various hormonal and no hormonal molecules [19].

This form of mechanotransduction would be responsible for a number of physiological processes in the body, including proprioception, effects on bone

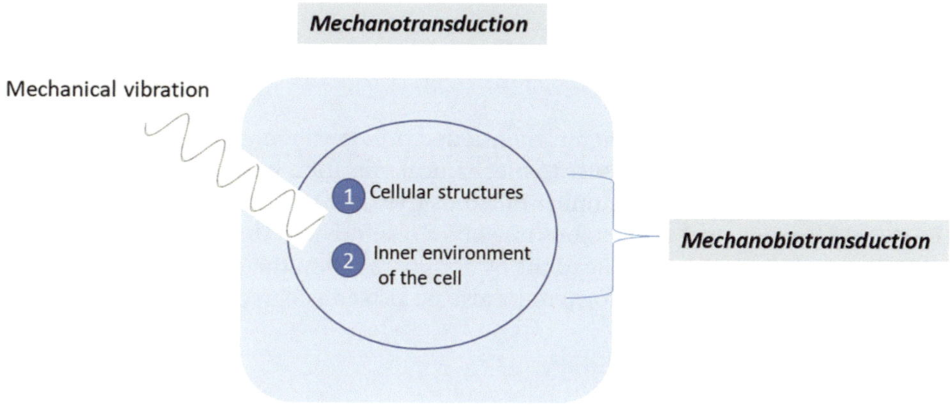

Figure 4.
Interaction of the mechanical vibration with the cell and the mechanobiotransduction.

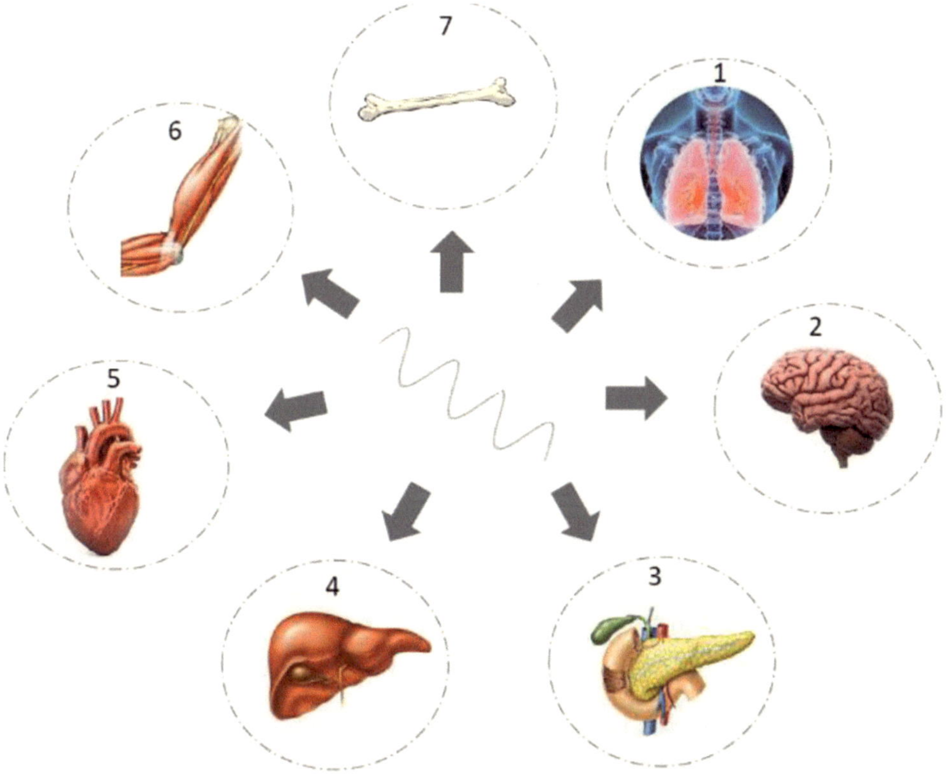

Figure 5.
Some targets of the mechanical vibration in the body related to proprioception (2, 6, 7), effects on bone mineral density (6) and in the metabolism (3, 4), endocrine (2, 3, 4), and immunity systems (2, 7), muscle (6) and vital functions (1, 5), balance (2, 6, 7), and functionality (2, 6, 7).

mineral density and in the metabolism, endocrine and immunity systems, muscle and vital functions, balance, and functionality. The mechanical vibration would be a physical agent that would lead to mechanobiomodulation of the physiological phenomena in various organs or systems as it is suggested in **Figure 5**. Mechanical vibration could act as an agent that promotes the modulation of biological effects through specific signaling pathways, as various hormonal and other substances. Vibration therapy might be considered a complementary intervention that can be used in the management of individuals with different health conditions.

3.1 Vibration therapy

In vibration therapy, parameters mentioned previously must be considered. Additionally, the time of exposure to mechanical vibration in a session, the total time of the intervention, the number of exposures, rest time in each session, and the weekly frequency of the sessions must be considered. In the case of whole-body vibration exercise generated due to the Systemic vibration therapy, the person's position in relation to the platform must also be also considered [8].

3.1.1 Devices used in vibration therapy

3.1.1.1 Local vibration therapy

The devices used in local vibration therapy are relatively simple and are small, and in general, are portable devices device that applies vibration directly over the muscle or the tendon [20]. Buttons are available for selecting the operational conditions of the intervention characteristics, which consider the frequency of mechanical vibration. Local vibration therapy is very important for several individuals that are in long-term immobilization, immobilization by a cast, or being in the early rehabilitation period after surgery [10, 20].

3.1.1.2 Systemic vibration therapy

The device used in Systemic vibration therapy is a vibrating platform. Systemic vibration therapy is a clinical intervention in which mechanical vibration generated on a vibrating platform is transmitted to the entire body of the person who is in contact with the base of the platform producing the whole-body vibration exercise in the individual [8, 12, 16].

There are two main types of vibrating platforms, which are shown in **Figure 6A** and **B**. **Figure 6A** represents a vibrating platform where the base performs a movement with vertical displacement as a result of the force applied. The oscillating of this base can be vertical or triplane way. **Figure 6B** has demonstrated the side alternating vibrating platform, where the base performs side alternating movements (up and down) [8, 12, 16].

In the side alternating vibrating platform, the base rests on a central fulcrum. When turned on, while the right side of the base goes up, the left side goes down, generating mechanical vibration, like a seesaw. The mechanical vibration is then transmitted to the individual who is in contact with the base, and this platform is called the side alternating platform [8, 12, 16].

In the vertical platform, the whole base of the platform goes up and down which is called the vertical displacement type. This vertical displacement may be due to a simple displacement of the base, lowering and raising. In this case, the vibrating

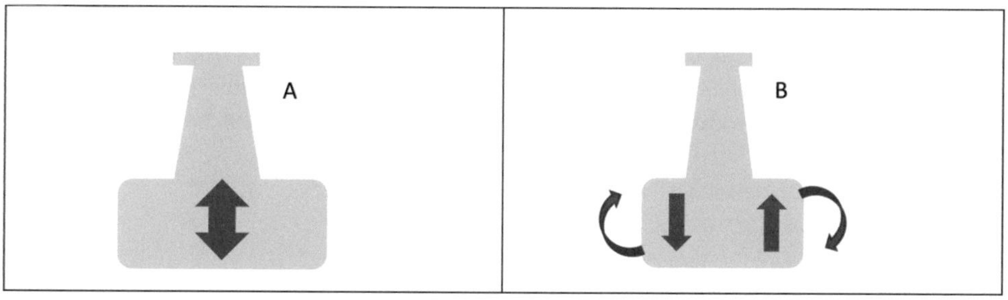

Figure 6.
Vibrating platforms and oscillation of their bases.

platform is called a synchronous vertical type of platform. This vertical displacement can also be a result of the base displacement in three planes. In this case, the platform is named the triplane vertical platform [8, 12].

It is easy to verify that, associated with the mechanical vibration, a force is generated, which is responsible for the displacement of the base of the vibrating platform, and it is transmitted to the person's body. This force arises from the action of the acceleration imposed by the vibrating platform on the body, which has a certain mass [8, 12, 16].

3.2 Local vibration therapy

Local vibration therapy could be an alternative form of vibration training for individuals that are unable to perform systemic vibration therapy. The main interest of Local vibration therapy compared to Systemic vibration therapy is that it does not necessarily require any active contribution from the participant. Local vibration therapy is not an entirely novel concept and in fact, it has been used for a long time in the field of neuroscience. Indeed, Local vibration therapy applied to the tendon can induce several physiological effects such as a tonic vibration reflex or muscle movement illusion depending on the experimental setup [10, 20, 21].

3.3 Systemic vibration therapy

In Systemic vibration therapy, the mechanical vibration produced on the vibrating platform is transmitted to the person generating an exercise throughout the whole body of the individual, the whole-body vibration exercise. Typically, the person has their feet positioned on the base of the vibrating platform, being in an orthostatic position with knees bent or sitting in an ancillary chair positioned in front of the platform [8].

There is a scientific evidence that Systemic vibration therapy can (i) improve muscle strength and potency, sleep quality, peripheral blood circulation, flexibility, functionality, balance, postural control, and quality of life; (ii) reduce pain, muscle fatigue, the risk of falling, and (iii) increase muscle fiber recruitment and bone mineral density [8, 12, 16, 22].

4. Conclusion

In this chapter, we discussed the use of mechanical vibration as an intervention aimed to improve and optimize daily life. This vibration therapy can be used as a local application of mechanical vibration, to the whole body and as Systemic vibration therapy. Vibrational movements are present in our everyday life. Using these concepts of vibrational analysis, their understanding and optimization represent a challenge in bringing individuals to an original way of natural therapy.

Author details

Danúbia da Cunha de Sá-Caputo[1,2], Adérito Seixas[3,4], Redha Taiar[5] and Mario Bernardo-Filho[1]*

1 Laboratório de Vibrações Mecânicas e Práticas Integrativas, Departamento de Biofísica e Biometria, Instituto de Biologia Roberto Alcântara Gomes and Policlínica Piquet Carneiro, Universidade do Estado do Rio de Janeiro, Rio de Janeiro, RJ, Brazil

2 Faculdade de Ciências Médicas, Programa de Pós-Graduação em Fisiopatologia Clínica e Experimental,Universidade do Estado do Rio de Janeiro, Rio de Janeiro, RJ, Brazil

3 Escola Superior de Saúde Fernando Pessoa, Porto, Portugal

4 Faculdade de Desporto, LABIOMEP, INEGI-LAETA, Universidade do Porto, Porto, Portugal

5 GRESPI, University of Reims Champagne-Ardenne, France

*Address all correspondence to: bernardofilhom@gmail.com

References

[1] Espín J, Špacírová Z, Rovira J, Epstein D, Olry de Labry Lima A, García-Mochón L. Development of the European healthcare and social cost database (EUHCSCD) for use in economic evaluation of healthcare programs. BMC Health Services Research. 2022;**22**(1):405. DOI: 10.1186/s12913-022-07791-z

[2] Wu W, Zhang J, Yi R, Li X, Yu X. Cost-effectiveness of anti-retropulsive devices varies according to the locations of proximal ureteral stones: A retrospective cohort study. BMC Urology. 2022;**22**(1):43. DOI: 10.1186/s12894-022-00995-9

[3] Snowsill TM, Stathi A, Green C, Withall J, Greaves CJ, Thompson JL, et al. Cost-effectiveness of a physical activity and behaviour maintenance programme on functional mobility decline in older adults: An economic evaluation of the REACT (retirement in action) trial. The Lancet Public Health. 2022;**S2468-2667**(22):00030-00035. DOI: 10.1016/S2468-2667(22)00030-5

[4] Jarvis P, Carra I, Jafari M, Judd SJ. Ceramic vs polymeric membrane implementation for potable water treatment. Water Research. 2022;**215**:118269. DOI: 10.1016/j.watres.2022.118269

[5] Feldman MD, Petersen AJ, Karliner LS, Tice JA. Who is responsible for evaluating the safety and effectiveness of medical devices? The role of independent technology assessment. Journal of General Internal Medicine. 2008;**23**(Suppl. 1):57-63. DOI: 10.1007/s11606-007-0275-4

[6] Alotaibi YK, Federico F. The impact of health information technology on patient safety. Saudi Medical Journal. 2017;**38**(12):1173-1180. DOI: 10.15537/smj.2017.12.20631

[7] Sampietro-Colom L, Lach K, Pasternack I, Wasserfallen JB, Cicchetti A, Marchetti M, et al. Guiding principles for good practices in hospital-based health technology assessment units. International Journal of Technology Assessment in Health Care. 2015;**31**(6):457-465

[8] van Heuvelen MJG, Rittweger J, Judex S, Sañudo B, Seixas A, Fuermaier ABM, et al. Reporting guidelines for whole-body vibration studies in humans, animals and cell cultures: A consensus statement from an International Group of Experts. Biology (Basel). 2021;**10**(10):965. DOI: 10.3390/biology10100965

[9] Sañudo B, Seixas A, Gloeckl R, Rittweger J, Rawer R, Taiar R, et al. Potential application of whole body vibration exercise for improving the clinical conditions of COVID-19 infected individuals: A narrative review from the world Association of Vibration Exercise Experts (WAVex) panel. International Journal of Environmental Research and Public Health. 2020;**17**(10):3650. DOI: 10.3390/ijerph17103650

[10] Souron R, Besson T, Millet GY, Lapole T. Acute and chronic neuromuscular adaptations to local vibration training. European Journal of Applied Physiology. 2017;**117**(10):1939-1964. DOI: 10.1007/s00421-017-3688-8 Epub 2017 Aug 1. Erratum in: Eur J Appl Physiol. 2017; PMID: 28766150

[11] Cardinale M, Wakeling J. Whole body vibration exercise: Are vibrations good for you? British Journal of Sports Medicine. 2005;**39**(9):585-589. DOI: 10.1136/bjsm.2005.016857

[12] Rittweger J. Vibration as an exercise modality: How it may work, and what its potential might be. European Journal of Applied Physiology. 2010;**108**(5):

877-904. DOI: 10.1007/s00421-009-1303-312

[13] Abercromby AF, Amonette WE, Layne CS, McFarlin BK, Hinman MR, Paloski WH. Vibration exposure and biodynamic responses during whole-body vibration training. Medicine and Science in Sports and Exercise. 2007;**39**(10):1794-1800. DOI: 10.1249/mss.0b013e3181238a0f

[14] Abercromby AF, Amonette WE, Layne CS, McFarlin BK, Hinman MR, Paloski WH. Variation in neuromuscular responses during acute whole-body vibration exercise. Medicine and Science in Sports and Exercise. 2007;**39**(9):1642-1650. DOI: 10.1249/mss.0b013e318093f55

[15] Kim D, Kwon S. Vibrational stress affects extracellular signal-regulated kinases activation and cytoskeleton structure in human keratinocytes. PLoS One. 2020;**15**(4):e0231174. DOI: 10.1371/journal.pone.023117

[16] Prisby RD, Lafage-Proust MH, Malaval L, Belli A, Vico L. Effects of whole body vibration on the skeleton and other organ systems in man and animal models: What we know and what we need to know. Ageing Research Reviews. 2008;**7**(4):319-329. DOI: 10.1016/j.arr.2008.07.004

[17] Rauch F, Sievanen H, Boonen S, Cardinale M, Degens H, Felsenberg D, et al. Reporting whole-body vibration intervention studies: Recommendations of the International Society of Musculoskeletal and Neuronal Interactions. Journal of Musculoskeletal & Neuronal Interactions. 2010;**10**(3):193-198 PMID: 20811143

[18] Bernardo-Filho M, Bemben D, Stark C, Taiar R. Biological consequences of exposure to mechanical vibration. Dose Response. 2018;**16**(3):1559325818799618. DOI: 10.1177/1559325818799618

[19] Sá-Caputo DC, Marconi EM, Costa-Cavalcanti RG, Domingos L, Giehl PM, Paiva DN, et al. Alterations on the plasma concentration of hormonal and non hormonal biomarkers in human beings submitted to whole body vibration exercises. Scientific Research and Essays. 2015;**10**(8):287-297

[20] Lapole T. Pérot C effects of repeated Achilles tendon vibration on triceps surae force production. Journal of Electromyography and Kinesiology. 2010;**20**(4):648-654

[21] Lapole T, Temesi J, Gimenez P, Arnal PJ, Millet GY. Petitjean M Achilles tendon vibration-induced changes in plantar flexor corticospinal excitability. Experimental Brain Research. 2015;**233**(2):441-448

[22] Oroszi T, MJG v H, Nyakas C, van der Zee EA. Vibration detection: Its function and recent advances in medical applications. F1000Res. 2020;**9**:F1000. Faculty Rev-619. DOI: 10.12688/f1000research.22649

Chapter 13

Methods and Tools for Assessing Muscle Asymmetry in the Analysis of Electromyographic Signals

Kamala Pashayeva and Namiq Abdullayev

Abstract

The generalized information about the possibilities of assessing asymmetry and the prospects of research tools is presented. The important role of the choice of different methods for processing electromyographic signals, the results of which can be considered as an objective criterion for assessing the asymmetry of the muscles of the extremities, is noted, such as the asymmetry coefficient, a widely used parameter in statistical analysis, which characterizes the asymmetry of the statistical distribution. Also applied is the segmental method of studying the body to obtain estimates of the composition and differences between individual body segments. The isokinetic test method, which makes it possible to assess asymmetry in measuring muscle strength, relies on the randomness of the dynamic processes of the biological system. Use of nonlinear dynamics, the theory of dynamic chaos, and fractal analysis allows for determining the fractal properties of biosignals, and from the classical methods used correlation analysis.

Keywords: electromyography, asymmetry coefficient, multifractal analysis, isokinetic test, correlation analysis

1. Introduction

The connection between the evolutionary processes of complex systems, which include biological ones, is associated with the phenomenon of symmetry breaking. This leads to the need to study the indicators of asymmetry in the study of the behavior of complex systems [1]. Asymmetry is used as the best method for displaying possible variations when examining the limbs of the skeletal system. The observed asymmetry of the limbs of the skeletal system is associated with mechanical and genetic factors. Electromyography (EMG) research has grown in popularity over the past few years. Progressive understanding of the human body, increased awareness to explore the benefits of interdisciplinary research, advances in sensory technology, and the exponential growth of the computational power of computers are all factors contributing to the expansion of EMG research (relevant references will be explained in detail). Functional asymmetry is an integral feature of the human brain, which manifests itself in various forms of human behavior and motor activity [2]. The study of functional asymmetry and lateral preferences is important not only from a theoretical but also from a practical point of view, since both the effectiveness of the fulfillment of sports motor actions and the likelihood of injury can depend on its severity [3, 4]. It is these areas of research on motor asymmetry in sports that remain the most relevant. The aim of the study in [5] was to study the general and individual features of the asymmetry of the speed-strength indicators of the muscles of the knee joint in Paralympic basketball players and its relationship with the results in jumping exercises.

There are different approaches to assessing the asymmetry of different human organs. The asymmetry coefficient was calculated as the ratio of the difference between the minimum and maximum EMG values of symmetrical muscles to a larger value [5]. The Electroencephalography (EEG) method was used to assess the asymmetry of the normalized quantitative indicator—the coefficient of asymmetry [6]. When visualizing the reconstructed cardiac signal, the asymmetry coefficient was also used and estimated [7].

2. Estimation of the asymmetry of electromyographic signals using the statistical distribution of asymmetry coefficients

Functional asymmetry is an integral feature of the human brain, which is manifested in various forms of human behavior and motor activity [8].

There are different approaches to assessing the asymmetry of different human organs. The asymmetry coefficient (KAs) was calculated as the ratio of the difference in EMG values of symmetrical muscles on the side of its minimum (X1) and maximum (X2) decrease to a larger value [5]:

$$K_{As} = \frac{(X_1 - X_2) * 100\%}{X_1}. \tag{1}$$

The method of a normalized quantitative indicator, the asymmetry coefficient, was used to assess the EEG asymmetry [9, 10]. What is universal for its calculation is the formula

$$(\text{А} - \text{Б})/(\text{А} + \text{Б})\text{x}100\%, \tag{2}$$

where A is the numerical characteristic of the EEG of the left hemisphere, and B is the right one.

2.1 Method

The skewness coefficient is a widely used parameter in statistical analysis that characterizes the skewness of a statistical distribution.

The central moment of distribution can be calculated by the formula [11]:

$$m_k^{(0)} = E(\xi - m_i)^k = \begin{cases} \int (x - m_i)^k f(x)dx, \textit{if } \xi \textit{ uninterrupted}; \\ \sum\limits_i (x_i^0 - m_i)^k p_i, \textit{ if discret.} \end{cases} \tag{3}$$

Here k is order; ξ is a discrete random variable with possible values $\boldsymbol{x_i}$ and probabilities of their realization $\boldsymbol{p_i}$, $(\boldsymbol{i} = \mathbf{1, 2, 3}, \ldots .)$.

By formula (1), it is easy to understand that if the density $\boldsymbol{f}_\xi(\boldsymbol{x})$ (or the sequence of probabilities $\boldsymbol{P}\{\xi = \boldsymbol{x_i^0}\}$ is symmetric with respect to the mean value $\boldsymbol{m_1} = \boldsymbol{E}\xi$ (i.e. $\boldsymbol{f}(\boldsymbol{m_1} - \boldsymbol{x}) \equiv \boldsymbol{f}(\boldsymbol{m_1} + \boldsymbol{x})$), then all odd central moments (if they exist) $\boldsymbol{x_{2k+1}^{(0)}}$ are equal to zero. Therefore, any odd, non-zero torque can be considered as a characteristic of the asymmetry of the corresponding distribution. The simplest of these characteristics is $m_3^{(0)}$ and is taken as the basis for calculating the so-called asymmetry coefficient γ_1—a quantitative characteristic of the degree of skewness of the distribution [10]:

$$\gamma_1 = \frac{\frac{1}{N}\sum_{i=1}^{N}(S_i - m_x)^3}{\sigma^3} \tag{4}$$

where $m_x = \frac{1}{N}\sum_{i=1}^{N} S_i$ – sample mean, $\sigma^2 = \frac{1}{(N-1)}\sum_{i=1}^{N}(S_i - m_x)^2$ - sample variance, $S_i, \overline{1:N}$ - time series.

All symmetric distributions will have zero skewness. Probability distributions with the "long part" of the density curve located to the right of the top are characterized by positive asymmetry, and distributions with the "long part" of the density curve located to the left of its top are negatively skewed [10].

The range of variability of the asymmetry coefficient is determined from −3 to +3.

At the same time, it is generally accepted that asymmetry above 0.5 (regardless of sign) is significant and less than 0.25 is insignificant. With a symmetric distribution, the kurtosis coefficient Ek = 0. If Ek <0, then the distribution has a flat-topped character, and if Ek > 0, then it is peaked. We determined the fluctuation of qualitative features of the variational series by the total variance, based on the theorem of addition of the variance of the share of a feature.

Thus, the variation statistics for assessing the contractile properties of muscles is based on the asymmetry coefficient. By the degree of deviation of the asymmetry coefficient from the median, as a rule, one can judge the value of the Gaussian distribution density. The closer the skewness indicator is to the median, the higher the Gaussian distribution density. The deviation of the asymmetry from the median is determined by the standard deviation from the mean. For a normal distribution, 95% of the values are within two standard deviations of the mean and 68% are within one standard deviation [11].

2.2 Experimental part

For the experiment, 6 muscles of the lower extremities of a patient with a diagnosis of asymmetry were selected. Measuring signals were received from 12 leads, in pairs from the right and left parts of the limbs (**Table 1**).

To estimate the asymmetry coefficient, formula (4) was used and the skewness function was implemented by Matlab [12]. The experimental results obtained are given in **Table 2**.

As already noted, asymmetry above 0.5 (regardless of sign) is significant and less than 0.25 is insignificant. According to the results of the experiment, we can say that on the left side of the limbs for the muscles a-gm-lp, a-qfm-rf, there is a great tendency to asymmetry, and for a-bfm, both the left and right parts, there is a tendency to asymmetry. For the muscles a-qfm-vm, a-gm-mp, a slight asymmetry can be observed on the left side, and a tendency towards asymmetry for the right side.

To visualize the results, you can present them in the form of a histogram (**Figure 1**).

To assess the method used, the results obtained are compared with the values obtained by the Myograph, which are given in **Figure 2**.

Based on the results in **Figure 2**, we can say that the patient has left-sided asymmetry in the a-qfm-vl muscles, since the highest voltage is observed on the

##	Muscles	Abbreviation
1	Biceps femoris muscle	a-bfm
2	Gastrocnemius muscle – lateral part	a-gm-lp
3	Quadriceps femoris muscle – rectus femoris	a-qfm-rf
4	Quadriceps femoris muscle – vastus lateralis	a-qfm-vl
5	Quadriceps femoris muscle – vastus medialis	a-qfm-vm
6	Gastrocnemius muscle – medial part	a-gm-mp

Table 1.
Measuring muscle signals used in the experiment.

##	Muscles	The asymmetry coefficients	
		Left (L)	Right (R)
1	a-bfm	0.3516	0.3936
2	a-gm-lp	0.4484	0.3735
3	a-qfm-rf	0.4518	0.1304
4	a-qfm-vl	0.0681	0.4413
5	a-qfm-vm	0.2507	0.3110
6	a-gm-mp	0.0709	0.3532

Table 2.
The value of the asymmetry coefficient depending on the location of the muscles.

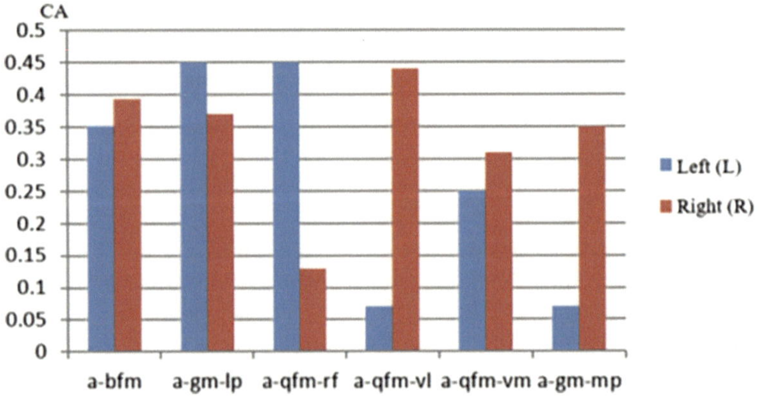

Figure 1.
Diagram of the asymmetry coefficient of paired muscles.

right side (from the bottom of the fourth drain). It is also not very convenient to compare this value with the value of the paired muscles (second line from the top).

The experimental data help not only to conveniently compare the results, but also to give a predictive conclusion about the possibility of the expected muscle pathology. The value between the interval $0.25 < x < 0.5$ can be used as the bias towards asymmetry.

It is also possible to use the difference in the asymmetry coefficients for convenient observation of the results (**Figure 3**).

The results in **Figure 3** show the positions of the asymmetry during the measurement and may allow immediate observation.

DOI: http://dx.doi.org/10.5772/intechopen.103061

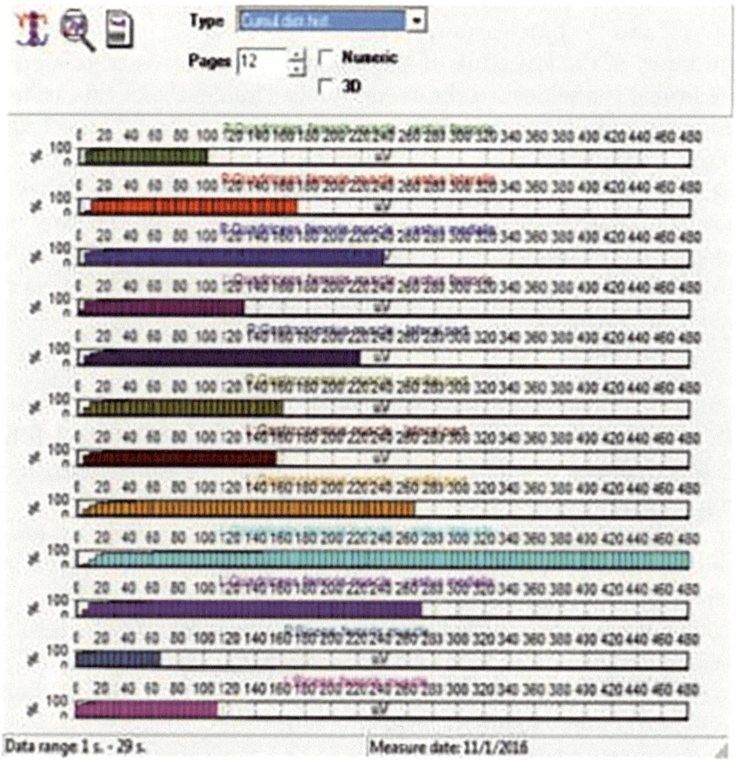

Figure 2.
Measurement results with myograph.

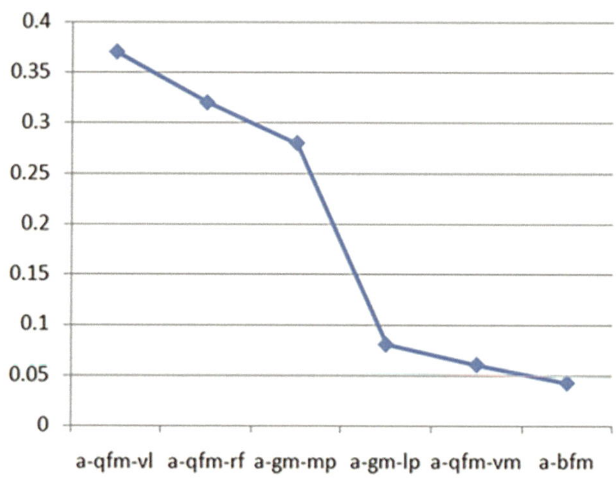

Figure 3.
The difference in the coefficient of asymmetry of paired muscles.

3. Assessment of the degree of asymmetry by the measured muscle strength of the limbs

The main purpose of segmental body examination methods is to obtain estimates of the composition and differences of individual body segments. Such analysis can be performed both statically and dynamically to investigate the differences between segments under various influences. The body segments analyzed are usually the limbs and trunk, and in some cases the head.

The asymmetry of the structure of the human body, expressed to a greater extent in the limbs, is a widespread phenomenon. The degree of this asymmetry is affected by the way of life, the experience of a person's professional activity, which is manifested in the aggregate of signs of inequality in the functions of arms, legs, halves of the body, and face during the formation of general motor behavior.

Even in relatively uniform cross-sectional areas of the body, the musculoskeletal mass is unevenly distributed. For example, in the overwhelming majority of the world's population, the right hand is superior to the left in strength. This symmetry is expressed by the formula

$$A = S/D,$$

where D - muscle strength of the right, S - muscle strength of the left hand [13]. This ratio is less than one for right-handers, more than one for the left, and equal to one for ambidextra.

There are different methods and means for assessing asymmetry (anthropometric, bioimpedance analysis, assessment of strength indicators, etc.), which allow such comparisons to be made both quantitatively and visually [14–17].

To assess the asymmetry of the limbs of the studied patients, the results of in vivo experiments were used using a 12-channel ME6000-EMG device. We studied the biopotentials of three muscles of the lower extremities, two of them lateral and one medial direction (**Table 3**). Measurement time - 30 sec.

For the studied muscle types, 6 leads were used, thus six signals were recorded for the right (R) and left (L) sides. **Table 4** shows the values for three examples of the maximum amplitudes of biopotentials in microvolts, the values of which are proportional to the muscle strength of the objects under consideration.

For the corresponding leads for the left and right sides, the difference in the maximum amplitude values of the signals can be estimated as follows, for example:

$$\Delta A(QFM.rf) = QFM.rf_{max}(L) - QFM.rf_{max}(R)$$

For one and the same derivation, when calculating the average value of the difference in amplitudes (AVDA), it is necessary to take into account the difference of all measured values. For instance,

$$\text{AVDA} = \Big(\Delta A_{\text{прим. }1}(QFM.rf) + \Delta A_{\text{прим. }1}(QFM.vl) + \Delta A_{\text{прим. }1}(QFM.vm) + \Delta A_{\text{прим. }1}(QM.lp) + \Delta A_{\text{прим. }1}(\text{QM.mp}) + \Delta A_{\text{прим. }1}(BFM)\Big)/6$$

Muscles	Abbreviation
Quadriceps femoris muscle – rectus femoris	QFM-rf
Quadriceps femoris muscle – vastus lateralis	QFM-vl
Quadriceps femoris muscle – vastus medialis	QFM-vm
Gastrocnemius muscle – lateral part	QM-lp
Gastrocnemius muscle – medial part	QM-mp
Biceps femoris muscle	BFM

Table 3.
Studied biopotentials.

Muscles	Measurement values, μV					
	example 1		example 2		example 3	
	L	R	L	R	L	R
Quadriceps femoris muscle – rectus femoris	130	100	165	175	200	235
Quadriceps femoris muscle – vastus lateralis	480	170	135	160	255	205
Quadriceps femoris muscle – vastus medialis	270	240	480	230	290	300
Gastrocnemius muscle – lateral part	150	220	140	175	120	140
Gastrocnemius muscle – medial part	260	160	180	165	175	225
Biceps femoris muscle	110	70	70	100	110	165

Table 4.
The values for three examples of the maximum amplitudes of biopotentials.

Muscles	QFM-rf	QFM-vl	QFM-vm	QM-lp	QM-mp	BFM	C3PA
Example 1	0.3	3.1	0.25	0.7	0	0.4	0.79
Example 2	0.1	0.25	2.5	0.35	0.15	0.3	0.61
Example 3	0.35	0.5	0.1	0.2	0.5	0.55	0.37
...	...	...	...	...	...	...	...

Table 5.
The difference in the maximum amplitudes of the received signals (in percentage terms).

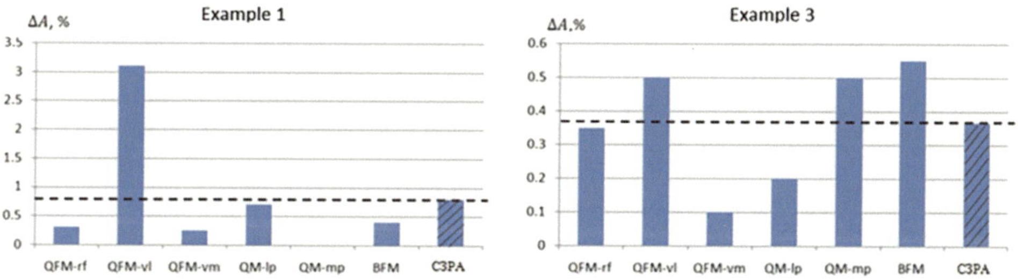

Figure 4.
Comparison of the average values of the measured signals for different leads for two examples.

For the corresponding leads, the difference in the maximum amplitudes of the received signals (in percentage terms), as well as the difference in the average values of the measured signals, are shown in **Table 5**.

Comparison of the average values of the measured signals for different leads for two examples (in the form of histograms) is shown in **Figure 4**.

For example 1, it can be seen that only for one muscle QFM-vl there is a pronounced asymmetry, and for other muscles relative to the mean value there is no tendency to asymmetry. In example 3, the maximum asymmetry is observed in lead BFM; however, there is a tendency to asymmetry in leads QFM-vl and QM-mp. In this case, the average value of the difference in amplitudes can be used as the degree of asymmetry A, since this value is with the difference in muscle strength measured from the corresponding muscle of the limbs.

It is possible to conventionally accept the range of variation of A from 0 to 1. If we accept the degree of asymmetry equal to 0.5 as an average level, then the value <0.5 is estimated as a low degree, and the value >0.5 as a high degree of asymmetry. For the examples shown, the degree of asymmetry can be assessed according to the following scale (**Figure 5**).

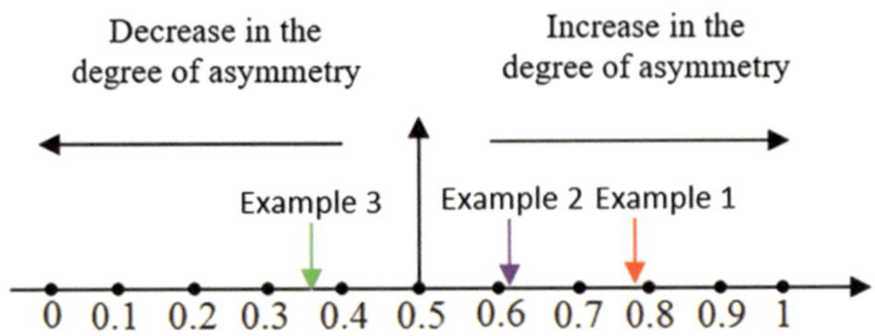

Figure 5.
Scale of the degree of asymmetry.

The proposed approach makes it possible to quantitatively assess the severity of the asymmetry of the studied limbs.

If you use directly the measurement results using the 12-channel ME6000-EMG device, then the measurement results are reflected in the protocol—**Figure 6** (for two examples).

For the leads used (left and right), 12 signals of the studied muscle are recorded during the period of innervation and reinnervation. In this case, the assessment of the measurement results is carried out visually to the values of biopotentials, proportional to the muscle strength of the object under study. As can be seen from **Figure 3**, these values are maximum for the Quadriceps femoris muscle - vastus lateralis.

For the first example, the maximum value of muscle strength corresponds to the 9th line, for the second example it is the 3rd line. However, it is impossible to establish the degree of asymmetry of the studied muscle in a particular patient from the given measurement protocol. It is possible to group the results of measurements of muscle strength for different muscles of patients—**Figure 7a, b**. The obtained histograms for the left and right sides of the studied muscles of patients do not make it possible to assess the degree of asymmetry and the magnitude of this asymmetry, since the maximum values for different leads (QFM-vl and QFM-vm) can be maximum.

Thus, in comparison with the results of direct measurements and with the subsequent visualization of the obtained protocol, the proposed method for assessing the degree of asymmetry, and then the severity of asymmetry of the muscles under study, is more acceptable.

To obtain reliable and reproducible results on the example of 30 patients, all requirements of the measurement procedure were met.

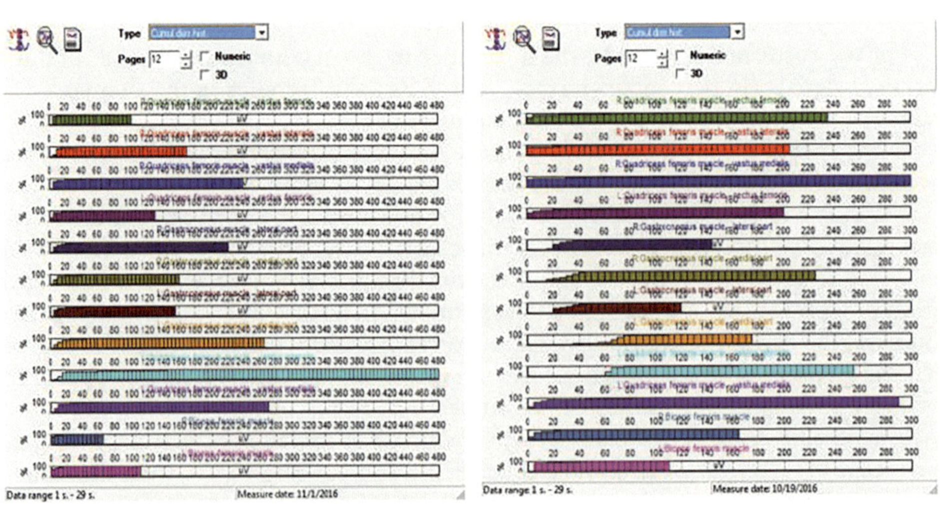

Figure 6.
The measurement results using the 12-channel ME6000-EMG device.

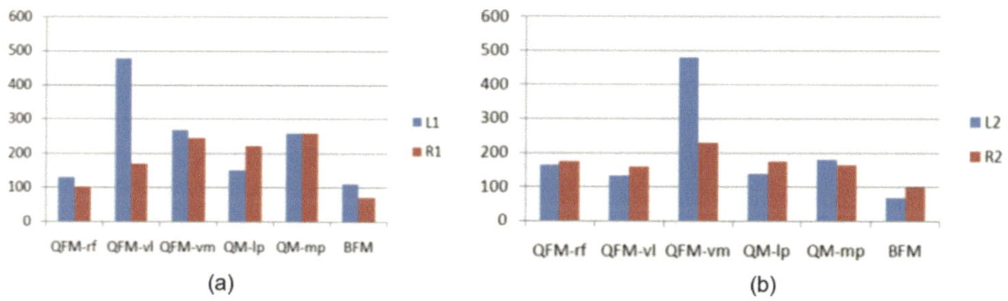

Figure 7.
Grouping results of measurements of muscle strength for different muscles of patients.

Assessment of the degree of asymmetry of muscle strength according to the proposed method allows an expert doctor to accurately assess the differences in the biopotentials of the studied muscles of the limbs and effectively use the treatment method to reduce the degree of asymmetry.

4. Assessment of asymmetry in permanent muscles based on isokinetic test results

The asymmetry observed in the skeletal system can be caused by both mechanical effects and genetic factors. Asymmetry is used in the skeletal system as a method that best reflects the variations that may occur in the study of the limbs. Asymmetry, especially in the upper extremities, is due to the fact that there is more freedom of movement. On the other hand, if the symmetry of the upper extremities is broken in favor of one side, the contralateral side is superior and advanced in the lower extremities. Numerous experiments on the upper extremities have shown that the main cause of bilateral asymmetry is side choice [18–20].

Asymmetry in the muscles can damage not only the esthetic structure, but also health. Muscles of different strengths can cause damage to the spine and other structures by creating completely different pressure points.

This condition is most often seen in people who have an inversely proportional shortness on one side of the hamstring muscles.

In isokinetic compression, the rate of skeletal muscle contraction is constant. In isokinetic compressions, each movement is performed at a constant speed due to the destination. On the contrary, in isotonic compression, it is impossible to keep the speed constant in a certain motion.

In isokinetic compressions, motion occurs in three separate phases.

a. acceleration phase: acceleration phase of motion;

b. isokinetic loading: the phase at which the motion is performed at a constant speed and equal resistance;

c. deceleration phase: the deceleration phase before the movement is completed.

Since the speed is not constant during the acceleration and deceleration phases, the physical activity performed at this stage cannot be considered isokinetic. Since the optimal test speeds for each joint movement are not known, it is important to find the angular velocities with the isokinetic loading range of the joints. In this regard, the estimates made with an isokinetic dynamometer calculate the peak torque, work, and power parameters corresponding to the isokinetic range.

As the speed of the dynamometer increases, the time of the compression and deceleration phases increases, and the phase time with the main isokinetic load decreases. Studies have shown that serious errors in assessment can occur if these three phases are not taken into account during flexion-extension movements performed at different angular velocities. Therefore, the assessment of the isokinetic loading phase, especially at high angular velocities, may be important for the correct interpretation of the data.

With the development of technology, as in many areas, there have been developments in the field of strengthening and rehabilitation of human muscles. In general, isometric and isotonic (concentric- eccentric) compression types are used to strengthen the muscle. This is especially important in the assessment of dynamic neuromuscular capabilities in sports and in the quantitative assessment of outcomes. In order to determine the muscle capacity that can occur during dynamic muscle contraction (construction), it is necessary to measure the force and force exerted at a certain angular velocity. These values are quantified with an isokinetic dynamometer [21–24].

The purpose of the research and the problem statement.

Formulas used in the calculation of muscle strength and research-related terms.

Force (F) is defined as a physical quantity that stops motion or turns stagnation into motion, the unit of which is Newton (N).

Work (W) is the force applied at a certain distance; the unit is the Newton-meter (Nm) or Coul. The work done does not depend on time. Mathematical formula: $W = F \cdot d$ (where d is the distance).

The moment of force (torque) is the force that creates a rotation by applying a point or axis, the unit of which is the Newton-meter.

Power (P) is the work done in a single time; the unit is Watt (W).

$$P = W/\ t;\ \ P = F \cdot d/t;\ \ P = F \cdot t.$$

Angular velocity is the distance traveled in a single time; the unit is degrees/second (°/sec).

Factors affecting measurements when measuring muscle strength.

Personal characteristics:

- Age: As opposed to an age, person's body mass (fat-free) decreases. As getting older, type II fibers decrease, so muscle strength decreases. Age is an important factor in assessing the torque, speed, and strength characteristics of skeletal muscles.

- Height

- Body mass

- Sex

- Sports past

- Dominant party

- Damage condition

- Action features

- Joint angle: Depending on the length-tension relationship and the biomechanical properties of the joint, the force is different for each joint.

Muscle movement: With isokinetic devices, force, work and force can be measured in both concentric and eccentric compressions. Most studies have shown that the force at eccentric compression is greater than that at concentric compression. This is because in eccentric compression, both contractile and non-contractile elastic components are involved in the formation of force, while in concentric compression only contractile structures are involved.

Test type: Isometric, isotonic, or isokinetic compression types are measured with an isokinetic dynamometer.

Bicycle ergometer is used for the lower extremity and arm ergometer for the upper extremity for warm-up (muscle training) (**Table 6**).

The experiments are warm-up exercises for 5 minutes on a bicycle ergometer with 55 ± 5 rpm. Warm-up loads are regulated according to a person's heart rate, and the heart rate is recorded by a telemetry monitor (S810, Polar, Finland) that visualizes the heartbeat. During the warm-up period, the heart rate is maintained between 100 and 120 beats per minute. The arm ergometer is used in the same way for the upper circumference. Stretching exercises are performed for 5 minutes before and after the test to prevent possible injuries.

As shown in **Table 1**, a protocol of test results is prepared. To allow individuals to adapt to the isokinetic measurements, the test is repeated on the isokinetic dynamometer at 210°/sec and 180°/sec at five maximum positions, with 45 seconds rest between repetitions. Concentric peak values of torque of the Working and power variables. Using a Cybex Norm dynamometer, the angular velocity is measured three times with an increase of 30°/s in each set from 30°/s to 450°/s. There is a time of 30 seconds for a break between measurements. Which of the three iterations has the highest peak torque is used in data analysis.

Angular velocity (degree/sec)	Number of repetitions	Break time (second)
210	5	45
180	5	45
30	3	30
60	3	30
90	3	30
120	3	30
150	3	30
180	3	30
210	3	30
240	3	30
270	3	30
300	3	30
330	3	30
360	3	30
390	3	30
420	3	30
450	3	30

Table 6.
Test protocol.

Angular velocity	Normalized power	
	Right foot (thigh) abduction	**Left leg (thigh) abduction**
30	30	30
60	50	50
90	80	60
120	70	75
150	110	80
180	90	90
210	90	85
240	80	65
270	105	80
300	80	72
330	65	74
360	70	70
390	65	72
420	65	65
450	60	70

Table 7.
Foot-thigh abduction.

Foot (thigh) abduction: The movement is performed with 59.00 ± 8.2 degrees of articular movement (**Table** 7).

4.1 Discussion of the obtained results

According to **Table 2**, we construct the following graphs to assess the asymmetry in the muscles. The graph shows the results according to the angular values on the horizontal axis and the results according to the power values on the vertical axis (**Figure 8**). As can be seen from the graph, the muscle strengths in the right and left legs differ from each other at certain angular velocity values during abduction. At some angular velocity values, the muscle forces in the right and left legs are the same (30°/sec, 60°/sec, 180°/sec, 360°/sec), and these values indicate that there is no asymmetry. We do not take these prices into account. At different values of angular velocity, the asymmetry

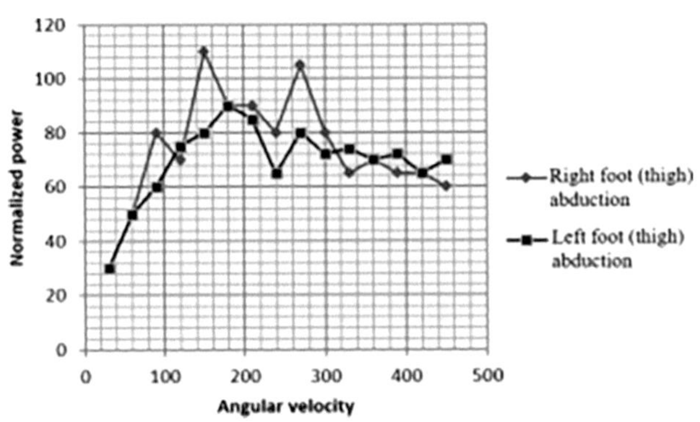

Figure 8.
Abduction of the right and left leg (thigh).

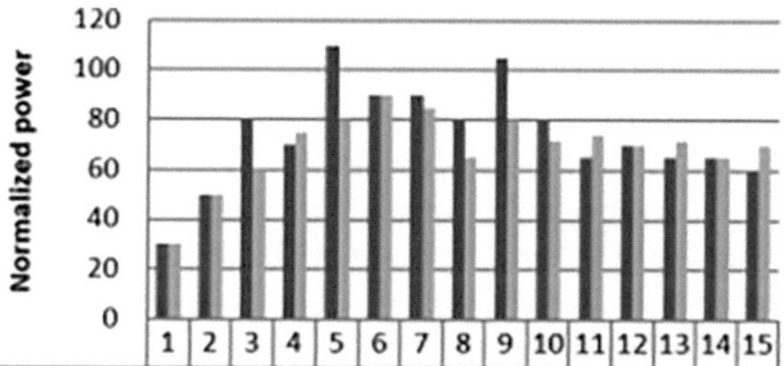

	1	2	3	4	5	6	7	8	9	10	11	12	13	14	15
Right foot (thigh) abduction	30	50	80	70	110	90	90	80	105	80	65	70	65	65	60
Left foot (thigh) abduction	30	50	60	75	80	90	85	65	80	72	74	70	72	65	70

Figure 9.
Histogram for asymmetry assessment during right and left leg abduction.

between the right and left foot is also different. At some values, the asymmetry is less noticeable (120°/sec, 210°/sec, 300°/sec, 330°/sec, 390°/sec, 450°/sec). At some values, there is a sharp asymmetry (90°/sec, 150°/sec, 240°/sec, 270°/sec).

The histogram of the results is shown in **Figure 9**.

4.2 The result

The minimum difference between right and left muscle strength is 5 W/kg, and the maximum difference is 30 W/kg. Given that the difference between these values is 25 W/kg, the difference in power values of 12 + 5, i.e. 17 W kg and below, in the assessment of asymmetry during abduction between the right and left arm is a natural asymmetry, and values above 17 W/kg it would be more correct to accept the existing asymmetry.

The minimum difference between right and left muscle strength is 5 W/kg, and the maximum difference is 70 W/kg. Since the difference between these values is 65 W/kg, differences in muscle strength of 32 + 5, i.e. 37 W/kg and below, can be considered as a natural asymmetry, and differences in muscle strength greater than 37 W/kg can be considered as existing asymmetry.

5. Evaluation of limbs muscle asymmetry on the basis of the method of multifractal fluctuation analysis

The study of signals of biological systems should be carried out with an account of such important factors as the existence of nonlinear interrelationships between different physiological indicators and between reports of organic biological signals. Their non-stationary nature is limited to the application of classical methods of analysis of biological signals.

Chaosticity of dynamic processes of biological systems and fractal properties of biosignals obtained from different structures of the organism require descriptions of the processes occurring in these systems with the use of nonlinear analogical dynamics, theories of dynamism. Based on the application of such methods of analysis, it is possible to obtain diagnostic information indicators, which come from each of the methods that can serve as an early predictor of disease of a particular organ.

In this article, the assessment of fluctuation of random processes using the method of fluctuation analysis of electromyographic signals is considered. The meaning of these signals is represented in the form of a dynamic time series to assess the asymmetry of the limbs of the human body [25–28].

There are not a large number of publications in science-based databases using multifractal approaches for the analysis of myographic signals. The author used fractal analysis to assess the morphological complexities of the surface of the connecting parts, scanned by a 3D scanner [29]. The possibility of predicting the asymmetry of electromyographic signals from the ends (arms and legs) was tested by the method of multifractal multiplicity [16]. The Higuchi fractal size was used to establish the imbalance of the jaw and the loss of muscle strength in the hands by helping the surface electromyography [17].

In the work are given examples of changes in the fluctuation functions of the electromyographic signal for different levels of load on a specific muscle [30].

Electromyographic signals are considered in this work, comparable to the ends: the right and left part of the hip muscle. In contrast to the classical approach to the assessment of asymmetry with the use of a single point (maximum) of the measured signal, we consider the multiplicity of the measured signals of the finite points as heterogeneous unevenly distributed fractional points. To assess the chaosticity of myographic signals, it is possible to use the characteristics of fractal multiplicity, such as the fractal size of Hausdorff, the indicator of Herst, generalized size, correlation, and information size [31–34].

5.1 Materials and methods

In the current period, in clinical conditions, the assessment of asymmetry is carried out at the maximum value of the amplitude of the muscles. This process includes in itself "maximum contraction of the muscle - the achievement of the peak in the maximum relaxation of the muscle", is the informative result and considered only the value of the peak. If you consider the whole process as a dynamic time series, then in order to make a decision it is necessary to include all the elements of the coincidence that creates this process. To examine all the data in a dynamic range and the minimum step size of a window in one report it is necessary to ensure the frequency of record lengths and window sizes. This segmentation is performed in two passages, performed in opposite directions.

The calculation algorithm consists of the following steps.

Initially from the series x(k), k = 0,1,2 ... N allocate the total fluctuation (or fluctuation profile)

$$Y(i) = \sum_{k=1}^{i} [x(k) - \overline{x}], \quad i = 1, 2 \ldots N, \tag{5}$$

where $\overline{\boldsymbol{x}}$ - is the average arithmetic series x(κ).

Divide the full interval $[\mathbf{1}, \boldsymbol{N}]$ by $\boldsymbol{N_s} = [\boldsymbol{N}/s]$ segments, each of which contains s values. The elements of the new interval will be $\boldsymbol{x}_{(\nu-1)s+1}, \ldots, \boldsymbol{x}_{\nu,s}$, $\nu = 1, \ldots$, Ns. It follows that in the case of $\boldsymbol{s} > \boldsymbol{N}/\mathbf{4}$ the function of the deformed variance loses statistical informativeness due to the small number of $\boldsymbol{N_s} < \mathbf{4}$, used in the medium. At the same time it is necessary to fulfill the inequality s $< \mathbf{10}$ [35–37].

After changing the random variable $\boldsymbol{Y(i)}$ we add $\boldsymbol{y_\nu(i)} \neq \mathbf{0}$ to find the polynomial for this function using the method of the least squares, and calculate the variance in the interval ν:

$$F^2(\nu, s) = \frac{1}{s} \sum_{i=1}^{s} \{y[(\nu - 1)s + i] - y_\nu(i)\}^2 \tag{6}$$

for segments $\nu = \mathbf{1}, \mathbf{2}, \ldots \boldsymbol{N_s}$, in the case of fragmentation is performed in the direct direction, and for the reverse sequence $\nu = \boldsymbol{N_s} + \mathbf{1}, \ldots, \mathbf{2}\boldsymbol{N_s}$ we use the equation

$$F^2(\nu, s) = \frac{1}{s}\sum_{i=1}^{s}\{y[N-(\nu-N_s)s+i]-y_\nu(i)\}^2 \quad (7)$$

Conduct the distribution of deformed dispersions at intervals

$$F_q(s) = \left\{\frac{1}{2N_s}\sum_{\nu}^{2N_s}\left[F^2(\nu,s)\right]^{q/2}\right\}^{1/q} \quad (8)$$

Coefficient 2 in the signifier and in the upper limit of the sum used only for reflation of the algorithm with two passes.

At zero value of the order q this equilibrium contains indefiniteness, and then by definition

$$F_0(s) = \exp\left\{\frac{1}{4N_s}\sum_{\nu=1}^{2N_s} ln\left[F^2(\nu,s)\right]\right\} \quad (9)$$

To find the dependence $\boldsymbol{F_q(s)}$ we change the time scale s with the fixed indicator $\boldsymbol{q}$ and represent it in binary logarithmic coordinates.

If the studied series corresponds to a similar number ($s \to 0$), then the scaling relationship is fulfilled

$$F_q(s) \sim s^{h(q)}, \quad (10)$$

where $\boldsymbol{h(q)}$ is a generalized index of Herst [35]. For stationary time series h (2) = H is the known index of the degree of Hearst, which with one side does not depend on $\boldsymbol{q}$, and with the other variance is the same for all segments. In the positive/negative value q, $\boldsymbol{h(q)}$ indicates the scaling behavior of segments with large/small fluctuations [35].

For small values of s, $\boldsymbol{h(q)}$ we determine the linear regression [36].

$$F_q(s) = h(q) \cdot \ln(s) \quad (11)$$

The standard representation of the scaling properties of the temporal series assumes a transition from the indicator Hearst $\boldsymbol{h(q)}$ to the mass indicator $\boldsymbol{\tau(q)}$ and the spectral function f (α), the size of Rennie, which are in [37].

Mass index is calculated by the formula:

$$\tau(q) = qh(q) - 1 \quad (12)$$

The spectral function has a connection with the mass indicator and the indicator Hearst:

$$\alpha(q) = \frac{d\tau(q)}{dq} = h(q) + q\frac{dh}{dq}$$

$$f(\alpha) = 1 + q(\alpha)[\alpha - h(q(\alpha))] \quad (13)$$

where $\boldsymbol{\alpha}$ is an indicator of Gelder, which estimates the probability of the occurrence of the element of fractal multiplicity in the ν-th fragment.

The size of Rennie is determined by the equilibrium of spectral function and (12)

$$D_q = \frac{qh(q) - 1}{q - 1}, \tag{14}$$

Apparently the equation is not fulfilled when q = 1. For this value according to the rules of Lopital (14), we use the dependence:

$$D(1) = h(1) + \left.\frac{\partial h}{\partial q}\right|_{q=1} \tag{15}$$

5.2 Discussion of results

With the purpose of demonstration of the possibility of using this method for quantitative assessment of asymmetry of the patient's muscle. Conduct testing of the expressed method on EMG signals. Calculation is carried out separately for each multiplicity.

The experiments used muscle signals: Quadriceps femoris muscle - rectus femoris, Quadriceps femoris muscle - vastus lateralis, Quadriceps femoris muscle - vastus medialis, Gastrocnemius muscle - lateral part, Gastrocnemius muscle - medial part, and biceps femoris muscle.

In accordance with the above-mentioned algorithm for the computational experiment, medical records were used of the quadriceps femoris muscle-vastus lateralis, obtained with a 16-channel electromyograph ME6000 in lateral and right medial and medial lobes.

Signals are marked $\mathbf{x}_l(\boldsymbol{k})$ - for the separation of the left part, $\mathbf{x}_r(\boldsymbol{k})$ - for the separation of the right part. Each signal was broken down into 5 segments ($\boldsymbol{N}_s = 5$). In the time series in both directions $\mathbf{x}_l(\boldsymbol{k})$ s = 83 and in $\mathbf{x}_r(\boldsymbol{k})$ s = 83.

Dependence $\boldsymbol{F}_q(\boldsymbol{s})$ for differential values $\boldsymbol{q} = \overline{\mathbf{1, 9}}$ obtained after accounting trend in formulas (6) and (7) – **Figure 10**. When the values $\boldsymbol{q} < 0$ and $\boldsymbol{q} > 4$ are so different that it is possible to say that they are repeated (**Figure 10**) and with these values they lose their significance. It is found and in the values of the indicator Renée calculated using (12) (**Figure 11**).

The results of the indicator Hersta are shown in **Figure 12**. At $\boldsymbol{q} > 2$ values it is possible to observe well-marked value of the indicator, which gives an opportunity to use it as an information indicator. Between the values of $\boldsymbol{h}(\boldsymbol{q})$ is determined by the relationship $\boldsymbol{h}^L_{(q)} > \boldsymbol{h}^R_{(q)}$ and this is observed at positive values of $\boldsymbol{q}$.

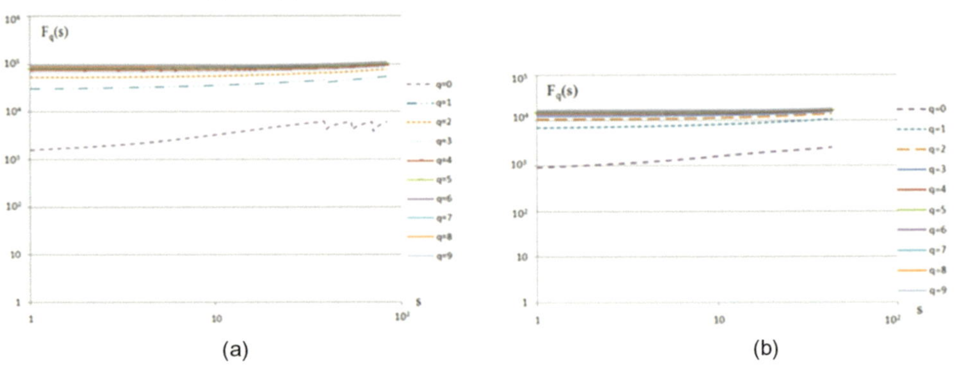

(a) (b)

Figure 10.
The dependence of the variance of the quadriceps femoris muscle-vastus lateralis on the size of the segment s ((a) - s = 83; (b) - s = 43) at different values of the deformation parameter q (q = 1–9).

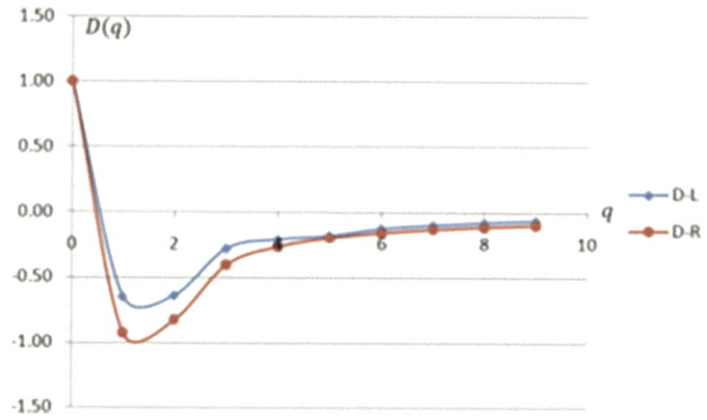

Figure 11.
Rennie's graphics for the right and left parts.

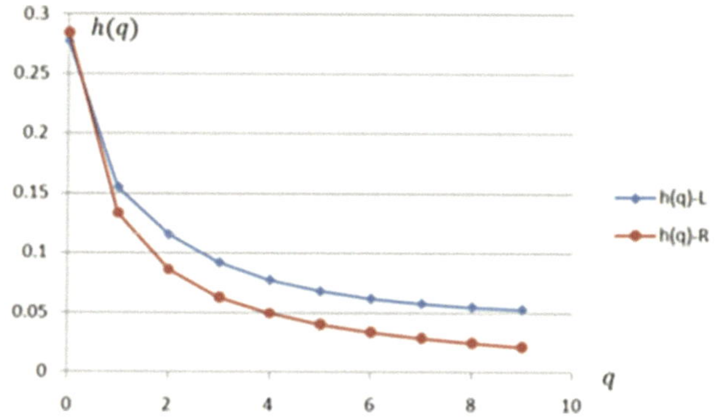

Figure 12.
Herst's indicator graphics are for the left and right parts.

Defining $\boldsymbol{D_q^{(L)} andD_q^{(R)}}$ parameter $\boldsymbol{D_q}$ obtained from the left and right parts of the Quadriceps femoris muscle-vastus lateralis muscle of the patient. From **Figure 12** easily determines the relationship

$$D_q^{(L)} > D_q^{(R)}$$

This inequality is fulfilled for $0 < q < 4$, and for other values we get repetitive values (it can be seen from the graphs), which lose their diagnostic value

$$D_q^{(L)} = D_q^{(R)}$$

The numerical value of the spectral function f (α) is shown in **Figure 13**.

As in the graphs of the indicator Hersta (**Figure 12**) here is also found good correlation in the values $\boldsymbol{q}$ >2. With the increase of the value of q in the signals of the left part of the mouse, the value of f(α) is increased in comparison with the value of the right part

$$f_q^{(L)} > f_q^{(R)}$$

5.3 The conclusion

The results show that the proposed method of acceptance and for the analysis of the detection of asymmetry of human extremities. It is possible to consider that the

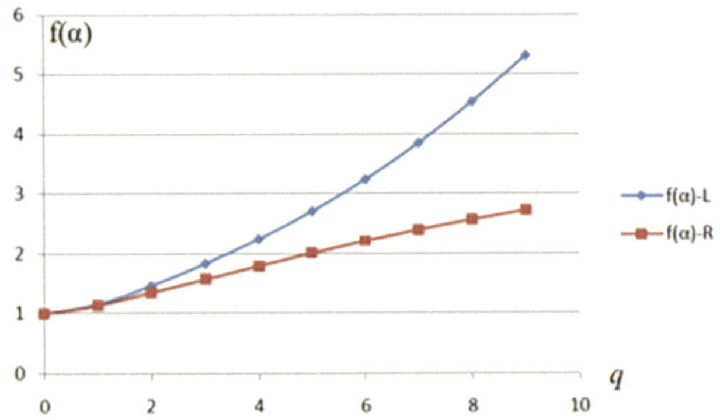

Figure 13.
Graphs of the spectral function f(α) for the right and left parts.

magnitudes that are used as the main characteristics of multifractals are informative signs that can be used to detect violations of the asymmetry of the ends. The results obtained show that in order to reveal the asymmetry of the finite points it is necessary to use the indicator Hearst and the value of the spectral function, as the informational range is wider than that of the indicator Reny.

6. Use of correlation analysis to assess the level of asymmetry in muscles

Electromyography is the only objective and informative method of studying the leading diseases of the nervous system, the functional state of the peripheral nervous system. Electromyography allows not only to determine the nature of the disease and its topical diagnosis, but also to objectively monitor the effectiveness of treatment and predict the time and stages of the recovery process [38].

Although symmetry is considered ideal in the body, this is not the case. In other words, the muscle mass of a healthy person's limbs has a slightly different mass and strength compared to the opposite side. One method of determining asymmetry is the analysis of EMG signals received by surface electrodes [25, 39].

The application of various methods to the processing of EMG signals, including mathematical, statistical, and complex, can be found in numerous literature sources [16, 29, 40–42]. It should be noted that despite the widespread use of complex mathematical processing methods in recent decades to increase the accuracy of calculations and reliability of diagnostic results, the development of processing devices based on the application of such methods is weak in terms of processing algorithms and constructive implementation. In this regard, the application of classical processing methods does not lose its relevance.

Correlation functions characterize the stable statistical characteristics of EMG. Some of these features have a functional or phenomenological value in the interpretation of EMG, but some of them open up new interesting ways in the neurophysiological analysis of the neuromotor apparatus.

In [43], the authors used a correlation analysis method to recognize the movement of the limbs. The obtained measurement results are compared with the EMG placed in the database and the signals are classified. The method of mutual correlation was used in [44] to analyze the process of renewal of the unit of movement of the nervous-muscular system. [45] examined the correlation between the age of patients with Packerson's disease and the frequency of tremor.

The maximum value of the correlation function (correlation coefficient) characterizes the relationship of processes over time, their degree of class.

Interference EMF is the result of a large number of potentials located in the separation area. However, then it is impossible to separate the action potentials of individual units of action. The dispersion of loads over time passing through motoneurons is not so great. Therefore, the statistical determination of the phase relationship of the two interfering EMGs allows to reveal the relationship of the action potentials of the two groups of units of motion over time (if these two EMGs reflect the loads of different HV). Based on this, cross-correlation analysis has opened up great opportunities in the study of synchronization of motoneuron charges.

6.1 Problem solving methods and approbation

In the mutually correlated analysis of EMG, the integral of the derivatives of two different functions is found. If they are not completely dependent and the phase ratios are random, the mutual correlation function will be equal to 0 for any τ. If the processes are related and the phases of any of the two curves at τ often overlap, then the mutual correlation function τ will be positive at the considered value.

In order for the value of the correlation function not to depend on the change in EMG or amplification of the electromyograph, it is normalized, ie it is expressed as part of the average power of both processes [46]:

$$R_{norm}(\tau) = \frac{\frac{1}{T}\int_0^T f_1(t) f_2(t+\tau)dt}{\sqrt{\frac{1}{T}\int_0^T f_1^2(t)dt}\sqrt{\frac{1}{T}\int_0^T f_2^2(t)dt}} \tag{16}$$

As a result of normalization, the correlation value is relative (it indicates the share of class electrical events in total electrical activity).

It is not advisable to use the correlation analysis method to measure the duration of the waves, as this quantity can be obtained by a simple instrument or by visual means.

The maximum of the mutual correlation function is accompanied not only by the value of $\tau = 0$, but also by a slip.

This shift indicates that there is a connection between the two EMFs. But one of them is late compared to the other. The average value of this delay is characterized by the value of the landslide, ie it is possible to speculate on which EMG delay is based on its direction. A small displacement may be due to a difference in the path of excitation from one electrode to another. Therefore, significant landslides greater than 3–4 ms are considered.

If we imagine the human body divided into two parts from the center, it is not difficult to see that most organs are symmetrical and consist of right and left parts: limbs (hands, feet), cerebral hemispheres, lungs, kidneys, and so on. Even the only visible organs in the general system consist of two symmetrically divided parts, such as the heart (right and left atrium, right and left ventricle), and so on.

Some pathological changes, working conditions, habits, and some sports form asymmetries that can cause serious complications in the body. This leads to the pathology of the part that consumes more energy after a certain period.

Various methods and tools are used in clinics and hospitals to identify such deficiencies. **Figure 14** shows the measurement results recorded using the ME6000-EMQ - 12-channel electromyograph.

In this example, 12 measurements are made without separation, and the results reflect the muscle strength in the form of a graph or figure. In this device, muscle

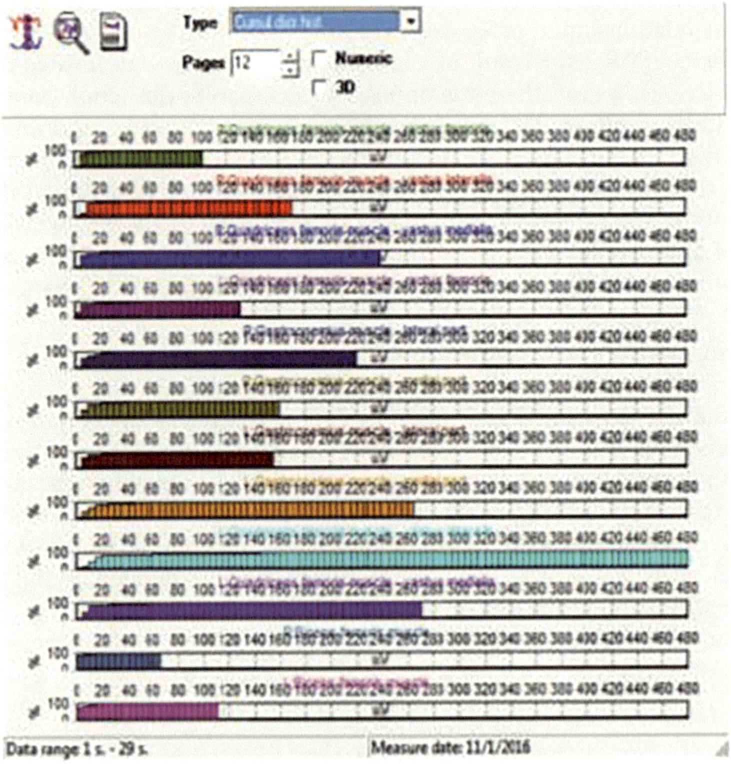

Figure 14.
Measurement result recorded using ME6000-EMQ device.

strength is recorded on a scale equal to 480 μV. The measurement time is 30 seconds. Here, the value is taken as the result of an indicator equal to the maximum amplitude. That is, for example, **Figure 1** shows the maximum value of muscle strength in the quadriceps femoris muscle - vastus lateralis, and this muscle is considered to have undergone asymmetry. However, it is not possible to see the level of asymmetry in other muscles here.

The muscles being measured are the main muscles that control the movement of the lower extremities. Muscles used in experiment are the same, and are given in **Table 1**.

The measurement results are collected in the form of a file with.dbf, .xls, .m, or any other possible extensions for further processing. An example is **Figure 15**. Here L and R show the left and right parts as the corresponding muscle.

The appropriate sequence of operations is then performed to calculate the correlation function or correlation coefficient of the corresponding pair of signals.

Computer modeling of calculations was performed in the Excel software package. The results of the calculated correlation coefficient are shown in **Table 8**, and the histogram of the results for muscles is shown in **Figure 3**.

As can be seen from the table, the results obtained (correlation coefficients) are the value of the correlation dependence of the muscle pair on each other (right or left) and not on the environment. This result does not show the difference between a muscle in one area and another, but the relationship between a pair of muscles over time. On the other hand, this approach allows us to determine how weak or strong the degree of class failure in the muscles is, and thus which muscle mass is more prone to asymmetry. These can be seen more clearly visually in **Figure 16**.

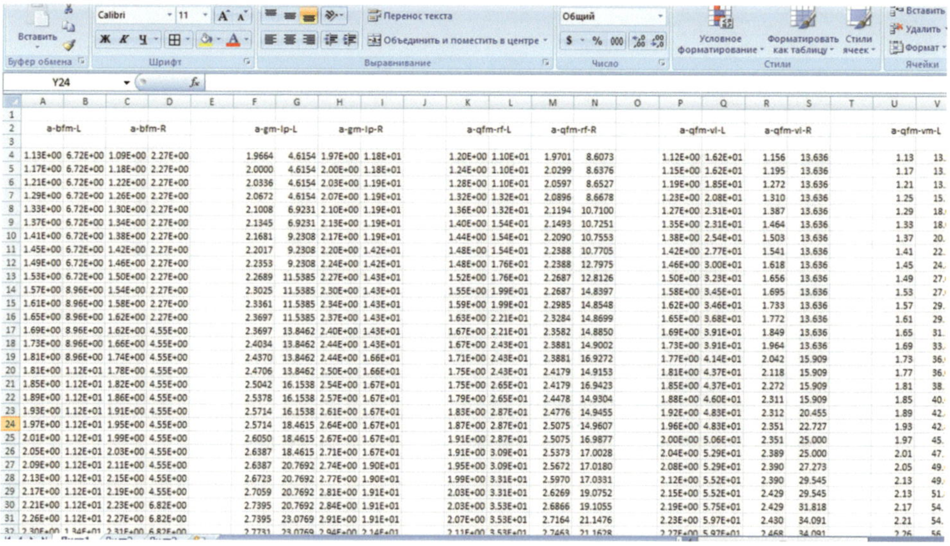

	A	B	C	D	F	G	H	I	K	L	M	N	P	Q	R	S	U	V
2	a-bfm-L		a-bfm-R		a-gm-lp-L		a-gm-lp-R		a-qfm-rf-L		a-qfm-rf-R		a-qfm-vl-L		a-qfm-vl-R		a-qfm-vm-L	
4	1.13E+00	6.72E+00	1.09E+00	2.27E+00	1.9664	4.6154	1.97E+00	1.18E+01	1.20E+00	1.10E+01	1.9701	8.6073	1.12E+00	1.62E+01	1.156	13.636	1.13	13.
5	1.17E+00	6.72E+00	1.18E+00	2.27E+00	2.0000	4.6154	2.00E+00	1.18E+01	1.24E+00	1.10E+01	2.0299	8.6376	1.15E+00	1.62E+01	1.195	13.636	1.17	13.
6	1.21E+00	6.72E+00	1.22E+00	2.27E+00	2.0336	4.6154	2.03E+00	1.19E+01	1.28E+00	1.10E+01	2.0597	8.6527	1.19E+00	1.85E+01	1.272	13.636	1.21	13.
7	1.29E+00	6.72E+00	1.26E+00	2.27E+00	2.0672	4.6154	2.07E+00	1.19E+01	1.32E+00	1.32E+01	2.0896	8.6678	1.23E+00	2.08E+01	1.310	13.636	1.25	15.
8	1.33E+00	6.72E+00	1.30E+00	2.27E+00	2.1008	6.9231	2.10E+00	1.19E+01	1.36E+00	1.32E+01	2.1194	10.7100	1.27E+00	2.31E+01	1.387	13.636	1.29	18.
9	1.37E+00	6.72E+00	1.34E+00	2.27E+00	2.1345	6.9231	2.13E+00	1.19E+01	1.40E+00	1.54E+01	2.1493	10.7251	1.35E+00	2.31E+01	1.464	13.636	1.33	18.
10	1.41E+00	6.72E+00	1.38E+00	2.27E+00	2.1681	9.2308	2.17E+00	1.19E+01	1.44E+00	1.54E+01	2.2090	10.7553	1.38E+00	2.54E+01	1.503	13.636	1.37	20.
11	1.45E+00	6.72E+00	1.42E+00	2.27E+00	2.2017	9.2308	2.20E+00	1.42E+01	1.48E+00	1.54E+01	2.2388	10.7705	1.42E+00	2.77E+01	1.541	13.636	1.41	22.
12	1.49E+00	6.72E+00	1.46E+00	2.27E+00	2.2353	9.2308	2.24E+00	1.42E+01	1.48E+00	1.76E+01	2.2388	12.7975	1.46E+00	3.00E+01	1.618	13.636	1.45	24.
13	1.53E+00	6.72E+00	1.50E+00	2.27E+00	2.2689	11.5385	2.27E+00	1.43E+01	1.52E+00	1.76E+01	2.2687	12.8126	1.50E+00	3.23E+01	1.656	13.636	1.49	27.
14	1.57E+00	8.96E+00	1.54E+00	2.27E+00	2.3025	11.5385	2.30E+00	1.43E+01	1.55E+00	1.99E+01	2.2687	14.8397	1.58E+00	3.45E+01	1.695	13.636	1.53	27.
15	1.61E+00	8.96E+00	1.58E+00	2.27E+00	2.3361	11.5385	2.34E+00	1.43E+01	1.59E+00	1.99E+01	2.2985	14.8548	1.62E+00	3.46E+01	1.733	13.636	1.57	29.
16	1.65E+00	8.96E+00	1.62E+00	2.27E+00	2.3697	11.5385	2.37E+00	1.43E+01	1.63E+00	2.21E+01	2.3284	14.8699	1.65E+00	3.68E+01	1.772	13.636	1.61	29.
17	1.69E+00	8.96E+00	1.62E+00	4.55E+00	2.3697	13.8462	2.40E+00	1.43E+01	1.67E+00	2.21E+01	2.3582	14.8850	1.69E+00	3.91E+01	1.849	13.636	1.65	31.
18	1.73E+00	8.96E+00	1.66E+00	4.55E+00	2.4034	13.8462	2.44E+00	1.43E+01	1.67E+00	2.43E+01	2.3881	14.9002	1.73E+00	3.91E+01	1.964	13.636	1.69	33.
19	1.81E+00	8.96E+00	1.74E+00	4.55E+00	2.4370	13.8462	2.44E+00	1.66E+01	1.71E+00	2.43E+01	2.3881	16.9272	1.77E+00	4.14E+01	2.042	15.909	1.73	36.
20	1.81E+00	1.12E+01	1.78E+00	4.55E+00	2.4706	13.8462	2.50E+00	1.66E+01	1.75E+00	2.43E+01	2.4179	14.9153	1.81E+00	4.37E+01	2.118	15.909	1.77	36.
21	1.85E+00	1.12E+01	1.82E+00	4.55E+00	2.5042	16.1538	2.54E+00	1.67E+01	1.75E+00	2.65E+01	2.4179	16.9423	1.85E+00	4.37E+01	2.272	15.909	1.81	38.
22	1.89E+00	1.12E+01	1.86E+00	4.55E+00	2.5378	16.1538	2.57E+00	1.67E+01	1.79E+00	2.65E+01	2.4478	14.9304	1.88E+00	4.60E+01	2.311	15.909	1.85	40.
23	1.93E+00	1.12E+01	1.91E+00	4.55E+00	2.5714	16.1538	2.61E+00	1.67E+01	1.83E+00	2.87E+01	2.4776	14.9455	1.92E+00	4.83E+01	2.312	20.455	1.89	42.
24	1.97E+00	1.12E+01	1.95E+00	4.55E+00	2.5714	18.4615	2.64E+00	1.67E+01	1.87E+00	2.87E+01	2.5075	14.9607	1.96E+00	4.83E+01	2.351	22.727	1.93	42.
25	2.01E+00	1.12E+01	1.99E+00	4.55E+00	2.6050	18.4615	2.67E+00	1.67E+01	1.91E+00	2.87E+01	2.5075	16.9877	2.00E+00	5.06E+01	2.351	25.000	1.97	45.
26	2.05E+00	1.12E+01	2.03E+00	4.55E+00	2.6387	18.4615	2.71E+00	1.67E+01	1.91E+00	3.09E+01	2.5373	17.0028	2.04E+00	5.29E+01	2.389	25.000	2.01	47.
27	2.09E+00	1.12E+01	2.11E+00	4.55E+00	2.6387	20.7692	2.74E+00	1.90E+01	1.95E+00	3.09E+01	2.5672	17.0180	2.08E+00	5.29E+01	2.390	27.273	2.05	49.
28	2.13E+00	1.12E+01	2.15E+00	4.55E+00	2.6723	20.7692	2.77E+00	1.90E+01	1.99E+00	3.31E+01	2.5970	17.0331	2.12E+00	5.52E+01	2.390	29.545	2.13	49.
29	2.17E+00	1.12E+01	2.19E+00	4.55E+00	2.7059	20.7692	2.81E+00	1.91E+01	2.03E+00	3.31E+01	2.6269	19.0752	2.15E+00	5.52E+01	2.429	29.545	2.13	51.
30	2.21E+00	1.12E+01	2.23E+00	6.82E+00	2.7395	20.7692	2.84E+00	1.91E+01	2.03E+00	3.53E+01	2.6866	19.1055	2.19E+00	5.75E+01	2.429	31.818	2.17	54.
31	2.26E+00	1.12E+01	2.27E+00	6.82E+00	2.7395	23.0769	2.91E+00	1.91E+01	2.07E+00	3.53E+01	2.7164	21.1476	2.23E+00	5.97E+01	2.430	34.091	2.21	54.
32	2.30E+00	1.34E+01	2.31E+00	6.82E+00	2.7731	23.0769	2.94E+00	2.14E+01	2.11E+00	3.53E+01	2.7463	21.1628	2.27E+00	5.97E+01	2.468	34.091	2.26	56.

Figure 15.
Measurement results from 12 muscles (sets Xn and Yn).

##	Abbreviation	Correlation coefficient
1	a-bfm	0.769
2	a-gm-lp	0.878
3	a-qfm-rf	0.952
4	a-qfm-vl	0.553
5	a-qfm-vm	0.995
6	a-gm-mp	0.774

Table 8.
Results of the calculated correlation coefficient.

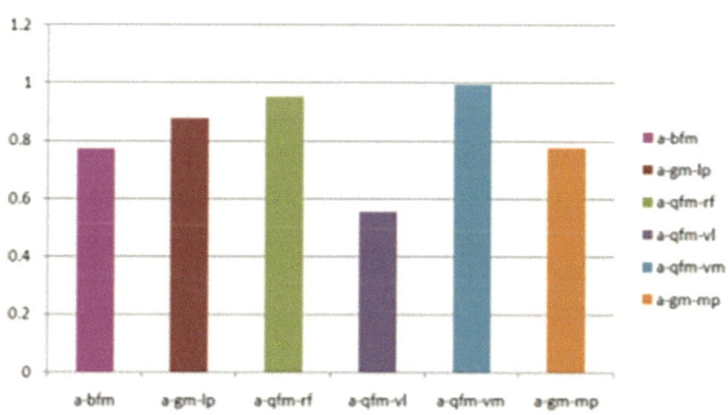

Figure 16.
Histograms of muscle-dependent values of correlation coefficients.

6.2 Application of the obtained results

Figure 17 shows a comparative interpretation of the results obtained from the measurement of muscle strength and the correlation analysis of the measurement results using the available apparatus of the EMG signals.

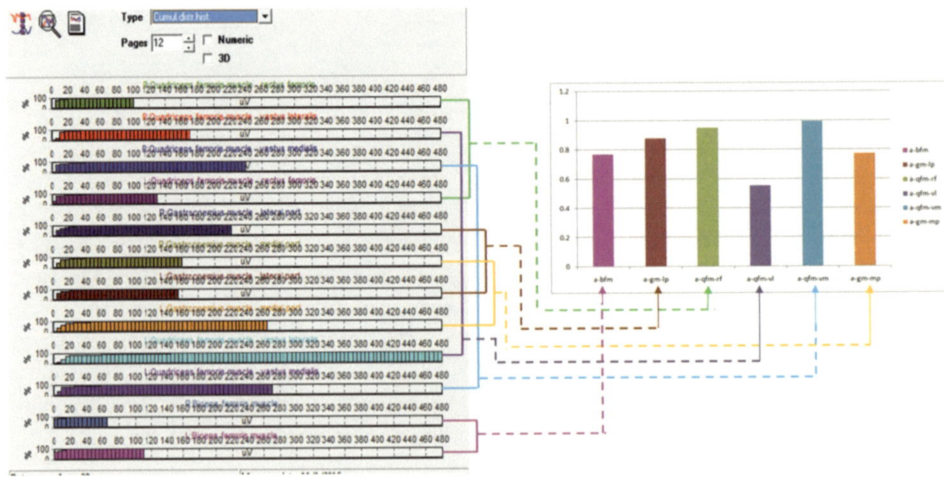

Figure 17.
Comparison of the results obtained from the measurement of muscle strength and the correlation analysis of the measurement results of the EMG signals using the existing apparatus.

As can be seen from the figure, in the first case, the measurement results are presented separately for each muscle in the form of histograms or graphs. However, sometimes the results obtained from the right or left side of the same muscle are inconsistent, making this comparison difficult. On the other hand, because the diagnosis is based on the maximum value, it is difficult to observe and compare the tendency to asymmetry in other muscles. This is also reflected in the comparison of different measurement results.

The results obtained by calculating the correlation coefficient are not only simpler in terms of visual observation, but also easier to compare. It can be easily deduced from the graph that the biceps femoris muscle and the gastrocnemius muscle are already prone to asymmetry in the medial part muscles (**Figure 17**), and this is important information in determining subsequent treatment procedures.

6.3 The result

A correlation analysis method has been proposed that allows the determination of this asymmetry on the basis of EMG signals and the judgment of its level in different measurements. For this purpose, 12 signal results from three main muscle types covering the lower extremity were used, and the asymmetry was determined by calculating the correlation coefficient of the samples. This allows to easily compare the results from a visual point of view, as well as to determine the level of asymmetry in other muscles.

7. Conclusion

Muscles are one of the main constituents of the human body and are complex and numerous. In this regard, complementary methods are needed in the diagnosis of neuromuscular diseases and the choice of treatment methods.

The results of the study show that assessment of the degree of asymmetry of muscle strength allows an expert doctor to accurately assess the differences in the biopotentials of the studied muscles of the limbs. The segmental method also gives informative values about the composition and differences between individual body segments. The multifractal nature of human allows use of the quantities used as key features of multifractals as an informative sign that can be used to detect a violation of the asymmetry of the limbs. The isokinetic test results help to assess asymmetry in measuring muscle strength, relying on the randomness of the dynamic processes of the biological system, which again contains informative parameters. Research and practical calculations show that these methods can be used to assess asymmetry and are used as a complementary tool in making diagnostic decisions.

Author details

Kamala Pashayeva[1]* and Namiq Abdullayev[2]

1 Baku Higher Oil School, Baku, Azerbaijan

2 Azerbaijan Technical University, Baku, Azerbaijan

*Address all correspondence to: is_kamalya@yahoo.com

References

[1] Nikitin O, Kislyakov A. Indicators of symmetry in cluster analysis of complex systems. Vladimir-Suzdal: Proceedings of the XIV International Conference "Physics and Radio Electronics in Medicine and Ecology" FREME'2020; July 1-2, 2020, book 1. pp. 168-172

[2] Functional asymmetries. Available from: http://oddandeven.narod.ru/FunctionalAsymmetryOfHuman/104.htm [Accessed: March 8, 2020]

[3] Tsvetkov M, Fishman B. The use of descriptive statistics methods to assess the concise properties of the muscle on the basis of given single contractions in athletes of different specialization. Bulletin of Novgorod State University. 2005;**232**:26-30

[4] Bezgodkov Y, Fedotov A, Abolin A and others. Method of assessment of functional shortening of the lower extremities. Patent RU2532880 C1 published. 2014. Availale from: http://gpma.ru/science/nauka/pat-2010-2014.pdf. [Accessed: February 27, 2020]

[5] Kolesnikov S, Saifutdninov M, Chegurov O, Kolesnikova E. Dynamics of the functional state of the muscles of the lower extremities in patients after endoprosthesis of the pelvic joint under the conditions of application of soft-spoken manual technique. Modern problems of science and education. 2015;**2**:124

[6] Guidance on functional interdisciplinary asymmetry. - M: Научный мир, 2009. 836 с. Available from: http://www.cerebral-asymmetry.narod.ru/Rukovod_book.htm [Accessed: March 10, 2020]

[7] Isakovich D, Isakovich V. Cardioagenoscope - a new useful model of ECG processing. Pero Publishing House; 2014. p. 138

[8] Functional asymmetries. Available from: http://oddandeven.narod.ru/FunctionalAsymmetryOfHuman/104.htm [Accessed: March 10, 2020]

[9] Guidance on functional interstitial asymmetry. - M: Научный мир, 2009. 836 с. Available from: http://www.cerebral-asymmetry.narod.ru/Rukovod_book.htm [Accessed: March 10, 2020]

[10] Cardioagenoscope. Useful model 128470R. Available from: http://bankpatentov.ru/node/378077 [Accessed: March 12, 2020]

[11] Tsvetkov MS, Fishman BB. The use of descriptive statistics methods to assess the comparative properties of the muscle on the basis of given single contractions in athletes of different specialization. Bulletin of the Novgorod State University. 2005;**232**:26-30

[12] MATLAB in examples and tasks. Textbook, The MathWorks, Inc. 2013

[13] Functional asymmetries. Available from: http://nsicu.ru/books/34/chapters/540 [Accessed: February 23, 2020]

[14] Abolin AB et al. Method for assessing functional shortening of the lower limb. Available from: www.findpatent.ru/patent/253/2532880.html [Accessed: March 12, 2020]

[15] Nikolaev D, Smirnov V, Bobrinskaya I, Rudnev S. Bioimpedance analysis of the human body composition. –M.: Nauka; 2009. 392 p. DOI: 10.20538/1682-0363-2018-2-121-132

[16] Stephen D, Hajnal A. Transfer of Calibration Between Hand and Foot: Functional Equivalence and Fractal Fluctuations. Attention, Perception, & Psychophysics. 2011;**73**:1302-1328. DOI: 10.3758/s13414-011-0142-6

[17] Dang K, Minh H, et al. Analyzing surface EMG signals to determine relationship between jaw imbalance and arm strength loss. Bio Medical Engineering Online. 2012;**55**:55. DOI: 10.1186/1475-925X-11-55

[18] Croisier J, Foidart-Dessalle M, Tinant F, Crielaard J, Forthomme B. An isokinetic eccentric program for the management of chronic lateral epicondylar tendinopathy. BJSM. 2007; **41**(4):269-275. DOI: 10.1136/bjsm.2006.033324

[19] Brown L, Whitehurst M. The effect of short-term isokinetic training on force and rate of velocity development. Journal of Strength and Conditioning Research. 2003;**17**(1):88-94. DOI: 10.1519/1533-4287(2003)017<0088:teosti>2.0.co;2

[20] Bompa T. Periodization, Training Structure and Method. Ankara: Bağırgan Yayınevi; 2003

[21] Cheung C, Hong Y. Isokinetic specific tension of quadriceps in sprinters, distance runners and normal young adults. Available from: http://coachesinfo.com/category/athletics/217/ [Accessed: January 15, 2020]

[22] Palmer A, Strobeck C. Fluctuating asymmetry analysis revisited. In: Polak M, editor. Developmental instability: Causes and consequences. Oxford University Press. 2003. p. 488

[23] Zatsiorsky VM, Biomechanics in Sport. United Kingdom: Blackwell Science; 2005. p. 56. http-2 Delsys, surface electromyography: detection and recording. Available from: http://serveroersted.dtu.dk/personal/jw/Courses/31654/pdf/semgintro.pdf. [Accessed: March 10, 2020]

[24] Tugba A. Determination of load range for differences in measurements made with isokinetic dynamometer. Adana: Physiological Anabilim Branch, Çukurova University, Institute of Health Sciences; 2008

[25] Rynkiewicz M, Rynkiewicz T, Zurek P, Zicmann E, Szymanik R. Asymmetry of muscle mass distribution in tennis players. Trends in Sport Sciences. 2013;**1**(20):47-53

[26] Available from: http://www.bonamedica.ru/assimmetrii-cheloveka/ [Accessed: November 5, 2019]

[27] Goldberger E, Ригни D, West Б. Chaos and fractals in human physiology. Feb 1990;**262**(2):42-49. DOI: 10.1038/scientificamerican0290-42. Available from: https://pubmed.ncbi.nlm.nih.gov/2296715/ [Accessed: December 12, 2020]

[28] Isaeva B. Fractal and chaotic patterns in the morphology of animals. Proceedings of the Institute of Zoology of the Russian Academy of Sciences Appendix No 1; 2009. pp. 199-218. UDC 573.2; 573.4

[29] Zumwalt A. New Method for Quantifying the Complexity of Muscle Attachment Sites. The Anatomical Record (Part B: New Anat.). 2005;**286B**:21-28. DOI: 10.1002/ar.b.20075

[30] Bogachev M, Gromova K, Klionsky D, and others. Fluctuation analysis of physiological signals. Radioelectronics. 2012;**6**(6):37-45

[31] Paitgen H, Jurgens H, Saupe D. Chaos and fractals: New frontiers of science. New York: Springer-Verlag; 1992. p. 984

[32] Feder E. Fractal. –M: Mir, 2001. p. 260

[33] Gorshenkov AA, Klikushin YN. Methods of estimating chaos signals. Polzunovsky Herald. 2011;**3**(1):30-33. DOI: UDC 621.317.08; 621.317.1; 621.317.6

[34] Kantelhardt J, Zschienger S, Koscielny-Bumde E, Havlin S,

Bumde A, Stanley H. Multifractal detrended fluctuation analysis of non-stationary time series. Physica A. 2002; **316**:87-114. DOI: 10.1016/S0378-4371 (02)01383-3

[35] Mali P, Mukhopadhyay A. Multifractal characterization of gold market: A multifractal detrended fluctuation analysis. Physica A: Statistical Mechanics and its Applications. 2014;**413**:361-372. DOI: 10.1016/j.physa.2014.06.076

[36] Абдуллаев N, Dyshin O, Khasmamedova G. Diagnosis of the state of the cardiovascular system on the basis of fractal analysis RR-intervalogram. Biomedical Radio Electronics. 2010;**12**:25-29

[37] Olemskoy A, Borisyuk B. Multifractal analysis of time series. Bulletin of Sum SU. 2008;**2**:70-81

[38] Geht B. Theoretical and Clinical Electromyography. L.: Nauka. 1990. p. 229

[39] Functional asymmetries. Available from: http://oddandeven.narod.ru/FunctionalAsymmetryOfHuman/104.htm [Accessed: August 5, 2021]

[40] Abdullaev N, Ismailova K. Application of neural networks for recognition of pathological changes in the stimulated electromyogram. //Медицинская техника, –M. 2011; **6**(270):1-7

[41] Abdullaev N, Dyshin O, Ismailova K. Analysis of spontaneous activity of muscle fibers and motor units on the basis of wavelet-packet processing electromyogram. Biomedical Radioelectronics. 2011;**12**: 42-48

[42] Abdullaev N, Ismailova K. Assessment of information reliability of diagnostic conclusions in electromyography with the help of the method of indeterminate logical derivation. Information-measuring and control systems. 2012;**10**(4):60-67

[43] Burhade S, Kanwade A. Correlation analysis of electromyogram signals. International Journal for Modern Trends in Science and Technology. 2016;**2**(07): 117-122

[44] Stashuk D, De Luca C. Update on the decomposition and analysis of EMG signals. Computer Aided Electromyograhy and Expert Systems: Elsevier Science Publishers; 1989. pp. 39-53. DOI: 10.1152/jn.00009.2006

[45] Ivanova E, Fedin P, Brutyan A, Ivanova-Smolenskaya I, Illarioshkin S. Clinical and electrophysiological analysis of trembling hyperkinesia with essential tremor and Packirson's disease. Neurological Journal. 2013;**5**:21-26

[46] Zaichenko K, Zharinov O, Kulin A, Kulygina L, Orlov A. Collection and processing of bioelectric signals. SPbGUAP: SPb; 2001. p. 140